Venous Thrombosis: Principles and Practice

Venous Thrombosis: Principles and Practice

Editor: Miley Humes

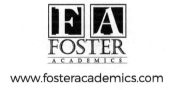

www.fosteracademics.com

www.fosteracademics.com

Cataloging-in-Publication Data

Venous thrombosis : principles and practice / edited by Miley Humes.
   p. cm.
Includes bibliographical references and index.
ISBN 978-1-64646-601-6
1. Thrombophlebitis. 2. Phlebitis. 3. Thrombosis. 4. Thrombophlebitis--Risk factors. I. Humes, Miley.
RC696 .V46 2023
616.145--dc23

Foster Academics,
118-35 Queens Blvd., Suite 400,
Forest Hills, NY 11375, USA

ISBN 978-1-64646-601-6 (Hardback)

Contents

Preface

Over the recent decade, advancements and applications have progressed exponentially. This has led to the increased interest in this field and projects are being conducted to enhance knowledge. The main objective of this book is to present some of the critical challenges and provide insights into possible solutions. This book will answer the varied questions that arise in the field and also provide an increased scope for furthering studies.

Thrombosis refers to the formation of blood clots in the blood vessels, i.e, veins and arteries. Venous thrombosis refers to the formation of blood clots in veins whereas arterial thrombosis refers to condition when blood clots block an artery. Thrombosis may be caused due to factors such as surgical procedures, immobility, inherited predisposition to blood clots, use of oral contraceptives, and underlying health conditions. Medical conditions such as cancer, pregnancy, inflammatory bowel disease, obesity, and certain rheumatic diseases can increase the risk of venous thrombosis. Deep vein thrombosis (DVT) and superficial venous thrombosis are the two common forms of venous thrombosis. DVT is a condition that leads to the formation of blood clots in the veins located deep in the human body. Some common tests for diagnosing venous thrombosis are duplex venous ultrasound, venography, magnetic resonance imaging (MRI), and computed tomography (CT) scan. The main treatment for venous thrombosis is anti-coagulant medication that helps to control the formation of blood clots in the body. This book provides significant insights into venous thrombosis. It consists of contributions made by international experts. Those in search of information to further their knowledge will be greatly assisted by this book.

I hope that this book, with its visionary approach, will be a valuable addition and will promote interest among readers. Each of the authors has provided their extraordinary competence in their specific fields by providing different perspectives as they come from diverse nations and regions. I thank them for their contributions.

Editor

Predictive risk factors of venous thromboembolism (VTE) associated with peripherally inserted central catheters (PICC) in ambulant solid cancer patients

Osamah Al-Asadi[1,2,3]* ⓘ, Manar Almusarhed[1,2,4] and Hany Eldeeb[1,2]

Abstract

Aims: Peripherally inserted central catheters(PICC) lines are becoming increasingly popular in solid cancer patients for the administration of chemotherapy. This study aims looking at the incidence of PICC line related and distant thromboembolism associated with these catheters and exploring risk factors.

Methods: Records were reviewed for 158 patients who underwent PICC line insertion over the two years period in the medical oncology unit, Milton Keynes University Hospital. The Incidence PICC line related Deep Venous Thrombosis (DVT) which is defined as upper extremity DVT at the site of PICC line insertion was documented after checking reports of ultrasound Doppler of all symptomatic patients to confirm the presence of thrombo-embolism and Computed Tomography(CT)scan or Computed Tomography Pulmonary Angiography (CTPA) to confirm the presence Pulmonary Embolism(PE).

Results: 23(13%) symptomatic patients with confirmed diagnosis by ultrasound Doppler were found to have PICC line related DVT and similar number of patients developed distant VTE, namely PE and lower limbs DVT. Average time to thrombo-embolism from the insertion of PICC line was 13 days and 51 days in distant VTE. Statistically significant results have been identified in the term of risk factors leading to VTE events during the period of PICC line insertion.

Conclusions: VTE is a common complication in medical oncology patients who underwent insertion PICC line insertion for chemotherapy. Risk of distant VTE is high as well as the PICC line related DVT and the risk of the PICC line related DVT is higher in the first two weeks after PICC insertion. We concluded that high BMI,high PLTs count and Fluropyrimidine containing chemotherapy are all significant risk factors for VTE events recorded while smoking and high BMI are significantly contributing to the high rate of the PICC line related DVT.

Introduction

The use of PICC line has grown significantly in hospitalized patients in comparison with central venous catheters reflecting their clinical advantages besides avoiding iatrogenic complications frequently associated with central venous catheters [1, 2]. As the PICC line terminated in central veins, they can be used for the infusion of chemotherapy in an outpatient setting for cancer patients [3, 4].However, accumulating evidence suggests that PICC lines are associated with important complications, including upper-extremity DVT,PE, loss of Intravenous access and post thrombotic syndrome [5–11]. The PICC line related DVT in patients with cancer leads to increasing morbidity and mortality [12]. Unfortunately, no much work has been conducted to look at the incidence and risk factors for VTE in cancer patients following the insertion of PICCs as published

* Correspondence: aksaakirq@gmail.com
[1]Department of Oncology, Milton Keynes University Hospital, Milton Keynes, UK
[2]School of Medicine, University of Buckingham, Buckingham, UK
Full list of author information is available at the end of the article

researches had focused on all central venous catheters of which just 15% were PICCs [13]. The incidence of PICC related VTE varies widely in different studies, with the symptomatic VTE in this scenario is reported to be varying around 6% to up to 18% and in few studies, it was around 25% [1, 3] while the rate of asymptomatic thrombosis has been reported to be up to 35–71.9% [14–18]. Many of these studies use a retrospective design and the actual rate of PICC related DVT is still not well defined. It is very important to further explore the incidence and risk factors for PICC line related venous thrombosis. In our study we analyse our experience with PICC insertion in the ambulatory solid cancer patient's population and measure the incidence of local, distant VTE events and relative risk factors.

Aims

To assess the incidence of PICC related VTE in solid cancer patients in the ambulatory setting who underwent PICC line insertion in Macmillan Unit, Milton Keynes university hospital in two years. We also aim to identify any patient related or catheter related risk factors. Also, we measure the incidence of distant VTEs like PE and lower-limbs DVT that developed during the period of PICC line insertion.

Method

All patients with solid cancers who received chemotherapy through the PICC line for the period January 2016 to December 2017 were included. Electronic patient records were reviewed for their age, gender, history of antiplatelet or anticoagulation, pervious risk factor for VTE, chemotherapy type, smoking, Body Mass Index(BMI), White Blood Cell(WBC) count, Platelet (PLT) count, prior PICC line insertion in the last 6 months, pathological diagnosis and treatment setting such as early (neoadjuvant and adjuvant) vs palliative setting. The Incidence of PICC line related DVT which is defined as upper extremity DVT at the site of PICC line insertion and distant VTE were confirmed on ultrasound Doppler in all symptomatic patients and CT scan or CTPA.

Statistical analysis

Data analysis was made using SPSS software, version 22 (IBM Corp., Armonk, NY, USA). Descriptive statistics for continuous variables included mean, median and range. The number and proportions of the categorical data were used to characterize the demographics and baseline of the study population. A multivariate logistic regression model was conducted to examine the association between risk factor and development of VTE events. Multicollinearity was assessed using variance inflation factors and spearman correlations. In all analysis, the null hypothesis was rejected at 5% as a cut of the point for Significance (two-tailed) testing.

Results

Total of 180 patients were retrospectively evaluated for PICC insertion. 22 patients have been excluded due to incomplete data.158 patients with completed data were found eligible for analysis. The PICC line related DVT was identified in 23 (13%) of symptomatic patients with confirmed diagnosis by ultrasound Doppler while distant VTE was identified in 23(13%) of patients in the cohort; two of them had the PICC line related DVT already. The distribution of distant VTE was 18(78%) patients as PE while the lower limbs DVT recorded in only 5(22%) patients. The mean age of the participants at the time of PICC insertion was 57 with a range of 27 to 80. 102 (64%) patients were female. The primary diagnosis was Colorectal cancer ($n = 78$, 49.4%), followed by breast cancer ($n = 63$, 39.9%) and pancreatic cancer ($n = 9$, 5.7%). Only 13 (8.2%) had prior PICC insertion in the last 6 months. Regarding the treatment intention, 96 (60.7%) were on palliative treatment, 41 (26%) were on adjuvant treatment, and 21 (13.3%) were on neoadjuvant. Smokers represent 18.9% (30 patients)of the cohort. The previous risk factor for VTE was found in 25 patients (15.9%) of the cohort. Twelve (7.6%) patients had a previous VTE event. Fluropyrimidine containing chemotherapy was given in 80% of the patients. The baseline characters are shown in the Table 1. After PICC insertion, the median time required for PICC line related DVT development was 13 days 95% CI (12, 32) and 51 days 95% CI (45, 77) in distant VTE.

Table 2 shows the logistic regression model that included all potential predictive factors for VTE events. This model indicated that smoking increased the risk of PICC related DVT by four.

fold (Odds Ratio [OR] 3.9, 95% Confidence Interval [CI] 1.01, 13.98). Also, Body mass index was a significant predictor (Odds Ratio [OR] 1.11, 95% Confidence Interval [CI] 1.01, 1.23). Regarding distant VTE predictors, only BMI was identified as significant risk factor (Odds Ratio [OR] 1.12, 95% Confidence Interval [CI] 1.00, 1.23). When considering all VTE events together, BMI (Odds Ratio [OR] 1.13, 95% Confidence Interval [CI] 1.05, 1.22) and PLT count (Odds Ratio [OR] 1.13, 95% Confidence Interval [CI] 1.05, 1.22) were significant. Using Fluoropyrimidine chemotherapy increased the risk by 10-fold (Odds Ratio [OR] 10.06, 95% Confidence Interval [CI] 1.60, 63.05). No other significant predictors were found considering all VTE events. Figure 1 shows the summary of odds ratios of all potential predictive factors. For PICC line related DVT prediction, the

Table 1 Baseline characteristics and patient demographic of the study cohort

Characteristic	All patients (n = 158)	PICC-related DVT (n = 23)	Distant VTE (n = 23)
Age (Mean)	57	52	62
Gender			
Male	56 (35.4%)	7 (12.5%)	9 (16%)
Female	102 (64.6%)	16 (15.7%)	14 (13.7%)
Primary cancer			
Breast	63 (39.9%)	14 (22.2%)	2 (3.1%)
Colorectal	78 (49.4%)	8 (10.2%)	17 (21.8%)
Pancreas	9 (5.7%)	1 (11.1%)	3 (33.3%)
Other	8 (5%)	0	1 (12.5%)
Treatment intention			
Neoadjuvant	21 (13.3%)	6 (28.6%)	0
Adjuvant	41 (26%)	8 (19.5%)	1 (2.4%)
Palliative	96 (60.7%)	9 (9.3%)	22 (23%)
History of antiplatelet or anticoagulation	14 (8.9%)	2 (14.3%)	2 (14.3%)
Previous VTE event	12 (7.6%)	2 (16.7%)	1 (8.3%)
Smoking	30 (18.9%)	7 (23.3%)	2 (6.6%)
Pervious risk factor for VTE	25 (15.9%)	2 (8%)	4 (16%)
Chemotherapy type			
Fluropyrimidine containing	127 (80.3%)	21 (16.5%)	21 (16.5%)
Fluropyrimidine non-containing	31 (19.7%)	2 (6.4%)	2 (6.4%)
Prior PICC line in last 6 months	13 (8.2%)	1 (7.7%)	4 (30.8%)

PICC peripherally inserted central catheter, *PRDVT* PICC related *DVT*, *VTE* vascular thromboembolism

exploratory logistic regression model was made on the items of Michigan score variables, and no significant predictors were found.

Discussion

A common problem for cancer patients which could interrupt or delay cancer systemic treatment and affect the morbidity significantly is the PICC-related DVT. Our study found the symptomatic PICC related DVT incidence is 13%. Many retrospective design studies reported an incidence of symptomatic PICC-related thrombosis, ranging from 1% to 18 with few studies hit the limit of 28% [3, 4, 14–16, 19].However, there were several prospective studies reporting higher asymptomatic or incidental PICC -related DVT incidence, ranging from 27 to 71% [4, 14, 17, 20, 21].The possible causes for the wide variation in reported incidence may be related to study population, study design, the diagnosis method (Doppler US or venography), screening population (symptomatic or asymptomatic), the inconsistency in the definition of the VTE events (the difficulty in distinguishing mural thrombosis from central venous catheter occlusion by the catheter sleeve) and differences in the quality of patient surveillance. Implanted ports were associated with roughly 60% a relative risk reduction in cancer related thrombosis (OR = 0.43; 95% CI, 0.23–0.80) compared with PICC lines [13]. The possible explanation might be related to the relative less risk of endothelial injury because there is less movement of the catheter with port devices and the lower incidence of infection.

Physiologically speaking, this adverse event is not surprising. The PICC line is occupying much of the cross-sectional diameter of peripheral veins of the arm which predispose to venous stasis [22]. Peripherally inserted central catheter tips often displace and injure endothelium as they are prone to migration [23]. The infusion of chemotherapy is also carrying prothrombotic risk and with all above factors, PICC line often creating the perfect media for thrombosis [24]. Risk factors of catheter-associated thrombosis can be categorized to three types although they reported in different studies with great variation:

1) Chemotherapy type and use of prophylactic anticoagulant.
2) Patient's factor like recent trauma or surgery, cancer, history of VTE, older age and renal failure
3) Catheter size, type, tip location, insertion site, numbers of venous insertions, and the catheter dwell time [25].

Table 2 Logistic regression model of factors with potential predictive value

Parameter	PRDVT		Distant VTE		All VTE	
	Odds Ratio (95%CI)	P value	Odds Ratio (95%CI)	P value	Odds Ratio (95%CI)	P value
Age on insertion	0.97 (0.92, 1.02)	0.270	1.02 (0.97, 1.08)	0.393	1.00 (0.96, 1.04)	0.971
Female	0.29 (0.54, 1.59)	0.155	2.50 (0.75, 8.33)	0.135	1.81 (0.65, 5.04)	0.254
Primary cancer type						
Breast	N/A	N/A	1.18 (0.04, 31.75)	0.922	2.76 (0.169, 45.00)	0.746
Colorectal	N/A	N/A	0.84 (0.03, 26.54)	0.923	1.07 (0.09, 13.65)	0.959
Pancreas	N/A	N/A	0.82 (0.02, 42.66)	0.920	2.82 (0.137, 58)	0.502
Intention to treatment						
Adjuvant	1.16 (0.25, 5.42)	0.851	N/A	N/A	1.43 (0.33, 6.198)	0.629
Palliative	1.33 (0.12, 15.32)	0.187	N/A	N/A	4.62 (0.57, 37.56)	0.153
Ongoing antiplatelet or anticoagulation therapy	1.31 (0.21, 8.22)	0.777	2.91 (0.34, 24.76)	0.329	1.30 (0.30, 5.69)	0.730
Previous VTE event	1.28 (0.17, 9.77)	0.814	0.27 (0.02, 2.91)	0.277	0.77 (0.16, 3.61)	0.740
Smoking	3.90 (1.09, 13.98)	0.036*	0.29 (0.05, 1.66)	0.166	1.61 (0.59, 4.40)	0.351
Pervious risk factor for VTE	0.40 (0.07, 2.42)	0.315	0.66 (0.12, 3.36)	0.612	0.54 (0.15, 1.95)	0.348
Fluropyrimidine containing chemotherapy	5.87 (0.69, 50.22)	0.106	6.80 (0.21, 224.50)	0.283	10.06 (1.6, 63.05)	0.014*
BMI ≥ 30	1.11 (1.01, 1.23)	0.026*	1.12 (1.00, 1.23)	0.033*	1.13 (1.05, 1.22)	0.001*
WBC count	0.86 (0.69, 1.08)	0.202	1.08 (0.95, 1.23)	0.218	1.01 (0.91, 1.12)	0.865
Platelet count	1.01 (1.00, 1.01)	0.103	1.00 (1.00, 1.01)	0.245	1.00 (1.00, 1.01)	0.034*
Prior PICC line in last 6 months	0.74 (0.08, 7.14)	0.791	3.97 (0.80, 19.78)	0.092	2.16 (0.58, 8.03)	0.252

DVT deep vein thrombosis, *PICC* peripherally inserted central catheter, *PRDVT, PICC related DVT, VTE* vascular thromboembolism, *CI* confidence interval, WBC white blood cells, *BMI* body mass index, *N/A* not applicable
*= $P < 0.05$ statistically significant

A recent study looked at PICC related thrombosis in all hospital patients found a number of significant risk factors for developing a PICC related DVT which included PICC size, previous DVT and surgery lasting more than one hour [10]. Another study identified that DVT risk correlated to catheter diameter, with DVT rates of 0,1and 6.6% per catheters sized < 3-F, 4-F and 5-F respectively [26]. The importance of lumen size was further highlighted in a follow-on study [27]. In our study the catheter size used was uniform of 4-F and all PICC insertions were conducted by interventional radiologist under fluoroscopy guidance. One study identified that the inappropriate choice of central venous access device and insertion technique as important risk factors for post-procedure complications, particularly in critically ill patients [28].However, one study that conducted on cancer patients with PICC line, none of the above-mentioned variables were predictive of PICC line related DVT and reported that co-morbidities such as diabetes, COPD and advanced cancer did predict DVT [3]. Lee et al. identified previous catheterization, more than one insertion attempt and ovarian cancer as being associated with an increased incidence of DVT [29].

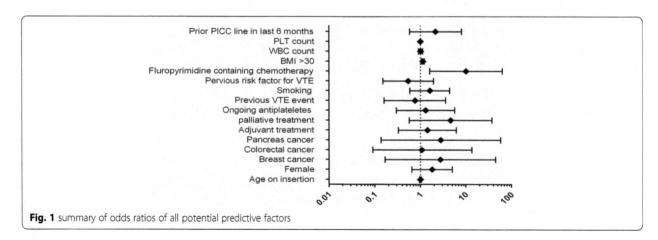

Fig. 1 summary of odds ratios of all potential predictive factors

In our study the median time required for PICC line related DVT development was 13 days 95% CI (12, 32). A large prospective study in the USA reported that 70% of thrombosis events occurred in the first week of insertion while 30% developed in the second week, after which no thromboses were identified [30]. These findings are similar to other studies conclusion in this aspect like one study which found PICC-related thrombosis forming at a mean-time of 12.4 ± 11 days while other studies also reported a mean thrombosis forming time of 15 days [16, 31, 32].Our finding is concords with previous literature reports and suggested the significance of prevention in the first 2 weeks after PICC insertion.

Significant risk factors in our study have been identified by multivariable logistic regression analyses which are smoking and high BMI with significant correlation to the PICC line related DVT while high PLT count and Fluropyrimidine containing chemotherapy found to have a significant relationship to all VTE events. In a large meta-analysis, involving 32 observational studies, found an increased risk of VTE with smoking independent of other risk factors [33]. Possible biological explanations for this relationship are procoagulant state, higher level of plasma fibrinogen and inflammation status which all may underlie the association between smoking and VTE risk [34–36]. Also, it has been shown that the fibrinogen concentration decreased quickly after smoking cessation [37, 38]. A high PLT count at the time of catheter insertion seems to be correlated with the rate of thrombotic complications in cancer patients which was demonstrated in one study that reported a lower risk of central venous catheter-related DVT in cancer patients with a low PLT count [39]. The influence of chemotherapy upon the rate of all VTE events in our cohort might relate to the increase risk for VTE in general with chemotherapy which is around more than two-fold [40]. In our study, 5-fluorouracil containing chemotherapy was associated with an increased risk of type VTE. This effect could be explained by the well-known pro-thrombotic and endothelial effects of 5-fluorouracil [41].

Compared with previous studies, our study had some advantage by exploring the distant VTE events during the period of PICC line insertion which showed a similar incidence of 23(13%) patients of the cohort; two of them had the PICC line related DVT already. The distribution of distant VTE was 18(78%) patients as PE while the lower limbs DVT recorded in only 5(22%) patients. The incidence of PE associated with the central venous catheter in cancer patients ranging from 15 to 25% [4].Two studies measured the incidence of symptomatic CTPA proven PE in cancer patients with the central venous catheter -related DVT and the incidence was 25 and 30%, respectively. However, both studies are of small size [42, 43].

The recorded symptoms in our study for patients who developed PICC line related DVT included swollen upper arm, forearm, axilla with discomfort or pain over the upper limb with inserted PICC line. Of note, some patients had veins engorgement over the affective side. In a meta-analysis, doppler ultrasound with compression was reported to have a pooled sensitivity of 91% and specificity of 93% in diagnosing upper extremity venous thrombosis [44].It is safe,low cost, non-invasive and fast making it the ideal method for diagnosis.

The current guidance does not recommend thromboprophylaxis in the setting of a long-term PICC line in cancer patients as no current evidence suggests that thromboprophylaxis is helpful to prevent these events despite a number of randomized controlled trials(RCT) [45, 46]. Moreover, a recent meta-analysis of 12 clinical trials assessing either primary prophylaxis dose heparins or low dose Warfarin in cancer patients with central venous catheters failed to show any benefit on the primary endpoints studied [47].

But there were still limitations in our study like determination of catheter tip position in those patients who developed the PICC line related DVT prior to its removal and assessing the vein lumen to catheter dimension ratio which considered as risk factors for PICC related DVT. The position of the tip at the junction of the superior vena cava and the right atrium may be a protective measure due to a greater dilutional effect when chemotherapeutic agents are infused or because the likelihood that the tip of the catheter will be in direct contact with the endothelium is a lower. Finally, due to the relatively small number of patients, we were unable to do internal validation For the Michigan score which is a PICC line related DVT prediction module.

Conclusion

VTE is a common complication in medical oncology patients who underwent insertion PICC line insertion for chemotherapy. Risk of distant VTE is high as well as the PICC line related DVT and the risk of the PICC line related DVT is higher in the first 2 weeks after PICC insertion. We concluded that high BMI,high PLTs count and Fluropyrimidine containing chemotherapy are all significant risk factors for VTE events recorded while smoking and high BMI are significantly contributing to the high rate of the PICC line related DVT. There is no consensus on the role of prophylactic anticoagulation to reduce its incidence. Further study is required to generate risk prediction models to identified patients at higher risk for PICC line related DVT.

We recommend keeping a low threshold to arrange a Doppler ultrasound in any cancer patient with the PICC line with presentation such as pain and/or swelling in the same arm with PICC line, as the incidence is high.Further research on risk factors and the consequences of PICC thrombosis would also be very helpful. As our study identified some reversible risk factors that significantly associated with the PICC related DVT(smoking and high BMI), further patient education is advisable and probably prospective study after these risk factors modification will consolidate our finding. We recommend also further validation for the new Michigan Risk Score for PICC-Related Thrombosis which might be useful for estimation the risk of catheter-related thrombosis prior to inserting a PICC, support testing for thrombosis in patients with vague symptoms and can help about the anticoagulation period in patients with confirmed DVT related to PICC with a higher score. Finally, the consideration of Port-a-cath instead of PICC line in cancer patient with high risk of DVT is still not a standard option in the UK despite the lower risk of line related thrombosis and infection which worth further research.

Abbreviations

BMI: Body Mass Index; CI: Confidence Interval; CRT: Clinical Randomised Trial; CT: Computed Tomography; CTPA: Computed Tomography Pulmonary Angiography; DVT: Deep Venous Thrombosis; OR: Odd Ratio; PE: Pulmonary Embolism; PICC: Peripheral Inserted Central Catheter; PLT: Platelet; VTE: Venous Thromboembolism; WBC: White Blood Cell

Acknowledgements

Not applicable.

Author details

[1]Department of Oncology, Milton Keynes University Hospital, Milton Keynes, UK. [2]School of Medicine, University of Buckingham, Buckingham, UK. [3]College of medicine, Al-Mustansiriyah University, Baghdad, Iraq. [4]College of medicine, Babylon University, Babylon, Iraq.

References

1. O'Brien J, et al. Insertion of PICCs with minimum number of lumens reduces complications and costs. J Am Coll Radiol. 2013;10:864–8.
2. Gibson C, et al. Peripherally inserted central catheters: use at a tertiary care pediatric center. J Vasc Interv Radiol. 2013;24:1323–31.
3. Aw A, et al. Incidence and predictive factors of symptomatic thrombosis related to peripherally inserted central catheters in chemotherapy patients. Thromb Res. 2012;130(3):323–6.
4. Verso M, Agnelli G. Venous thromboembolism associated with long-term use of central venous catheters in cancer patients. J Clin Oncol. 2003;21(19): 3665–75.
5. Chopra V, et al. The problem with peripherally inserted central catheters. JAMA. 2012;308:1527–8.
6. Chopra V, et al. Risk of venous thromboembolism associated with peripherally inserted central catheters: a systematic review and meta-analysis. Lancet. 2013; 382:311–25.
7. Lobo BL, et al. Risk of venous thromboembolism in hospitalized patients with peripherally inserted central catheters. J Hosp Med. 2009;4:417–22.
8. Liem TK, et al. Peripherally inserted central catheter usage patterns and associated symptomatic upper extremity venous thrombosis. J Vasc Surg. 2012;55(3):761–7.
9. Sperry BW, Roskos M, Oskoui R. The effect of laterality on venous thromboembolism formation after peripherally inserted central catheter placement. J Vasc Access. 2012;13(1):91–5.
10. Evans RS, et al. Risk of symptomatic DVT associated with peripherally inserted central catheters. Chest. 2010;138(4):803–10.
11. Winters JP, et al. Central venous catheters and upper extremity deep vein thrombosis in medical inpatients: the medical inpatients and thrombosis (MITH) study. J Thromb Haemost. 2015;13(12):2155–60.
12. Fallouh N, et al. Peripherally inserted central catheter-associated deep vein thrombosis: a narrative review. Am J Med. 2015;128(7):722–38.
13. Saber W, et al. Risk factors for catheter-related thrombosis (CRT) in cancer patients: a patient-level data (IPD) meta-analysis of clinical trials and prospective studies. J Thromb Haemost. 2011;9(2):312–9.
14. Chemaly RF, et al. Venous thrombosis associated with peripherally inserted central catheters: a retrospective analysis of the Cleveland Clinic experience. Clin Infect Dis. 2002;34(9):1179–83.
15. Cortelezzia A, et al. Central venous catheter-related complications in patients with hematological malignancies: a retrospective analysis of risk factors and prophylactic measures. Leuk Lymphoma. 2003;44(9):1495–501.
16. King MM, et al. Peripherally inserted central venous catheter-associated thrombosis: retrospective analysis of clinical risk factors in adult patients. South Med J. 2006;99(10):1073–7.
17. Paauw JD, et al. The incidence of PICC line-associated thrombosis with and without the use of prophylactic anticoagulants. JPEN J Parenter Enteral Nutr. 2008;32(4):443–7.
18. Itkin M, et al. Peripherally inserted central catheter thrombosis – reverse tapered versus nontapered catheters: a randomized controlled study. J Vasc Interv Radiol. 2014;25(1):85–91.
19. Loughran SC, et al. Peripherally inserted central catheters: a report of 2,506 catheter days. JPEN J Parenter Enteral Nutr. 1995;19(2):133–6.
20. Kamphuisen PW,et al. Catheter-related thrombosis: lifeline or a pain in the neck? Hematology Am Soc Haematol Educ Program. 2012;2012:638–44.
21. Liu Y, et al. Peripherally inserted central catheter thrombosis incidence and risk factors in cancer patients: a double-center prospective investigation 2015;11:153–160.
22. Nifong TP, McDevitt TJ. The effect of catheter to vein ratio on blood flow rates in a simulated model of peripherally inserted central venous catheters. Chest. 2011;140:48–53.
23. Song L, et al. Malposition of peripherally inserted central catheter: experience from 3012 cancer patients. Int J Nurs Pract. 2014;20:446–9.
24. Ackerknecht EH. Rudolf Virchow. Doctor, statesman, anthropologist. Madison, WI: University of Wisconsin, Madison; 1953.
25. Gallieni M, et al. Vascular access in oncology patients. CA Cancer J Clin. 2008;58(6):323–46.
26. Grove JR, et al. Venous thrombosis related to peripherally inserted central catheters. J Vasc Interv Radiol. 2000;11(7):837–40.
27. Evans RS, et al. Reduction of peripherally inserted central catheter-associated DVT. Chest. 2013;143(3):627–33.
28. Cotogni P, et al. Focus on peripherally inserted central catheters in critically ill patients. World J Crit Care Med. 2014;3(4):80–94.
29. Lee AY, et al. Incidence, risk factors, and outcomes of catheter-related thrombosis in adult patients with cancer. J Clin Oncol. 2006;24(9):1404–8.
30. Walshe LJ, et al. Complication rates among cancer patients with peripherally inserted central catheters. J Clin Oncol. 2002;20(15):3276–81.
31. Ng PK, et al. Peripherally inserted central catheters in general medicine. Mayo Clin Proc. 1997;72(3):225–33.
32. Ong B, et al. Peripherally inserted central catheters and upper extremity deep vein thrombosis. Australas Radiol. 2006;50(5):451–4.
33. Cheng YJ, Liu ZH, Yao FJ, et al. Current and former smoking and risk for venous thromboembolism: a systematic review and meta-analysis. PLoS Med. 2013;10(9):e1001515.
34. Lee KW, Lip GYH. Effects of lifestyle on hemostasis, fibrinolysis, and platelet reactivity: a systematic review. Arch Intern Med. 2003;163(19):2368–92.
35. Yarnell JW, Sweetnam PM, Rumley A, Lowe GD. Lifestyle and hemostatic risk factors for ischemic heart disease: the Caerphilly study. Arterioscler Thromb Vasc Biol. 2000;20:271–9.
36. Oger E, Lacut K, Van Dreden P, et al. High plasma concentration of factor VIII coagulant is also a risk factor for venous thromboembolism in the elderly. Haematologica. 2003;88:465–9.
37. Feher MD, Rampling MW, Brown J, et al. Acute changes in atherogenic and thrombogenic factors with cessation of smoking. J R Soc Med. 1990;83(3): 146–8.

38. Bakhru A, Erlinger TP. Smoking cessation and cardiovascular disease risk factors: results from the third National Health and nutrition examination survey. PLoS Med. 2005;2(6):e160.

39. Haire WD, et al. Hickman catheter-induced thoracic vein thrombosis: frequency and long-term sequelae in patients receiving high-dose chemotherapy and marrow transplantation. Cancer. 1990;66:900–8.

40. Blom JW, et al. Incidence of venous thrombosis in a large cohort of 66,329 cancer patients: results of a record linkage study. J Thromb Haemost. 2006; 4(3):529–35.

41. Polk A, et al. A systematic review of the pathophysiology of 5-fluorouracil-induced cardiotoxicity. BMC Pharmacol Toxicol. 2014;15:47.

42. Manuel Monreal. Upper-extremity deep venous thrombosis and pulmonary embolism. A prospective study Chest 1991; 99(2).

43. Monreal M. Pulmonary embolism in patients with upper extremity DVT associated to venous central lines--a prospective study. Thromb Haemost. 1994;72(4).

44. Chin EE, et al. Sonographic evaluation of upper extremity deep venous thrombosis. J Ultrasound Med. 2005;24(6):829–38.

45. Karthaus M, et al. Dalteparin for prevention of catheter-related complications in cancer patients with central venous catheters: final results of a double-blind, placebo-controlled phase III trial. Ann Oncol. 2006;17(2): 289–96.

46. Young AM, et al. Warfarin thromboprophylaxis in cancer patients with central venous catheters (WARP): an open-label randomised trial. Lancet. 2009;373(9663):567–74.

47. Akl EA, et al. Anticoagulation for people with cancer and central venous catheters. Cochrane Database Syst Rev. 2014;10:CD006468.

2

Evaluation of unmet clinical needs in prophylaxis and treatment of venous thromboembolism in high-risk patient groups: Cancer and critically ill

Benjamin Brenner[1*], Russell Hull[2], Roopen Arya[3], Jan Beyer-Westendorf[4,5], James Douketis[6,7], Ismail Elalamy[8,9], Davide Imberti[10] and Zhenguo Zhai[11]

Abstract

Background: Clinical practice shows that venous thromboembolism (VTE) presents a substantial burden in medical patients, and awareness and advocacy for its primary and secondary prevention remains inadequate. Specific patient populations, such as those with cancer and the critically ill, show elevated risk for VTE, bleeding or both, and significant gaps in VTE prophylaxis and treatment exist in these groups.

Objective: To present current expert insights and evidence on the unmet needs in thromboprophylaxis, and on the treatment of VTE in two high-risk patient groups: patients with cancer and the critically ill.

Methodology: To identify specific unmet needs in the management of VTE, a methodology was designed and implemented that assessed gaps in prophylaxis and treatment of VTE through interviews with 44 experts in the field of thrombosis and haemostasis, and through a review of current guidelines and seminal studies to substantiate the insights provided by the experts. The research findings were then analysed, discussed and consolidated by a multidisciplinary group of experts.

Results: The gap analysis methodology identified shortcomings in the VTE risk assessment tools, patient stratification approaches for prophylaxis, and the suboptimal use of anticoagulants for primary prophylaxis and treatment.

Conclusions: Specifically, patients with cancer need better VTE risk assessment tools to tailor primary thromboprophylaxis to tumour types and disease stages, and the potential for drug–drug interactions needs to be considered. In critically ill patients, unfractionated heparin is not advised as a first-line treatment option, low-molecular weight heparins remain the first choice for prophylaxis in critically ill and cancer patients due to their safety and efficacy profile, and the strength of evidence is increasing for direct oral anticoagulants as a treatment option over low-molecular-weight heparins. Herein we present novel insights and consolidated evidence collected from experts, clinical practice guidelines and original studies on the unmet needs in thromboprophylaxis, and on the treatment of VTE in patients with cancer and the critically ill.

Keywords: Venous thromboembolism, Cancer, Critically ill, Anticoagulants, Low-molecular-weight heparin

* Correspondence: b_brenner@rambam.health.gov.il
[1]Department of Hematology and Bone Marrow Transplantation, Rambam Health Care Campus, Haifa, Israel
Full list of author information is available at the end of the article

Background

Venous thromboembolism (VTE), which comprises deep vein thrombosis (DVT) and pulmonary embolism (PE), is a complex, multifaceted disease in which the clinical management in patients with cancer and the critically ill is challenging. Such patients are typically at increased risk for thrombosis and/or bleeding complications, and require special consideration for the prevention and treatment of VTE [1–3].

Despite the development of methodologically rigorous clinical practice guidelines that inform the prevention and treatment of VTE, adherence to such practices by healthcare professionals (HCP) is suboptimal. For example, although VTE-associated mortality has decreased considerably in surgical patients who receive postoperative thromboprophylaxis, in the high-risk patient groups identified above, thromboprophylaxis is commonly suboptimal and mortality rates remain high, with thrombosis being the second major cause of death in patients with cancer [4–7]. Moreover, overall survival of patients with cancer and VTE is shorter than those without VTE, even when accounting for tumour stage and cancer treatment [6, 7], and in critically ill patients, between 7 and 27% of deaths are due to PE [8].

Recent large, population-based studies show that anticoagulants are misused in terms of the appropriateness of the agent and dosing regimens administered [9]. In addition, despite the availability of risk stratification models for VTE and bleeding, they are complex, not optimally used in clinical practice and most require external validation [10, 11]. The alternative approach of systematically administering thromboprophylaxis to all at-risk medical patients in different clinical situations, for example in a post-hospitalisation period, without proper evaluation of VTE and bleeding risks could lead to unnecessary safety issues and has cost implications for healthcare systems [12].

Reduction of VTE incidence in medical patients is important to mitigate the risk of both initial VTE and VTE-associated sequelae comprising post-thrombotic syndrome [13] and chronic thromboembolic pulmonary hypertension [14]. In addition, VTE is associated with higher hospitalisation rates and longer in-hospital periods [15], resulting in a significant increase in the utilisation of healthcare resources.

Non-adherence to recommendations and guidance, or relying on expert opinion, remain important obstacles to the optimal administration of thromboprophylaxis [5]. Discrepancies between guideline recommendations, due to insufficient scientific evidence [16, 17], and differences in expert opinions highlight the need to review published evidence and clinical insights in order to identify unmet needs in prophylaxis and treatment of VTE, and potential ways to bridge these gaps between existing knowledge and practice.

Main text

Gap analysis methodology

The gap analysis methodology implemented involved qualitative research via telephone interviews, which took place from February to August 2017, with 44 experts from 12 countries or regions (Germany, France, Italy, Spain, UK, Brazil, Canada, China, Russia, Japan, Middle East and Africa). Using a pre-designed questionnaire [see Additional file 1], information was collected on prophylaxis and treatment of VTE in certain high-risk patient populations that were identified as those in which robust evidence and related practice guidelines were lacking or had considerable limitations. For the purpose of this paper, consolidated evidence collected from the interviews on gaps in the management of cancer and critically ill patients with VTE was supplemented through comprehensive quantitative research into published articles in PubMed and Cochrane Library from 2015 to 2017, and current guidelines published from 2015 until October 2018. Search terms included "cancer" or "tumour", "acutely ill" or "critically ill", and "venous thromboembolism". Literature searches were supplemented with identification of seminal studies in the field and relevant systematic reviews published at any time on VTE in patients with cancer or the critically ill. Evaluation of research findings and further insights were obtained through author discussions at the Thrombosis Think Tank [Paris, 28 February 2018] meeting, and the information gained on these two patient populations, cancer and critically ill, are reviewed in this paper.

Prevention and management of VTE in cancer

Despite an increase in the incidence of cancer in an ageing population around the world, survival of cancer patients is improving due to the introduction of novel therapies, improvements in existing treatment strategies and cancer prevention programmes. The annual incidence of VTE in patients with cancer ranges from 0.5 to 20% depending on the type of cancer, disease stage and associated treatment regimens, and is predicted to increase in the future [18], while VTE incidence in the general population remains unchanged [19]. Moreover, the risk of VTE is higher in more advanced stages of cancer, or with a metastatic disease, compared with less advanced cancer [20]. The association between VTE and cancer is also bidirectional, with 20% of all patients with VTE diagnosed with cancer, typically at the time that, or soon after, VTE is diagnosed [21–24]. The mortality rate in patients with cancer and concurrent VTE is 3-fold higher than that in cancer patients without VTE, and VTE is the second most common cause of death, after the malignancy itself, in patients with cancer [25]. Therefore, the primary and secondary prevention of

VTE presents an important unmet need in this patient population.

Epidemiology of VTE in patients with cancer

Current guidelines highlight lung, pancreatic, ovarian, gastrointestinal and brain tumours, as well as haematological malignancies, as those associated with the highest risk of thrombosis; lymphoid, gynaecological (other than ovarian) and bladder tumours as those carrying high risk of thrombosis; and breast, head and neck, and prostate cancers presenting with a lower risk of VTE [18, 26–28].

The incidence of VTE varies not only according to the type of cancer, but also within cancer types, specifically lung, ovarian, oesophageal, gastric, pancreatic and brain cancers, and chronic lymphocytic leukaemia. The incidence of VTE is particularly high in lung, pancreatic and brain cancers [29–31], and a paucity of data on how to manage these patients was noted by the experts who were interviewed, especially when patients are undergoing chemotherapy. For example, in a study of patients with lung cancer who received cancer treatment with curative intent, the cumulative incidence of VTE after 1 year reached 13.5% [29], while another study that examined VTE incidence in patients with non-small-cell lung cancer reported 6-month and 2-year rates of VTE of 4.2 and 6.4%, respectively [32]. In general, VTE incidence in lung cancer varies widely, from 1.3 to 21.5% [33–36], but the presence of VTE is consistently associated with a worse overall survival in such patients [36–38].

A systematic review and meta-analysis of VTE incidence rates reported a 2-year cumulative incidence rate of 11.2% in advanced pancreatic cancer [30], while in a more recent study the incidence of symptomatic and asymptomatic VTE was 16.5% in patients with pancreatic cancer [39]. In a meta-analysis of patients with brain tumours, the risk of VTE was found to be significantly related to glioma (risk ratio [RR] = 1.68, $P < 0.001$), high-grade glioma (RR = 1.70, $P < 0.001$) and glioblastoma multiforme (GBM) (RR = 1.74, $P < 0.001$) [31]. Overall data on risk for VTE according to the type of cancer and staging will guide clinical decisions on the use of thromboprophylaxis.

Clinical practice guidelines provide evidence-based recommendations for the primary prevention of VTE in patients with multiple myeloma (MM) who are undergoing treatment with cytotoxic chemotherapy and immunomodulatory imide drugs (IMiD) [40]. This evidence is based on the association of MM with VTE. At baseline the VTE rate is 3–4% in these patients, and this is further increased with exposure to risk factors, including treatment with high-dose dexamethasone, cytotoxic chemotherapy (doxorubicin), IMiDs (thalidomide and lenalidomide), erythropoiesis-stimulating agents, reduced mobility, fractures, and personal or family history of thrombosis [40, 41].

Chemotherapeutic regimens also contribute to the development of VTE, as the annual incidence of VTE in cancer patients treated with chemotherapy is 1 in 200, while in the general population it is 1 in 855 [42]. Outpatients receiving chemotherapy have a 6.5-fold increase in the risk of VTE compared to patients not treated with cytotoxic therapy [43], and the second most common cause of death in patients receiving outpatient chemotherapy is VTE [44].

In summary, expert opinion and a number of studies highlight the importance of identifying high-risk patients within cancer populations, who may benefit from thromboprophylaxis to prevent VTE and, in turn, decrease VTE-associated morbidity and mortality.

Risk assessment models and biomarkers for prediction of primary and recurrent VTE in patients with cancer

Guidelines from the British Committee for Standards in Haematology [45] recommend the Khorana risk score (KS) as a tool for categorising patients into very high VTE risk patients, such as those with gastric and pancreatic cancer, and high VTE risk patients, such as those with lung, gynaecological, bladder or testicular cancer, or lymphoma [45]. However, more recent evidence has shown that a high-risk score does not necessarily predict presence of VTE in patients with lung cancer, although it does associate with all-cause mortality [46]. Moreover, the KS has insufficient precision in stratifying patients with lung cancer who are receiving chemotherapy into high- and low-risk groups [47], and those with pancreatic cancer into high- and intermediate-risk groups [48, 49]. The latter high-risk patient group, however, could be identified by combining the KS or CONKO scores with an activated partial thromboplastin time [48]. In addition, the predictive value of the KS in cancer-associated thrombosis was higher when the analysis included platinum-based chemotherapy and the presence of distant metastases [50]. Another VTE risk assessment tool, the Ottawa score, considers the type of cancer, disease stage, gender and history of thrombosis, but it could not adequately predict recurrent VTE in patients receiving anticoagulants [51]. The risk of VTE fluctuates throughout a patient's disease course, and the type of cancer, stage and therapeutic regimens will have an impact on the level of VTE risk [52]. The experts recognise that there is an unmet need for improving VTE risk assessment tools for identifying cancer patients at risk, and for balancing those risks against anticoagulant-induced bleeding.

Current risk-assessment-based decisions that usually rely on clinical parameters as potential VTE biomarkers, including D-dimer and other biomarkers, are unlikely to have a significant impact on routine clinical practice in the foreseeable future [25]. However, a recent systematic review on biomarkers for prediction of thromboembolism in lung cancer demonstrated that D-dimer and epidermal growth factor receptor mutation were the most reproducible predictors of thromboembolism in this patient population [53]. Circulating tissue factor emerged as a potential biomarker in its highest quartile, where it was associated with the highest VTE recurrence rate in patients with cancer who were receiving anticoagulants, but this marker is not widely used in clinical practice [54].

Taken together, and with the experts advocating for personalised treatment based on risk-assessment models, these data demonstrate an urgent need to develop practical, realistic and useful risk assessment tools, which would be able to stratify cancer patients into high-, intermediate- and low-risk primary and recurrent VTE groups eligible for targeted thromboprophylaxis approaches.

Primary prevention of VTE in patients with cancer

Primary prophylaxis in patients with cancer should be considered, as the experts agreed on the importance of improving prevention of VTE, which presents a challenge in terms of recurrent thrombosis and clinically relevant bleeding. It was acknowledged that significant improvements in inpatient thromboprophylaxis have occurred over recent years; however, beyond hospitalisation the benefits of extended prophylaxis remain less well-defined and require further investigation as patients may remain at risk of VTE after hospital discharge. Current guidelines advise against routine thromboprophylaxis with low-molecular-weight heparin (LMWH) in ambulatory patients with active cancer receiving systemic anticancer therapy, such as adjuvant hormonal therapies or chemotherapy [45, 55, 56]. Primary prophylaxis may be indicated in specific subpopulations only, including those with pancreatic or lung cancer, ambulatory patients at high thrombotic risk [12, 27] and those receiving chemotherapy for prolonged periods of time [57]. However, antithrombotic therapy that extends beyond 6 months is controversial, but may be advised for patients with metastatic disease receiving chemotherapy, immunochemotherapy or radiotherapy [58]. It is also recommended that patients with cancer and reduced mobility who are admitted to hospital, or who are treated with thalidomide and lenalidomide combined with steroids or other systemic anticancer therapies, should receive prophylaxis with LMWH, unfractionated heparin (UFH) or fondaparinux [7, 59]. In at-risk patients, VTE prophylaxis should begin as soon as VTE risk has been identified [12], but administration of anticoagulants should consider comorbidities associated with cancer, the risk of bleeding and patient preferences [27].

In patients with metastatic disease and high risk of bleeding, LMWH is the preferred option over other anticoagulants, while vitamin K antagonist (VKA) should be avoided [6, 55]. However, in patients with renal failure, LMWH is not routinely recommended, as it increases

the risk of major bleeding [57]. In patients with MM at high risk of VTE, full-dose LMWH or adjusted-dose warfarin (targeted international normalised ratio ~1.5) are recommended, in contrast to MM patients with low-risk factors who are advised low-dose aspirin [7, 57]. A recent systematic review on MM patients who were treated with lenalidomide-based therapy and/or dexamethasone showed a reduction in VTE risk for patients on LMWH (1.4%) compared to patients on aspirin (10.7%) [60].

Clinical practice guidelines recommend LMWH for thromboprophylaxis in low-bleeding-risk patients with locally advanced or metastatic pancreatic cancer or lung cancer treated with systemic anticancer therapy [7]. The benefits of LMWH in reducing VTE risk were also demonstrated in the CONKO-004 trial, where the rates of symptomatic VTE reduced by 8.7% in patients with advanced-stage pancreatic cancer receiving primary prophylaxis with enoxaparin, compared to patients not receiving prophylaxis [61]. Fondaparinux should be considered in patients with previous heparin-induced thrombocytopenia (HIT) [6]. The role of direct oral anticoagulants (DOAC) for the prevention of VTE in cancer patients is uncertain [27]. Recent results from the CASSINI trial demonstrated the safety and efficacy of thromboprophylaxis with rivaroxaban in patients with cancer [62]. The study examined this DOAC for VTE prevention in ambulatory patients with various cancers and found that VTE and VTE-related deaths were significantly reduced during the on-treatment period, and major bleeding was low. However, the AVERT trial, which examined the safety and efficacy of apixaban to prevent VTE in high-risk cancer patients, found that although lower rates of VTE were observed in the apixaban group compared with the placebo group, major bleeding rates were much higher [63]. These contradictory results suggest that more trials are needed to consolidate future recommendations on the use of DOACs in this patient population [62].

Secondary prevention and treatment of VTE

In cancer patients who develop recurrent VTE despite appropriate anticoagulant therapy, expert opinion guidance suggests three treatment options, which include increasing the LMWH dose by 20–25%, switching therapy from VKA to LMWH, or inserting an inferior vena cava (IVC) filter in combination with anticoagulation therapy [7]. If a patient with cancer develops DVT or PE, treatment guidelines recommend initiating treatment with a once-daily LMWH regimen, with suggested pharmacological alternatives of fondaparinux for patients with ongoing or prior HIT, or UFH for patients with severe renal insufficiency or who are dialysis-dependent. An IVC filter should only be considered in selected patients with an absolute contraindication to anticoagulant therapy, given the prothrombotic stimulus of such foreign bodies [6, 7]. Finally, thrombolytic therapy should only be considered in patients with clinically massive DVT or PE, and with caution given the increased bleeding risk of patients with cancer [7]. A minimum of 3 months' anticoagulant therapy is recommended, with LMWH preferred over VKAs and with consideration given to at least 6 months of treatment, especially in patients who are receiving cancer treatment or with metastatic disease [7, 59, 64, 65]. However, the qualitative interviews highlighted a lack of consensus among physicians regarding treatment after the initial 6-month period. Indeed, the DALTECAN study examined the efficacy and safety of up to 12 months' treatment with dalteparin, and found that VTE recurrence and bleeding were clustered during the initial month after diagnosis, thereby supporting the long-term safety of LMWH therapy [66]. After 6 months' treatment, the need for ongoing anticoagulant therapy should be reassessed based on a risk versus benefit assessment in conjunction with patient values and preference [12].

The lack of published data on the benefits of VTE reduction through thromboprophylaxis versus the risks of bleeding was highlighted by the experts as one of the reasons why guideline recommendations are not routinely followed by physicians. Patients with GBM treated with lifelong anticoagulation have a reduced rate of recurrent VTE but, despite these findings, thromboprophylaxis is underutilised in such patients [67]. According to the experts interviewed, this may be partly due to differences in the views of oncology specialists regarding the need for treatment of established VTE compared to the role of primary thromboprophylaxis. In contrast, another study demonstrated that patients with cancer treated with anticoagulant therapy suffered a 3-fold higher incidence of intracranial haemorrhage [68]. The differences in the rate of VTE recurrence incidence and major bleeding events were linked to the type of cancer, as a study demonstrated that the rates of VTE recurrence and major bleeding events during the course of anticoagulation were similar in patients with breast or colorectal cancer, whereas a 2-fold higher rate of thromboembolic recurrences than the rate of major bleeding events was identified in patients with lung cancer, and a lower rate of VTE than bleeding was recorded in patients with prostate cancer [19]. These data underscore the importance of considering the type of cancer and associated comorbidities in order to weigh the potential benefits and risks of anticoagulant prophylaxis.

For the past two decades, LMWHs have been the preferred first-line treatment option for the management of cancer-associated VTE. This is supported by results from the qualitative survey, which found that 75% (33/44) of physicians interviewed use LMWH as standard of

care for thrombosis treatment. Several seminal studies have shown superior efficacy and safety of LMWHs over VKA. The CANTHANOX study reported 10.6% more patients experiencing one combined major outcome event, such as major bleeding or recurrent VTE within a 3-month period, in the warfarin group compared to the fixed-dose enoxaparin group [69]. The CLOT study demonstrated that a weight-adjusted dose of dalteparin was more effective in reducing the probability of recurrent VTE compared to a warfarin derivative over a 6-month treatment period [64]. Similarly, the LITE study found a greater number of VTE episodes in the VKA than the tinzaparin treatment group at 3 and 12 months, with largely similar minor bleeding complications [70], whereas the more recent CATCH study demonstrated a similar rate of recurrent VTE over a 6-month period with tinzaparin compared to warfarin, but a lower rate of relevant non-major bleeding was noted in the tinzaparin group [71]. The cumulative probability of being VTE-free at 6 months, as demonstrated by the ONCENOX study, was higher for the group receiving enoxaparin than for the group where treatment with enoxaparin preceded that with warfarin [72]. In summary, LMWHs seem to be preferred anticoagulants over VKAs.

More recently, DOACs have emerged as a potential alternative first-line treatment option for cancer-associated VTE, but with caveats. In general, the type of anticoagulant administered should be tailored according to patient and cancer type characteristics. The expert discussions and interviews highlighted that the advantages of LMWHs over DOACs include the ease of adapting the dose to the patient's body weight and anticoagulation need, no drug–drug interactions related to chemotherapy regimens, and flexibility around procedures and other clinical situations (e.g., thrombocytopenia) that require treatment interruption or dose reduction. However, the experts agreed that prolonged drug administration through subcutaneous injection was the most common disadvantage associated with LMWH treatment, followed, in certain countries, by the relatively high cost of LMWH. Currently, DOACs are used for treatment of VTE in patients with stable cancer who are not receiving anticancer therapy and when VKAs are unavailable [59]. Some published studies, specifically the AMPLIFY trial [73] and the Hokusai-VTE trial [74], demonstrate that DOACs have similar efficacy to that of LMWHs or warfarin. Nevertheless, the authors agreed that bleeding risk associated with DOACs should be addressed, as bleeding may be a more frequent cause of death than fatal VTE. The HOKUSAI-CANCER study compared dalteparin with edoxaban over a 12-month period and demonstrated a comparable rate of VTE recurrence in both groups, although a higher rate of major bleeding was observed in the edoxaban group [75]. In addition, in the recent SELECT-D study, patients treated with rivaroxaban displayed a lower cumulative VTE recurrence rate than those treated with dalteparin, but had a higher rate of major and clinically relevant non-major bleeding events in the 6-month period [65].

The experts noted that the administration of LMWHs and DOACs may become interchangeable, as patients with cancer have a complex clinical course and receive many different therapies; for example, it is possible to envisage that LMWHs will be used during hospitalisation and DOACs in out-of-hospital periods. The cost was considered to be one of the major reasons for insufficient adherence to guideline recommendations for the use of LMWHs. Among other reasons for the suboptimal use of LMWHs are inconvenience of LMWH injections and insufficient awareness of care givers regarding the importance of secondary prevention of VTE.

In conclusion, it is important to consider cancer site, stage of the disease and anticancer treatments given to patients to ensure the choice of an optimal anticoagulant and its dosage for secondary prevention of VTE.

Inadequate management of VTE in critically ill patients

VTE is a frequent cause of preventable morbidity and mortality in hospitalised acutely ill patients [76], and it is recognised that the main burden of disease occurs in an out-of-hospital setting when in-hospital thromboprophylaxis ceases upon discharge of these patients from hospital. DVT rates usually range from 13 to 31% in critically ill patients without thromboprophylaxis [77], and 26% of patients with undiagnosed or untreated PE will have a subsequent fatal embolic event [78, 79]. Moreover, a non-fatal recurrent embolic event will occur in another 26% of patients with PE [78, 79]. Continuous improvement in thromboprophylaxis in hospitalised acutely ill patients has occurred over the past decade, but expert consensus suggests prevention of VTE still remains a significant unmet need in medical patients compared to prevention of VTE and its management in surgical patients.

Stratification of VTE and bleeding risks in critically ill patients
At least one VTE risk factor is present in most hospitalised critically ill medical patients, and usually the risk of VTE remains in patients for several weeks after discharge from hospital [80]. Despite this problem, insufficient published data exist on the validity of risk scores for determining the risk level of VTE in critically ill patients. Some studies have investigated how to define subgroups of critically ill patients in which the benefit-to-risk ratio is in favour of thromboprophylaxis [81, 82]. The EXCLAIM study compared efficacy and safety of extended-duration thromboprophylaxis with enoxaparin

to placebo in acutely ill medical patients with prolonged reduced mobility [81]. The study found that extended administration of enoxaparin reduced the rate of VTE incidence from 4 to 2.5% but increased the rate of major bleeding events (0.8% versus 0.3% favouring placebo). However, the benefit of reduction of VTE incidence in some acutely ill medical patient subgroups, including patients with level 1 immobility, patients > 75 years of age and women, outweighed the risk of increase in major bleeding events [81]. The MAGELLAN trial demonstrated that D-dimer is an independent predictor of VTE risk (odds ratio 2.29) and a 3.5-fold greater incidence of VTE was detected in patients with D-dimer concentrations > 2-fold higher than the upper limit of normal (ULN) baseline value [82]. However, the experts agreed that D-dimer has little value as a biomarker of VTE in clinical practice and it is currently used for a purely scientific purpose. Decisions on prophylaxis are usually based on clinical parameters. Implementation of D-dimer in routine clinical practice for critically ill patients as part of a risk stratification model is difficult, as significant variation between the assays and protocols in different hospitals exists, thus making standardisation of the assay problematic. The experts noted that D-dimer is not a good marker for VTE for patients in the intensive care unit (ICU), as other factors, such as infection, can affect D-dimer levels. However, if D-dimer levels increase over a stay in hospital, then it could be indicative of thrombosis.

Moreover, the qualitative interviews highlighted limitations in carrying out assays in certain countries where samples had to be sent abroad for testing, or where patients lived in out-of-reach rural areas where general practitioners are in need of simple stratification methods for identifying high-risk patients. Indeed, 58% (14/24) of experts questioned considered that improved estimation of an individual's benefit-to-risk ratio required further experimental investigation to allow better patient stratification for personalised prophylactic anticoagulant therapy.

Prophylaxis and treatment regimens in critically ill patients
Thromboprophylaxis is recommended to all ICU patients, including high-risk patients with immobility until mobility is restored [83]. However, the experts agreed that there are no clear recommendations on how to identify patients at risk or on how to manage asymptomatic VTE, which is an underlying cause for symptomatic VTE. Moreover, in the recent APEX trial, acutely ill patients who were assessed for, and found to have, asymptomatic DVT had a 3-fold increased risk of short-term all-cause mortality [84].

LMWH is the anticoagulant of choice used in critical care units with a guideline-suggested enoxaparin dose of 40 mg once daily [12, 85]. The beneficial effects of enoxaparin given at 40 mg dose compared to placebo extend to a wide range of acutely ill medical patients, including patients with acute or chronic heart failure, acute or chronic respiratory failure, acute infectious disease, acute rheumatic disorder, cancer, a history of VTE or immobility [85]. The choice of a particular LMWH should be based on the magnitude of a clinical effect, level of evidence, approval by the regulatory authorities for each indication, and cost [79]. Consideration should be given as to whether LMWH should be administered once or twice per day depending on a specific clinical situation, while taking into account safety and a patient's renal function. Dalteparin and tinzaparin have safety advantages compared to enoxaparin when renal impairment manifests, i.e., when creatinine clearance is below 30 mL/min, because of differences in molecular weight and the LMWH clearance pathway, therefore prophylactic doses of dalteparin and tinzaparin in patients with impaired renal function are safe [86]. In contrast, fondaparinux is currently contraindicated in critically ill patients with severe renal disease [87].

Evidence suggests that LMWH should be a preferred option over UFH in critical care units, as the latter is linked to HIT and requires more frequent dosing [88]. The study of dalteparin and UFH efficacy and safety has demonstrated that proximal leg DVT rates are similar in the dalteparin and UFH groups, but treatment with dalteparin results in a significantly lower proportion of patients with PE when compared to treatment with UFH, while the rates of major bleeding or death in the hospital are similar between the groups [89]. The Avoid-Heparin Initiative proved additional benefits of using LMWH over UFH by demonstrating the decrease of the annual rate of suspected HIT by 42% ($P < 0.001$) and the annual rate of patients with a positive HIT assay by 63% ($P < 0.001$), where adjudicated HIT and HIT and thrombosis decreased by 79% ($P < 0.001$) and 91% ($P < 0.001$), respectively [88]. Moreover, hospital HIT-related expenditures decreased by US$266,938 per year in the avoid-heparin phase [88].

The duration of anticoagulant therapy may be restricted by the presence of individual risk factors for anticoagulant-induced bleeding. Thrombosis Canada guidelines note that patients > 75 years of age, those with renal or liver failure, patients with previous stroke history and those with cancer are at a higher risk of bleeding [76]. The International Stroke Trial, a large study of 14,578 patients with suspected acute ischaemic stroke, demonstrated that treatment with heparin was associated with an increased risk of haemorrhagic or serious extracranial haemorrhagic stroke. However, this was outweighed by a decrease in recurrent ischaemic stroke [90] and the American College of Physicians recommended the use of heparin for VTE prophylaxis in stroke

patients, provided evaluation of individual VTE and bleeding risks are carried out [79].

If pharmacological thromboprophylaxis is contraindicated due to high risk of bleeding, then application of elastic compression stockings or intermittent pneumatic compression is advised [91]. Mechanical compression is very effective in ICU patients and can be used in combination with pharmacological intervention [92], although the expert interviews suggest that compliance to mechanical compression is low in the ICU.

According to experts in countries where patients are expected to pay for medication, cost is a factor that restricts both prescription of prophylactic drugs and patient up-take of a prescribed medication. Prescriptions are limited to high-risk patients, those admitted to hospital for long periods or those undergoing surgical intervention. LMWH is available exclusively in special hospital units in these countries.

DOACs are not currently recommended by the guidelines for thromboprophylaxis in critically ill patients, and the authors agreed that LMWH is a preferred choice of an anticoagulant during hospitalisation, but after discharge from hospital a switch to DOACs may be recommended. In support of this statement, the APEX study demonstrated that a similar proportion of patients receiving extended thromboprophylaxis with betrixaban or standard-duration enoxaparin therapy achieved reduction in a composite of asymptomatic proximal DVT and symptomatic VTE without differences in frequency of major bleeding events [93]. Betrixaban also showed efficacy at an 80 mg dose versus standard-dose subcutaneous enoxaparin (40 mg once daily 10 ± 4 days) with a better primary efficacy outcome (6.27% versus 8.39%; relative risk reduction 0.26; $P = 0.023$). However, a greater risk of clinically relevant non-major bleeding compared to the enoxaparin group was observed [94]. The subpopulation analysis that involves patients with stroke also suggests benefits of betrixaban, as extended-duration treatment with betrixaban significantly reduced all-cause stroke and ischaemic stroke during a 77-day follow-up period [95]. The exploratory post-hoc analysis in patients with a history of VTE revealed that only 12 patients would need to be treated with betrixaban to prevent an additional VTE endpoint [96]. Extended thromboprophylaxis with betrixaban was more efficient compared with standard-duration enoxaparin, and resulted in reduced risk of VTE-related rehospitalisation at day 42 (0.25% versus 0.76%; hazard ratio [HR] 0.33) and at day 77 (0.46% versus 1.04%; HR 0.44) [96].

Extended prophylaxis beyond hospitalisation
According to our qualitative research, expert opinion on the benefits of extended prophylaxis is divided due to a lack of evidence and contradictory guidelines. The

experts stressed that acutely ill patients are exposed to an elevated risk of VTE after discharge from hospital, as VTE prophylaxis remains inadequate during this period, thus having an adverse effect on patient outcomes and presenting a financial burden on the healthcare system [80]. However, a prospective observational study reported that out of 5.5% of hospitalised critically ill patients who developed VTE, 74.1% of patients acquired VTE during hospitalisation and 25.9% following discharge, and the latter was affected by a history of VTE, recent surgery and pulmonary conditions [80]. ADOPT, EXCLAIM, MAGELLAN and APEX studies involved acutely ill hospitalised patients, examining efficacy and safety of extended-duration thromboprophylaxis with either enoxaparin or DOACs, including apixaban, betrixaban or rivaroxaban [81, 93, 97, 98]. These studies showed that following a 30-day or longer treatment period (up to 35 ± 4 days), VTE rates range from 2.5 to 5.7%, suggesting that significant VTE burden occurs well beyond hospitalisation [81, 93, 97, 98]. The ADOPT trial demonstrated an immediate increase in VTE risk when standard-duration (6–14 days) prophylaxis with enoxaparin was stopped [97]. Considering that acutely ill hospitalised patients are usually discharged before 5 days of hospitalisation and prophylaxis is discontinued post-discharge, VTE risk remains high in this period [97]. Extended-duration prophylaxis (28 ± 4 days) with enoxaparin administered to both hospitalised patients and outpatients was effective in reducing VTE incidence from 4 to 2.5% according to the EXCLAIM study [81]. The MAGELLAN study showed that rivaroxaban administered for an extended period (35 ± 4 days) was superior to standard-duration (10 ± 4 days) enoxaparin [98]. However, both the EXCLAIM and MAGELLAN studies showed an increase in major bleeding risk. The sub-analysis of the MAGELLAN study revealed that the high D-dimer (> 2-fold the ULN baseline level) group responded equally as well to enoxaparin or rivaroxaban at day 10, but rivaroxaban was superior to placebo at day 35 [82]. It has been noted that testing at the end of a 10-day prophylaxis regimen may identify individuals at greater risk of VTE who would benefit from extended therapy, but the impracticalities of collecting samples for laboratory tests on or after discharge from hospital have also been highlighted [82]. The APEX study demonstrates the benefits of extended prophylaxis with betrixaban in critically ill patients, but due to reduced length of hospital stay becoming more common and the discontinuation of these drugs post-discharge, thromboprophylaxis may remain inadequate [93].

While the above studies highlight the benefits of extended prophylaxis using enoxaparin or DOACs beyond the standard in-hospital therapy, they did not directly compare VTE rates in patients who received

anticoagulant therapy versus those who had no prophylaxis beyond the hospital stay. Recent results from the MARINER trial that directly evaluated the efficacy and safety of thromboprophylaxis – in this case with rivaroxaban, compared to a placebo – in preventing symptomatic VTE in high-risk medical patients from the start of hospital discharge to 45 days post-discharge found that extended thromboprophylaxis did not significantly lower the risk of VTE or death [99].

Based on findings from the APEX study, the US Food and Drug Administration (FDA) approved betrixaban for extended thromboprophylaxis in critically ill medical patients at risk of VTE due to moderate or severe restricted mobility [100]. However, this has not been the case in Europe where the Committee for Medicinal Products for Human Use found that on review of the data from APEX, the safety and efficacy of betrixaban was not robustly demonstrated [101]. In addition, recent guidelines published by the American Society of Hematology advise against extending pharmacological prophylaxis following hospital discharge [102]. Therefore, although post-discharge VTE prophylaxis may be warranted, a more liberal use of this concept outside of the selection criteria of APEX is not recommended.

Conclusions

In comparison to surgical patients, where VTE management has improved considerably, thromboprophylaxis for critically ill and cancer patients remains inadequate. This is partly due to a lack of relevant clinical trials in these patient populations, but may also be linked to the complication of comorbidities and a lack of understanding of HCPs on how to balance prophylaxis and bleeding risk. Despite an increase in survival rate of cancer patients, VTE incidence remains at an elevated level and is one of the major causes of mortality in this patient population. High VTE risk is linked to certain chemotherapeutic regimens and cancer or tumour types, therefore, the ability to stratify patients according to these criteria would improve VTE outcomes in cancer patients. However, biomarkers and risk assessment scores are inconsistent and in both critically ill and cancer patients, tests such as D-dimer may be affected by other factors related to the patient's illness, such as infection, rendering the test unreliable.

Due to its safety and efficacy profile, LMWH remains the first choice of prophylaxis in critically ill and cancer patients. VKA is not advised for patients with cancer and UFH is not recommended in critically ill patients due to the risk of HIT. The safety of DOACs due to the increased bleeding risk needs to be examined further before they can be used routinely in patients with cancer. However, a recent study and an FDA approval on the use of betrixaban for extended thromboprophylaxis in critically ill patients demonstrates the effectiveness of this DOAC in reducing VTE incidence.

Despite improvements in in-hospital thromboprophylaxis, post-discharge, the use of thromboprophylaxis needs to be clarified. In both critically ill and cancer patients, the risk of VTE extends outside the hospital stay, but out-of-hospital risk assessment is impractical and recent studies, FDA approval, European Medical Agency rejection and guideline recommendations on extended use of thromboprophylaxis following discharge are contradictory. Therefore, out-of-hospital thromboprophylaxis should be carefully considered according to a patient's benefit-to-risk profile.

Future studies need to examine methods of stratifying patients with cancer according to stage of disease, cancer site and cancer treatment, to improve knowledge regarding anticoagulant regimens in order to decrease the risk of bleeding and VTE recurrence. In critically ill patients, the burden of VTE lies outside the hospital setting and therefore, more studies are needed to examine practical means of risk assessing patients after discharge and to compare thromboprophylaxis options considering patient preferences, comorbidities and bleeding risk.

Abbreviations

DOAC: Direct oral anticoagulants; DVT: Deep vein thrombosis; FDA: US Food and Drug Administration; GBM: Glioblastoma multiforme; HCP: Healthcare professional; HIT: Heparin-induced thrombocytopenia; HR: Hazard ratio; ICU: Intensive care unit; IMiD: Immunomodulatory imide drugs; IVC: Inferior vena cava; KS: Khorana risk score; LMWH: Low-molecular-weight heparin; MM: Multiple myeloma; PE: Pulmonary embolism; RR: Risk ratio; UFH: Unfractionated heparin; ULN: Upper limit of normal.; VKA: Vitamin K antagonist; VTE: Venous thromboembolism

Acknowledgements

Editorial support was provided by Dr. Egle McDonald and Jane Juif, HealthCare21 Communications Ltd., Macclesfield, Cheshire, SK10 2XA, UK, and was supported by Sanofi.

Author details

[1]Department of Hematology and Bone Marrow Transplantation, Rambam Health Care Campus, Haifa, Israel. [2]Foothills Medical Centre and Thrombosis Research Unit, University of Calgary, Calgary, Canada. [3]King's Thrombosis Centre, Department of Haematological Medicine, King's College Hospital NHS Foundation Trust, London, UK. [4]Thrombosis Research Unit, Department of Medicine I, Division Hematology, University Hospital 'Carl Gustav Carus' Dresden, Dresden, Germany. [5]King's Thrombosis Service, Department of Haematology, King's College London, London, UK. [6]Department of Medicine, McMaster University, Hamilton, Ontario, Canada. [7]Thrombosis and Atherosclerosis Research Institute, Hamilton, Ontario, Canada. [8]I.M. Sechenov First Moscow State Medical University, Moscow, Russia. [9]Hematology and Thrombosis Center, Tenon University Hospital, Sorbonne University, Paris, France. [10]Haemostasis and Thrombosis Center, Hospital of Piacenza, Piacenza, Italy. [11]Department of Pulmonary and Critical Care Medicine, Center of Respiratory Medicine, China-Japan Friendship Hospital, National Clinical Research Center for Respiratory Diseases, Beijing, China.

References

1. Ay C, Kamphuisen PW, Agnelli G. Antithrombotic therapy for prophylaxis and treatment of venous thromboembolism in patients with cancer: review of the literature on current practice and emerging options. ESMO Open. 2017;2(2):e000188.
2. Thrombosis Canada (2017) Apixaban (Eliquis®). Available at: http://thrombosiscanada.ca/wp-content/uploads/2017/01/20.-Apixaban-2017 Jan13-FINAL.pdf. Accessed 8 Apr 2019.
3. Nicolaides AN, Fareed J, Kakkar AK, Comerota AJ, Goldhaber SZ, Hull R, et al. Prevention and treatment of venous thromboembolism--international consensus statement. Int Angiol. 2013;32(2):111–260.
4. Rocha AT, EFD P, Bernardo WM. Atualização em tromboembolismo venoso: profilaxia em pacientes clínicos – parte I. Revista da Associação Médica Brasileira. 2009;55:249–50.
5. Suh J, Desai A, Desai A, Cruz JD, Mariampillai A, Hindenburg A. Adherence to thromboprophylaxis guidelines in elderly patients with hospital acquired venous thromboembolism: a case control study. J Thromb Thrombolysis. 2017;43(2):172–8.
6. Farge D, Debourdeau P, Beckers M, Baglin C, Bauersachs RM, Brenner B, et al. International clinical practice guidelines for the treatment and prophylaxis of venous thromboembolism in patients with cancer. J Thromb Haemost. 2013;11(1):56–70.
7. Farge D, Bounameaux H, Brenner B, Cajfinger F, Debourdeau P, Khorana AA, et al. International clinical practice guidelines including guidance for direct oral anticoagulants in the treatment and prophylaxis of venous thromboembolism in patients with cancer. Lancet Oncol. 2016;17(10):e452–66.
8. Thrombosis Guidelines Group (2009) Thromboprophylaxis in acutely ill hospitalized medical patients. Available at: http://www.thrombosisguidelines group.be/. Accessed 8 Apr 2019.
9. Patil S, Ayad M, Maithili S, Patel B. Preventable vs non-preventable VTE in hospitalized patients. CHEST J. 2016;150(4):598A.
10. Lukaszuk RF, Dolna-Michno J, Plens K, Czyzewicz G, Undas A. The comparison between Caprini and Padua VTE risk assessment models for hospitalised cancer patients undergoing chemotherapy at the tertiary oncology department in Poland: is pharmacological thromboprophylaxis overused? Contemp Oncol. 2018;22(1):31–6.
11. Rosenberg D, Eichorn A, Alarcon M, McCullagh L, McGinn T, Spyropoulos AC. External validation of the risk assessment model of the international medical prevention registry on venous thromboembolism (IMPROVE) for medical patients in a tertiary health system. J Am Heart Assoc. 2014;3(6):e001152.
12. National Institute for Health and Care Excellence (2018) Venous thromboembolism in over 16s: reducing the risk of hospital-acquired deep vein thrombosis or pulmonary embolism. Available at: https://www.nice.org.uk/guidance/ng89. Accessed 8 Apr 2019.
13. Kahn SR. The post-thrombotic syndrome: the forgotten morbidity of deep venous thrombosis. J Thromb Thrombolysis. 2006;21(1):41–8.
14. Tapson VF. Acute pulmonary embolism. N Engl J Med. 2008;358(10):1037–52.
15. Winter MP, Schernthaner GH, Lang IM. Chronic complications of venous thromboembolism. J Thromb Haemost. 2017;15(8):1531–40.
16. Bates SM, Middeldorp S, Rodger M, James AH, Greer I. Guidance for the treatment and prevention of obstetric-associated venous thromboembolism. J Thromb Thrombolysis. 2016;41(1):92–128.
17. Engbers MJ, van Hylckama VA, Rosendaal FR. Venous thrombosis in the elderly: incidence, risk factors and risk groups. J Thromb Haemost. 2010;8(10):2105–12.
18. Horsted F, West J, Grainge MJ. Risk of venous thromboembolism in patients with cancer: a systematic review and meta-analysis. PLoS Med. 2012;9: e1001275.
19. Mahé I, Chidiac J, Bertoletti L, Font C, Trujillo-Santos J, Peris M, et al. The clinical course of venous thromboembolism may differ according to cancer site. Am J Med. 2017;130(3):337–47.
20. Louzada ML, Carrier M, Lazo-Langner A, Dao V, Kovacs MJ, Ramsay TO, et al. Development of a clinical prediction rule for risk stratification of recurrent venous thromboembolism in patients with cancer-associated venous thromboembolism. Circulation. 2012;126(4):448–54.
21. Heit JA, Spencer FA, White RH. The epidemiology of venous thromboembolism. J Thromb Thrombolysis. 2016;41(1):3–14.
22. Imberti D, Agnelli G, Ageno W, Moia M, Palareti G, Pistelli R. Clinical characteristics and management of cancer-associated acute venous thromboembolism: findings from the MASTER registry. Haematologica. 2008;93(2):273–8.

23. Guijarro R, de Miguel-Diez J, Jimenez D, Trujillo-Santos J, Otero R, Barba R. Pulmonary embolism, acute coronary syndrome and ischemic stroke in the Spanish National Discharge Database. Eur J Intern Med. 2016;28:65–9.

24. Monreal M, Falga C, Valdes M, Suarez C, Gabriel F, Tolosa C. Fatal pulmonary embolism and fatal bleeding in cancer patients with venous thromboembolism: findings from the RIETE registry. J Thromb Haemost. 2006;4(9):1950–6.

25. Sheth RA, Niekamp A, Quencer KB, Shamoun F, Knuttinen MG, Naidu S, et al. Thrombosis in cancer patients: etiology, incidence, and management. Cardiovasc Diagn Ther. 2017;7(Suppl 3):S178–85.

26. Hisada Y, Geddings JE, Mackman N. Venous thrombosis and cancer: from mouse models to clinical trials. J Thromb Haemost. 2015;13(8):1372–82.

27. Zamorano JL, Lancellotti P, Rodriguez Munoz D, Aboyans V, Asteggiano R, Galderisi M, et al. 2016 ESC position paper on cancer treatments and cardiovascular toxicity developed under the auspices of the ESC Committee for practice guidelines: the task force for cancer treatments and cardiovascular toxicity of the European Society of Cardiology (ESC). Eur Heart J. 2016;37(36):2768–801.

28. Walker AJ, Card TR, West J, Crooks C, Grainge MJ. Incidence of venous thromboembolism in patients with cancer - a cohort study using linked United Kingdom databases. Eur J Cancer. 2013;49:1404–13.

29. Li R, Hermann G, Baldini E, Chen A, Jackman D, Kozono D, et al. Advanced nodal stage predicts venous thromboembolism in patients with locally advanced non-small cell lung cancer. Lung Cancer. 2016;96:41–7.

30. Tun NM, Guevara E, Oo TH. Benefit and risk of primary thromboprophylaxis in ambulatory patients with advanced pancreatic cancer receiving chemotherapy: a systematic review and meta-analysis of randomized controlled trials. Blood Coagul Fibrinolysis. 2016;27(3):270–4.

31. Qian C, Yan H, Hu X, Zhang W, Liu H. Increased risk of venous thromboembolism in patients with brain tumors: a systematic review and meta-analysis. Thromb Res. 2016;137:58–63.

32. Lee YG, Kim I, Lee E, Bang SM, Kang CH, Kim YT, et al. Risk factors and prognostic impact of venous thromboembolism in Asian patients with non-small cell lung cancer. Thromb Haemost. 2014;111(6):1112–20.

33. Wang L, Baser O, Kutikova L, Page JH, Barron R. The impact of primary prophylaxis with granulocyte colony-stimulating factors on febrile neutropenia during chemotherapy: a systematic review and meta-analysis of randomized controlled trials. Support Care Cancer. 2015;23:3131–40.

34. Shahzad H, Wu R, Datta D. Does histologic type and stage of cancer impact the occurrence of VTE in lung cancer? Chest J. 2017;152(4):A637.

35. Delmonte A, Mariotti M, Scarpi E, Ulivi P, Gavelli G, Rossi A, et al. Venous thromboembolic events in advanced adenocarcinoma of the lung: impact on prognosis according to platinum therapies and presence of driver mutations. Ann Oncol. 2015;26(Suppl 6):vi73–89.

36. Kourelis TV, Wysokinska EM, Wang Y, Yang P, Mansfield AS, Tafur AJ. Early venous thromboembolic events are associated with worse prognosis in patients with lung cancer. Lung Cancer. 2014 Dec;86(3):358–62.

37. Steuer CE, Behera M, Kim S, Patel N, Chen Z, Pillai R, et al. Predictors and outcomes of venous thromboembolism in hospitalized lung cancer patients: a Nationwide inpatient sample database analysis. Lung Cancer. 2015;88(1):80–4.

38. Zer A, Moskovitz M, Hwang DM, Hershko-Klement A, Fridel L, Korpanty GJ, et al. ALK-rearranged non-small-cell lung cancer is associated with a high rate of venous thromboembolism. Clin Lung Cancer. 2017;18(2):156–61.

39. Kondo S, Sasaki M, Hosoi H, Sakamoto Y, Morizane C, Ueno H, Okusaka T. Incidence and risk factors for venous thromboembolism in patients with pretreated advanced pancreatic carcinoma. Oncotarget. 2018;9(24):16883–90.

40. Terpos E, Kleber M, Engelhardt M, Zweegman S, Gay F, Kastritis E, et al. European myeloma network guidelines for the management of multiple myeloma-related complications. Haematologica. 2015;100(10):1254–66.

41. Moreau P, San Miguel J, Sonneveld P, Mateos MV, Zamagni E, Avet-Loiseau H, et al. Multiple myeloma: ESMO clinical practical guidelines for diagnosis, treatment and follow-up. Ann Oncol. 2017;28(4):iv52–61.

42. Carrier M, Lazo-Langner A, Shivakumar S, Tagalakis V, Gross PL, Blais N, et al. Clinical challenges in patients with cancer-associated thrombosis: Canadian expert consensus recommendations. Curr Oncol. 2015;22:49–59.

43. Heit JA, Silverstein MD, Mohr DN, Petterson TM, O'Fallon WM, Melton LJ III. Risk factors for deep vein thrombosis and pulmonary embolism: a population-based case-control study. Arch Intern Med. 2000;160(6):809.

44. Khorana AA, Francis CW, Culakova E, Kuderer NM, Lyman GH. Thromboembolism is a leading cause of death in cancer patients receiving outpatient chemotherapy. J Thromb Haemost. 2007;5(3):632–4.

45. Watson HG, Keeling DM, Laffan M, Tait RC, Makris M. British Committee for Standards in H. guideline on aspects of cancer-related venous thrombosis. Br J Haematol. 2015;170(5):640–8.

46. Mansfield AS, Tafur AJ, Wang CE, Kourelis TV, Wysokinska EM, Yang P. Predictors of active cancer thromboembolic outcomes: validation of the Khorana score among patients with lung cancer. J Thromb Haemost. 2016;14(9):1773–8.

47. Noble S, Alikhan R, Robbins A, Macbeth F, Hood K. Predictors of active cancer thromboembolic outcomes: validation of the Khorana score among patients with lung cancer: comment. J Thromb Haemost. 2017;15:590–1.

48. Kruger S, Haas M, Burkl C, Goehring P, Kleespies A, Roeder F, et al. Incidence, outcome and risk stratification tools for venous thromboembolism in advanced pancreatic cancer - a retrospective cohort study. Thromb Res. 2017;157:9–15.

49. van Es N, Franke VF, Middeldorp S, Wilmink JW, Büller HR. The Khorana score for the prediction of venous thromboembolism in patients with pancreatic cancer. Thromb Res. 2017;150:30–2.

50. Petitto GS, Escalante CP, Richardson MN, Hernandez CR. Modified Khorana models for prediction of cancer-associated venous thromboembolism: an exploratory study. Blood. 2017;130(Suppl 1):4635 Accessed 04, March 2019. Retrieved from http://www.bloodjournal.org/content/130/Suppl_1/4635. Accessed 8 Apr 2019.

51. Alatri A, Mazzolai L, Font C, Tafur A, Valle R, Marchena PJ, et al. Low discriminating power of the modified Ottawa VTE risk score in a cohort of patients with cancer from the RIETE registry. Thromb Haemost. 2017;117(8):1630–6.

52. Ashrani AA, Gullerud RE, Petterson TM, Marks RS, Bailey KR, Heit JA. Risk factors for incident venous thromboembolism in active cancer patients: a population-based case-control study. Thromb Res. 2016;139:29–37.

53. Alexander M, Burbury K. A systematic review of biomarkers for the prediction of thromboembolism in lung cancer - results, practical issues and proposed strategies for future risk prediction models. Thromb Res. 2016;148:63–9.

54. Khorana AA, Kamphusien PW, Meyer G, Bauersachs R, Janas MS, Jarner MF, et al. Tissue factor as a predictor of recurrent venous thromboembolism in malignancy: biomarker analyses of the CATCH trial. J Clin Oncol. 2017;35(10):1078–85.

55. Konstantinides SV, Torbicki A, Agnelli G, Danchin N, Fitzmaurice D, Galie N, et al. 2014 ESC guidelines on the diagnosis and management of acute pulmonary embolism. Eur heart J. 2014;35(43):3033-3069, 3069a-3069k.

56. Al-Hameed F, Al-Dorzi HM, AlMomen A, Algahtani F, AlZahrani H, AlSaleh K, et al. Prophylaxis and treatment of venous thromboembolism in patients with cancer: the Saudi clinical practice guideline. Ann Saudi Med. 2015;35(2):95–106.

57. Mandalà M, Falanga A, Roila F, Group EGW. Management of venous thromboembolism (VTE) in cancer patients: ESMO Clinical Practice Guidelines. Ann Oncol. 2011;22(Suppl 6):vi85–92.

58. Easaw JC, Shea-Budgell MA, Wu CM, Czaykowski PM, Kassis J, Kuehl B, et al. Canadian consensus recommendations on the management of venous thromboembolism in patients with cancer. Part 2: treatment. Curr Oncol. 2015;22(2):144–55.

59. Lyman GH, Bohlke K, Khorana AA, Kuderer NM, Lee AY, Arcelus JI, et al. Venous thromboembolism prophylaxis and treatment in patients with cancer: American Society of Clinical Oncology clinical practice guideline update 2014. J Clin Oncol. 2015;33(6):654–6.

60. Al-Ani F, Bermejo JM, Mateos MV, Louzada M. Thromboprophylaxis in multiple myeloma patients treated with lenalidomide - a systematic review. Thromb Res. 2016;141:84–90.

61. Pelzer U, Opitz B, Deutschinoff G, Stauch M, Reitzig PC, Hahnfeld S, et al. Efficacy of prophylactic low-molecular weight heparin for ambulatory patients with advanced pancreatic cancer: outcomes from the CONKO-004 trial. J Clin Oncol. 2015;33(18):2028–34.

62. Khorana AA, Soff GA, Kakkar AK, Vadhan-Raj S, Riess H, Wun T, et al. Rivaroxaban Thromboprophylaxis in high-risk ambulatory Cancer patients receiving systemic therapy: results of a randomized clinical trial (CASSINI). Presented at ASH, 2018.

63. Carrier M, Abou-Nassar K, Mallick R, Tagalakis V, Shivakumar S, Schattner A, et al. Apixaban to prevent venous thromboembolism in patients with cancer. N Engl J Med. 2019;380(8):711–9.

64. Lee AY, Levine MN, Baker RI, Bowden C, Kakkar AK, Prins M, et al. Low-molecular-weight heparin versus a coumarin for the prevention of recurrent venous thromboembolism in patients with cancer. N Engl J Med. 2003;349(2):146–53.

65. Young AM, Marshall A, Thirlwall J, Chapman O, Lokare A, Hill C, et al. Comparison of an oral factor Xa inhibitor with low molecular weight heparin in patients with cancer with venous thromboembolism: results of a randomized trial (SELECT-D). J Clin Oncol. 2018;36(20):2017–23.

66. Francis CW, Kessler CM, Goldhaber SZ, Kovacs MJ, Monreal M, Huisman MV, et al. Treatment of venous thromboembolism in cancer patients with dalteparin for up to 12 months: the DALTECAN study. J Thromb Haemost. 2015;13(6):1028–35.

67. Edwin NC, Khoury MN, Sohal D, McCrae KR, Ahluwalia MS, Khorana AA. Recurrent venous thromboembolism in glioblastoma. Thromb Res. 2016;137: 184–8.

68. Zwicker JI, Karp Leaf R, Carrier M. A meta-analysis of intracranial hemorrhage in patients with brain tumors receiving therapeutic anticoagulation. J Thromb Haemost. 2016;14(9):1736–40.

69. Meyer G, Marjanovic Z, Valcke J, Lorcerie B, Gruel Y, Solal-Celigny P, et al. Comparison of low-molecular-weight heparin and warfarin for the secondary prevention of venous thromboembolism in patients with cancer: a randomized controlled study. Arch Intern Med. 2002;162(15):1729–35.

70. Hull RD, Pineo GF, Brant RF, Mah AF, Burke N, Dear R, et al. Long-term low-molecular-weight heparin versus usual care in proximal-vein thrombosis patients with cancer. Am J Med. 2006;119(12):1062–72.

71. Lee AYY, Kamphuisen PW, Meyer G, Bauersachs R, Janas MS, Jarner MF, et al. Tinzaparin vs warfarin for treatment of acute venous thromboembolism in patients with active cancer: a randomized clinical trial. JAMA. 2015;314(7): 677–86.

72. Deitcher SR, Kessler CM, Merli G, Rigas JR, Lyons RM, Fareed J, et al. Secondary prevention of venous thromboembolic events in patients with active cancer: enoxaparin alone versus initial enoxaparin followed by warfarin for a 180-day period. Clin Appl Thromb Hemost. 2006;12(4):389–96.

73. Agnelli G, Buller HR, Cohen A, Gallus AS, Lee TC, Pak R, et al. Oral apixaban for the treatment of venous thromboembolism in cancer patients: results from the AMPLIFY trial. J Thromb Haemost. 2015;13(12):2187–91.

74. The Hokusai-VTE Investigators. Edoxaban versus warfarin for the treatment of symptomatic venous thromboembolism. N Engl J Med. 2013;369:1406–15.

75. Raskob GE, van Es N, Verhamme P, Carrier M, Di Nisio M, Garcia D, et al. Edoxaban for the treatment of cancer-associated venous thromboembolism. N Engl J Med. 2018;378(7):615–24.

76. Thrombosis Canada (2016) Venous thromboembolism: duration of treatment. Available at: http://thrombosiscanada.ca/wp-content/uploads/2017/01/7.-VTE-Duration-of-Treatment-2016Dec07-FINAL-1.pdf. Accessed 8 Apr 2019.

77. Saigal S, Sharma JP, Joshi R, Singh DK. Thrombo-prophylaxis in acutely ill medical and critically patients. Indian J Crit Care Med. 2014;18(6):382–91.

78. Qaseem A, Snow V, Barry P, Hornbake ER, Rodnick JE, Tobolic T, et al. Current diagnosis of venous thromboembolism in primary care: a clinical practice guideline from the American Academy of family physicians and the American College of Physicians. Ann Fam Med. 2007;5(1):57–62.

79. Qaseem A, Chou R, Humphrey LL, Starkey M, Shekelle P. The clinical guidelines Committee of the American College of physicians. Venous thromboembolism prophylaxis in hospitalized patients: a clinical practice guideline from the American College of Physicians. Ann Intern Med. 2011;155(9):625–32.

80. Khalafallah AA, Kirkby BE, Wong S, Foong YC, Ranjan N, Luttrell J, et al. Venous thromboembolism in medical patients during hospitalisation and 3 months after hospitalisation: a prospective observational study. BMJ Open. 2016;6(8):e012346.

81. Hull RD, Schellong SM, Tapson VF, Monreal M, Samama MM, Nicol P, et al. Extended-duration venous thromboembolism prophylaxis in acutely ill medical patients with recently reduced mobility: a randomized trial. Ann Intern Med. 2010;153(1):8–18.

82. Cohen AT, Spiro TE, Spyropoulos AC, Desanctis YH, Homering M, Buller HR, et al. D-dimer as a predictor of venous thromboembolism in acutely ill, hospitalized patients: a subanalysis of the randomized controlled MAGELLAN trial. J Thromb Haemost. 2014;12(4):479–87.

83. Minet C, Potton L, Bonadona A, Hamidfar-Roy R, Somohano CA, Lugosi M, et al. Venous thromboembolism in the ICU: main characteristics, diagnosis and thromboprophylaxis. Crit Care. 2015;19:287.

84. Kalayci A, Gibson CM, Chi G, Yee MK, Korjian S, Datta S, et al. Asymptomatic deep vein thrombosis is associated with an increased risk of death: insights from the APEX trial. Thromb Haemost. 2018;118(12):2046–52.

85. Alikhan R, Cohen AT, Combe S, Samama MM, Desjardins L, Eldor A, et al. Prevention of venous thromboembolism in medical patients with enoxaparin: a subgroup analysis of the MEDENOX study. Blood Coagul Fibrinolysis. 2003;14: 341–6.

86. Atiq F, van den Bemt PM, Leebeek FW, van Gelder T, Versmissen J. A systematic review on the accumulation of prophylactic dosages of low-molecular-weight heparins (LMWHs) in patients with renal insufficiency. Eur J Clin Pharmacol. 2015;71(8):921–9.

87. Wahby KA, Riley LK, Tennenberg SD. Assessment of an extended interval fondaparinux dosing regimen for venous thromboembolism prophylaxis in critically ill patients with severe renal dysfunction using antifactor Xa levels. Pharmacotherapy. 2017;37(10):1241–8.

88. McGowan KE, Makari J, Diamantouros A, Bucci C, Rempel P, Selby R, et al. Reducing the hospital burden of heparin-induced thrombocytopenia: impact of an avoid-heparin program. Blood. 2016;127(16):1954–9.

89. Cook D, Meade M, Guyatt G, Walter S, Heels-Ansdell D, Warkentin TE, et al. Dalteparin versus unfractionated heparin in critically ill patients. N Engl J Med. 2011;364(14):1305–14.

90. International Stroke Trial Collaborative Group. The international stroke trial (IST): a randomised trial of aspirin, subcutaneous heparin, both, or neither among 19435 patients with acute ischaemic stroke. Lancet. 1997;349:1569–81.

91. Guyatt GH, Akl EA, Crowther M, Gutterman DD, Schuünemann HJ. The American College of Chest Physicians Antithrombotic Therapy and Prevention of thrombosis panel. Executive summary: antithrombotic therapy and prevention of thrombosis, 9th ed: American College of Chest Physicians evidence-based clinical practise guidelines. Chest. 2012;141(Suppl 2):S7–47.

92. Wan B, Fu HY, Yin JT, Ren GQ. Low-molecular-weight heparin and intermittent pneumatic compression for thromboprophylaxis in critical patients. Exp Ther Med. 2015;10(6):2331–6.

93. Cohen AT, Harrington RA, Goldhaber SZ, Hull RD, Wiens BL, Gold A, et al. Extended thromboprophylaxis with betrixaban in acutely ill medical patients. N Engl J Med. 2016;375(6):534–44.

94. Gibson CM, Halaby R, Korjian S, Daaboul Y, Arbetter DF, Yee MK, et al. The safety and efficacy of full- versus reduced-dose betrixaban in the acute medically ill VTE (venous thromboembolism) prevention with extended-duration Betrixaban (APEX) trial. Am Heart J. 2017;185:93–100.

95. Gibson CM, Chi G, Halaby R, Korjian S, Daaboul Y, Jain P, et al. Extended-duration betrixaban reduces the risk of stroke versus standard-dose enoxaparin among hospitalized medically ill patients: an APEX trial substudy (acute medically ill venous thromboembolism prevention with extended duration betrixaban). Circulation. 2017;135(7):648–55.

96. Yee MK, Nafee T, Daaboul Y, Korjian S, AlKhalfan F, Kerneis M, et al. Increased benefit of betrixaban among patients with a history of venous thromboembolism: a post-hoc analysis of the APEX trial. J Thromb Thrombolysis. 2018;45(1):1–8.

97. Goldhaber SZ, Leizorovicz A, Kakkar AK, Haas SK, Merli G, Knabb RM, et al. Apixaban versus enoxaparin for thromboprophylaxis in medically ill patients. N Engl J Med. 2011;365(23):2167–77.

98. Cohen AT, Spiro TE, Büller HR, Haskell L, Hu D, Hull R, et al. Rivaroxaban for thromboprophylaxis in acutely ill medical patients. N Engl J Med. 2013; 368(6):513–23.

99. Spyropoulos AC, Ageno W, Albers GW, Elliott CG, Halperin JL, Hiatt WR, et al. Rivaroxaban for thromboprophylaxis after hospitalization for medical illness. N Engl Med J. 2018;379:1118–27.

100. US Food and Drug Administration (FDA). FDA approved betrixaban (BEVYXXA, Portola) for the prophylaxis of venous thromboembolism (VTE) in adult patients. 2017. Available at: https://www.fda.gov/drugs/informationondrugs/approveddrugs/ucm564422.htm. Accessed 8 Apr 2019.

101. European Medicines Agency. Assessment report: Dexxience. International non-proprietary name: betrixaban. 2018. Available at: https://www.ema.europa.eu/documents/assessment-report/dexxience-epar-refusal-public-assessment-report_.pdf. Accessed 8 Apr 2019.

102. Schünemann HJ, Cushman M, Burnett AE, Kahn SR, Beyer-Westendorf J, et al. American Society of Hematology 2018 guidelines for management of venous thromboembolism: prophylaxis for hospitalized and nonhospitalized medical patients. Blood Adv. 2018;2(22):3198–25.

3

Chemoprophylaxis in addition to mechanical prophylaxis after total knee arthroplasty surgery does not reduce the incidence of venous thromboembolism

Jing Loong Moses Loh[1*] ⓘ, Stephrene Chan[2], Keng Lin Wong[3], Sanjay de Mel[4] and Eng Soo Yap[4*]

Abstract

Background: Venous thromboembolism (VTE) of the lower limbs is an important complication post total knee arthroplasty (TKA). Current guidelines recommend routine chemical prophylaxis to all patients undergoing this procedure but this is rarely done in Asia as it is believed that Asians have a lower risk of VTE. However, recent evidence suggests otherwise.

Aims: We evaluated the incidence of DVT after TKA in a multi-ethnic Asian population with and without pharmacological prophylaxis, as well as the management and outcome of patients with post-operative DVTs.

Methods: We conducted a retrospective study of consecutive patients who underwent TKA in our hospital from 1st January 2004 to 30th December 2014. All patients were on mechanical thromboprophylaxis via calf pumps after TKA with a postoperative day 3 to 5 doppler ultrasound (DUS) of bilateral lower limbs. 2258 (80.7%) patients did not receive additional chemoprophylaxis, while 540 (19.3%) received chemoprophylaxis on top of mechanical thromboprophylaxis. All patients who received chemoprophylaxis were administered the drug until they were ambulating, with a median administration duration of 6 days. Patients were followed up for a period of 3 months for recurrence of DVTs and 24 months for postoperative outcome scores.

Results: Two thousand nine hundred seventy-eight patients had DUS of the lower limbs with 134 diagnosed with DVT giving an incidence of 4.5%. Six of these patients had concurrent PEs. There were 26 (19.4%) proximal DVTs and 108 (80.6%) distal DVTs. After 3 months of follow up, no additional VTE occurred. None of the DVTs or PEs progressed.

All DVTs with accompanying PE were proximal. 102 out of 2200 patients (4.6%) without chemoprophylaxis developed DVT as compared to 32 out of 540 patients (5.9%) with chemoprophylaxis, which was not statistically significant ($p = 0.13$). 19 (0.8%) proximal and 83 (3.8%) distal DVT developed in the patient group without chemoprophylaxis while 4 (0.7%) proximal and 28 (5.2%) distal DVT developed in the patient group with ($p = 0.62$). Comparison of the incidence of PEs between the two groups, revealed a similar incidence with 5 out of 2200 patients (0.2%) without chemoprophylaxis developing PE as compared to 1 out of 540 patients (0.2%) with chemoprophylaxis ($p = 0.87$).

In addition, patients with chemoprophylaxis showed an association with higher post-operative outcome scores such as post op 6 months SF36 (PCS), post op 12 months SF36 (PCS), post op 12 months SF36 (MCS), post op 24 months SF36 (MCS) and post op 24 months WOMAC.

(Continued on next page)

* Correspondence: mosesloh1993@yahoo.com; Eng_Soo_YAP@nuhs.edu.sg
[1]Department of Orthopaedic Surgery, Singapore General Hospital, 20 College Road, Academia, Level 4, Singapore 169865, Singapore
[4]Department of Hematology-Oncology, National University Cancer Institute, National University Hospital, Singapore, Singapore
Full list of author information is available at the end of the article

(Continued from previous page)

Conclusion: In one of the largest Asian studies specifically investigating the incidence of DVT after TKA, we found that the incidence is low at 4.5%. This is in contrast to recent studies that showed higher post-operative VTE rates similar to Western populations. In addition, patients who were administered chemoprophylaxis did not have a statistically significant difference in incidence of VTE although it did show a correlation with higher post-operative outcome scores which may indicate better function. This was seen in functional outcome scores such as post op 6 months SF36 (PCS), post op 12 months SF36 (PCS), post op 12 months SF36 (MCS), post op 24 months SF36 (MCS) and post op 24 months WOMAC.

Introduction

There are over 1 million total hip and total knee replacement procedures performed each year in the United States alone [1]. Demand for hip and knee replacements is rising annually, and growth is expected to be substantial in the years to come due to various reasons including higher rates of diagnosis and treatment of advanced arthritis, as well as increasing demand for improved mobility and quality of life [1]. Venous thromboembolic events (VTE), including deep vein thrombosis (DVT) and pulmonary embolism (PE), are amongst one of the leading causes of morbidity and mortality associated with total knee arthroplasty (TKA) surgeries. 40–50% of patients with untreated symptomatic DVT will develop a PE within 3 months and 10% of patients with symptomatic PE die within an hour of onset [2]. In Caucasians, the DVT incidence following total knee arthroplasty (TKA) is reported at 41–85% and the incidence of pulmonary embolism (PE) of 1.5–10% [3]. The incidences of DVT reported in Asia following various orthopaedic procedures vary and have been reported to be as high as 53.3% [4–6]. In our local context, the reported rate of DVT after TKA is 14% [7].

The efficacy of chemical and mechanical thromboprophylaxis in preventing VTEs in this high-risk group of patients has been well demonstrated. The American Academy of Orthopaedic Surgeons (AAOS) recommends the use of pharmacologic agents and/or mechanical compressive devices for the prevention of venous thromboembolism in patients undergoing elective hip or knee arthroplasty, and who are not at elevated risk beyond that of the surgery itself for venous thromboembolism or bleeding [8]. Similarly, the American College of Chest Physicians (ACCP) states that in patients undergoing TKA, post-surgical chemical thromboprophylaxis with low-molecular-weight heparin (LMWH) or factor Xa inhibitors is recommended for a minimum of 10 to 14 days to reduce the risk and incidence of symptomatic deep vein thrombosis (DVT) and pulmonary embolism (PE) [9].

Despite this, chemoprophylaxis is generally underpractised in the Asian context [10], owing to concerns of bleeding, slow wound healing and prolonged wound drainage [11, 12]. In a recent paper, the bleeding from LMWH (enoxaparin) use after TKA in an Asian population was shown to be as high as 20% [13]. This reluctance to practise postoperative chemoprophylaxis is reinforced by the belief that the incidence of VTEs has been reported to be lower in the Asian population as compared to the Caucasian population [10]. This raises a debate about whether routine postoperative chemoprophylaxis is required in Asian patients [14].

The primary aim of this study is to determine the incidence of postoperative VTE following TKA in our local population with and without additional chemoprophylaxis in addition to routine mechanical prophylaxis in all patients. The secondary aims are to assess possible risk factors associated with VTE and to compare the 2 year functional outcomes of patients with and without postoperative VTE. We hypothesize that the rate of VTE in TKA patients is comparable to that of Western populations, and that there would be no differences in terms of functional outcomes between patients with and without postoperative VTE.

Materials and methods

We conducted a retrospective study of all patients who underwent elective TKA from 1st January 2004 to 31st December 2014 at an academic tertiary hospital for osteoarthritis of the knee. Ethics approval was obtained from the Institutional Review Board. Electronic and paper records were reviewed. The data was collected from case notes review, anaesthetic assessment chart reviews and electronic notes. Inclusion criteria were all patients who had underwent elective TKA during the specific time period. Patients who had total knee arthroplasty due to fractures, had unicompartmental knee arthroplasty and who were pre-operatively non ambulatory or minimally ambulatory, were excluded from the study.

Post-operative mobilisation and thromboprophylaxis protocol

Patients were allowed to stand on the first postoperative day and progressed to full-weight bearing activity with walking aids as tolerated. Each patient was provided with mechanical prophylaxis immediately post operation, which involved the use of both intermittent pneumatic compression pumps (ArjoHuntleigh Flowtron® Excel DVT pump system) and thromboembolic deterrent open toe knee length compression stockings (T.E.D™ Knee Length Anti- Embolism Stockings). Additional chemical thromboprophylaxis was administered, subject to the preference of the surgeon and the patient's risk profile. Mechanical prophylaxis was continued until patients were able to ambulate confidently with walking aids for two physiotherapy sessions on the same day. All patients underwent a DUS of both lower limbs within five days after their operation to detect DVT as part of a hospital wide protocol.

Data collection

Patient demographics including age, gender, significant co-morbidities, and pre-operative mobility status were recorded. Thrombotic risk factors such as hypertension, ischemic heart disease, Diabetes Mellitus, smoking habits, congestive heart failure, previous lower limb VTE and cancer were assessed.

The absence or presence of chemoprophylaxis use, in the form of subcutaneous low molecular weight heparin, was recorded for these patients, together with the presence or absence of VTE. The use of other anti-thrombotic agents postoperatively such as anti-platelet therapy was recorded The presence of DVT was defined as the lack of compressibility and impedance of normal blood in the affected veins, as seen on DUS, with the trifurcation point of the popliteal vein used as the demarcation between proximal and distal deep vein thrombosis. Patients who had symptoms suggestive of PE underwent computed tomography pulmonary angiogram (CTPA) for confirmation of PE, and the presence of symptomatic PE was also documented. Patients were followed up for three months to monitor for any recurrence of VTE.

All patients were followed up with outcome scores for 2 years post operation. Western Ontario and McMaster Universities Osteoarthritis Index [WOMAC] pain), and Short Form-36 (SF-36). Patient outcomes were recorded at six months, twelve months and twenty four months after surgery. These scores enable physicans to have an objective method of assessing the patient's function pre operation and postoperation, and can also be used to assess the patient's general wellbeing.. The WOMAC consists of 24 items divided into 3 subscales – Pain (WOMAC 1), Stiffness (WOMAC 2) and Physical Function (WOMAC 3). The 3 WOMAC subscales were normalized to 0–100 scales to correct for differences in scale range by using the methods recommended by Bellamy. The higher the score, the better the outcomes [15]. With regards to SF-36, the SF-36 is a 36-item patient-reported survey of patient health and reflects quality of life. It consists of eight scaled scores, which are the weighted sums of the questions in their section.

Each scale was transformed into a 0–100 scale on the assumption that each question carries equal weight. The higher the score, the less disability; a score of zero is equivalent to maximum disability and a score of 100 is equivalent to no disability. The eight sections are: vitality (SFVI), physical functioning (SFPF), bodily pain (SFBP), general health perceptions (SFGHP), physical role functioning (SFPRF), emotional role functioning (SFERF), social role functioning (SFSF) and mental health (SFMH) [16].

Patients who underwent therapeutic anti-coagulation therapy for DVT and/or PE were followed up for a minimum of 3 months to document any bleeding complications from anti-coagulation therapy.

Statistical analysis

Univariate analyses were performed to describe the presence of DVT in relation to the demographic variables, co-morbidities and surgical factors. Mann-Whitney U test was used for numerical prognostic factors, and chi-square test was used for categorical factors. As we noted differences in the age and sex of the patients, and the presence of cancer and previous VTE have been previously shown to demonstrate an increased risk in developing VTE, we adjusted our odds ratios for these four factors.

This was followed by multivariate logistic regression, performed using the variables identified as significant from the univariate analysis. A two-sided p-value of < 0.05 was used to select for these variables to be included in in multivariate logistic regression. Subsequent analysis also took a p-value of < 0.05 as unlikely to be due to chance. The logistic regression method used was Forward: Conditional, with an entry probability of 0.05 and a removal probability of 0.10.

Univariate analysis was also done to describe the type of prophylaxis in relation to functional outcome scores such as the post-op 6 month scores, post-op 12 months scores and post op 24 months scores.

All analysis was performed using IBM Statistical Package for Social Sciences (SPSS) Version 22.

Results

Using the above-mentioned criteria, 2978 patients were included in this 10-year study (2009 Chinese, 360 Malays, 390 Indians, 35 others). There were 725 men and 2073 women, with a mean age of 65.86. Mean body mass index was 27.85 kg/m2 (range, 24 to 31.5 kg/m2). This is illustrated in Table 1. All patients received mechanical thromboprophylaxis.

Two thousand two hundred fifty-eight (80.7%) patients did not receive additional chemoprophylaxis, while the remaining 540 (19.3%) received chemoprophylaxis along with mechanical thromboprophylaxis. All patients who received chemoprophylaxis were administered the enoxaparin

Table 1 Univariate analysis of Demographics, Comorbidities and Surgical Factors in relation to presence of DVT after TKR

Characteristic	Total	Presence of DVT		Odds Ratio (95% Confidence Interval)	P-Value	Adjusted Odds Ratio (95% Confidence Interval)	P-value
		Yes	No				
Demographic Variables							
Sex				1.77(0.91–1.86)	0.184		
Male	725	41 (5.7)	684 (94.3)				
Female	2073	150 (7.1)	1926 (92.9)				
Age (years)					0.671		
Median (range)		66.06 (40)	65.78 (58)				
Minimum and maximum	31 and 90						
Ethnicity				7.81 (7.21–8.456)	0.05	1.095 (0.89–1.349)	0.39
Chinese	2009 (72.7)	137 (6.8)	1872 (93.2)				
Malay	360 (11.8)	18 (5.0)	342 (95.09)				
Indian	394 (14.5)	27 (6.9)	367 (93.1)				
Others	35 (1.0)	6 (82.9)	29 (17.1)				
BMI				2.003 (1.783–2.412)	0.55	1.003 (0.973–1.035)	0.84
Median (range)		27.95 (28.63)	27.71 (52.46)				
Interquartile Range		5.45	5.92				
Comorbidities							
Hypertension				1.1.1.1 0.70 (0.60–1.09)	0.13	0.859 (0.602–1.224)	0.40
Y		111 (7.0)	1392 (93.0)				
N		80 (6.2)	1218 (93.8)				
Ischemic Heart Disease				1.1.1.1 1.00 (0.62–1.66)	0.99	1.000 (0.549–1.837)	0.99
Y		19 (6.7)	263 (93.3)				
N		172 (6.8)	2347 (93.2)				
Diabetes Mellitus				1.1.1.1 1.00 (0.69–1.48)	0.96	1.215 (0.78–1.893)	0.388
Y		34 (6.8)	468 (93.2)				
N		157 (5.8)	2539 (94.2)				
Cancer				0.65 (0.33–1.62)	0.42		
Y		7 (8.9)	71 (91.1)				
N		184 (8.3)	2036 (91.7)				
Smoking				0.06 (0.29–5.01)	0.81	1.29 (0.261–6.377)	0.755
Y		2 (5.7)	33 (94.3)				
N		189 (6.8)	2577 (93.2)				

Table 1 Univariate analysis of Demographics, Comorbidities and Surgical Factors in relation to presence of DVT after TKR (*Continued*)

Characteristic	Total	Presence of DVT		Odds Ratio (95% Confidence Interval)	P-Value	Adjusted Odds Ratio (95% Confidence Interval)	P-value
		Yes	No				
Consumption of Anti-Platelet Drugs				0.56 (0.47–1.45)	0.45	0.834 (0.400–1.738)	0.628
Y		14 (8.1)	159 (91.9)				
N		177 (6.7)	2451 (93.3)				
Consumption of NSAIDs				0.88 (0.72–2.00)	0.54	1.297 (0.697–2.415)	0.412
Y		17 (5.7)	273 (94.3)				
N		174 (6.9)	2337 (93.1)				
Previous Lower Limb VTE				9.85 (1.23–10.98)	0.00		
Y		5 (24.0)	16 (76.0)				
N		187 (6.7)	2592 (93.3)				
Family History of VTE				1.1.1.1.1 1.41 (0.02–1.66)	0.24	3.777 (0.063–22.518)	0.525
Y		1 (25.0)	4 (75.0)				
N		190 (6.8)	2606 (93.2)				
Surgical Factors							
Length of Stay		Y	N			1.152 (1.110–1.194)	0.000
Median (range)		9.33 (60)	6.42 (28)				
Interquartile Range		5	2				
Operation Time (minutes)				2.000 (0.954–3.025)	0.55	1.000 (0.996–1.005)	0.889
Median (range)		121 (213)	119 (353)				
Interquartile Range		43	28				

until they were ambulating, with a median administration duration of 6 days (minimum 2 days, maximum 30 days).

Overall rates of VTEs

Two thousand nine hundred seventy-eight patients had DUS of the lower limbs with 134 diagnosed with DVT with an incidence of 4.5%. There were 26 (19.4%) proximal DVTs and 108 (80.6%) distal DVTs. In addition, there were 6 PEs diagnosed on computer tomography of the chest. At 3 months of follow up, no additional VTE occurred.

Table 2 shows the sites of thrombi identified by the duplex Doppler ultrasound. All DVTs with accompanying PE were proximal.

Table 3 shows the method of treatment for the identified DVTs. Almost 50% were simply monitored while the other 50% were anticoagulated. Treatment of the DVTs was heterogeneous - in some cases, haematologists were consulted while in some cases, they were not. All proximal DVTs were anticoagulated. Out of the distal DVTs, only posterior tibial veins were not anticoagulated.

Subgroup analysis: comparison between patients with and without chemoprophylaxis

One hundred two out of 2200 patients (4.6%) without chemoprophylaxis developed DVT as compared to 32 out of 540 patients (5.9%) with chemoprophylaxis, which was not statistically significant ($p = 0.13$). 19 (0.8%) proximal and 83 (3.8%) distal DVT developed in the patient group without chemoprophylaxis while 4 (0.7%) proximal and 28 (5.2%) distal DVT developed in the patient group with ($p = 0.62$). Comparison of the incidence of PEs between the two groups, revealed a similar incidence with 5 out of 2200 patients (0.2%) without

Table 2 Sites of Lower Limb Venous Thromboses by Number and Percentage

Site	Number of Patients
Knees with no thrombi	2978
Knees with DVT	134 (100%)
Proximal DVT	26 (19.4%)
Superficial Femoral Vein	6
Popliteal Vein	20
Distal DVT	108 (80.6%)
Soleal	14
Peroneal	64
Posterior Tibial	30
Superfical Venous Thromboses	
Calf (Intramuscular)	27
Calf (Superficial)	2
Great Saphenous	15

Table 3 Type of Treatment for Patients with Lower Limb Venous Thromboses

Type of DVT Treatment	Number of Patients
Monitor	66
Anticoagulation	67

chemoprophylaxis developing PE as compared to 1 out of 540 patients (0.2%) with chemoprophylaxis ($p = 0.87$). 2 patients had bleeding complications – one from the group with chemoprophylaxis and one from the group without chemoprophylaxis.

Table 4 shows the comparison of the functional outcome scores with and without chemical prophylaxis. Post op 6 months SF36 (MCS), post op 12 months SF36 (MCS), post op 24 months SF36 (MCS), and post op 24 months WOMAC are statistically significant.

Table 5 shows the results of multivariate analysis using demographics, comorbidities, and surgical factors found to be significant on univariate analysis. For multivariate analysis, length of stay and previous lower limb VTE are significant.

Table 6 shows the results of multivariate analysis using the postoperative outcome scores which were found to be significant on univariate analysis. For multivariate analysis, post op 6 months SF36 (PCS) and post op 24 months SF36 (MCS) are significant. The analysis showed that the type of thromboprophylaxis was independently associated with post op 6 months SF36 (PCS), post op and post op 24 months SF36 (MCS).

Discussion

We showed that the incidence of DVTs in a multi-ethnic Asian population post elective total knee arthroplasty with mechanical prophylaxis is 4.6%. The use of mechanical and chemical prophylaxis did not lower the risk of developing DVT (incidence of 5.9%). Comparisons between the patient groups with and without chemoprophylaxis revealed that all DVT that developed with the use of chemoprophylaxis were proximal DVTs, suggesting that chemoprophylaxis could possibly have reduced the incidence of distal DVT more effectively than that of proximal DVT. This observation could also possibly explicate the relative ineffectiveness of chemoprophylaxis in reducing the incidence of pulmonary embolism, since pulmonary emboli were more strongly correlated with proximal DVT as found in our study. This observation has been noted in a few previous studies of total knee arthroplasty, where chemoprophylaxis has been found to be ineffective in reducing the incidence of PE [17, 18].

Patients who undergo total knee arthroplasty have been identified to have a high risk for VTE, leading to recommendations in international guidelines to use a

Table 4 Functional Outcome Scores of Patients with and without Chemoprophylaxis

Type of Outcome	With chemical prophylaxis	Without chemical prophylaxis	P-value
Post-Op 6 months SF-36 PCS	85.6	82.5	0.682
Post-Op 6 months SF-36 MCS	78.6	94.3	0.00
Post-Op 6 months WOMAC	82.6	83.0	0.914
Post-Op 12 months SF-36 PCS	76.0	74.4	0.118
Post-Op 12 months SF-36 MCS	82.4	68.8	0.00
Post-Op 12 months WOMAC	70.8	72.3	0.567
Post-Op 24 months SF-36 PCS	55.3	55.8	0.573
Post-Op 24 months SF-36 MCS	61.7	54.6	0.006
Post-Op 24 months WOMAC	51.9	56.5	0.08

combination of mechanical and chemical thromboprophylaxis before and after the procedure [19, 20].

Pharmacological thromboprophylaxis has been recommended to reduce the prevalence of postoperative DVT on the assumption that it will reduce the prevalence of PE, mortality, and thrombophlebitic syndrome [21, 22]. However, pharmacological thromboprophylaxis itself carries several risks such as the risk of bleeding, complications of blood loss, transfusion, transfusion-related transmission of disease, wound-healing problems, hematoma, slowed rehabilitation, wound drainage, and infection [23]. The practice of routine postoperative chemical thromboprophylaxis to prevent VTE has mainly been based on Western literature thus far, and the recent acknowledgement of studies which show a lower incidence of thromboembolism in Asia [24] has led to questions regarding the need for routine chemoprophylaxis for patients undergoing total knee arthroplasty.

Recent studies done in Asian populations however have shown otherwise, with the incidence of DVT being shown to be comparable in both Caucasian and Asian populations [25–27]. Treatment should ideally be individualized to the patient's risk profile, raising the question of Asian populations possibly following different guidelines for thromboprophylaxis after TKA. Current guidelines recommend differing modalities of

thromboprophylaxis depending on the patient's risk factors. The AAOS recommends that patients who have had a previous VTE should receive the combined modalities of pharmacologic prophylaxis and mechanical prophylaxis, such as thromboembolic deterrent (TED) stockings or intermittent pneumatic compressive devices (IPCD). In patients who have a known bleeding disorder (e.g., hemophilia) and/or active liver disease, only mechanical compressive devices should be used for preventing VTE [8]. This is identical to the ACCP which also advocates combined modalities for normal patients and solely mechanical prophylaxis or no prophylaxis for patients with an increased risk of bleeding [9]. Significantly, in a multicenter randomized controlled trial comparing IPCD against enoxaparin, Colwell et al. showed that IPCD was just as effective as enoxaparin in preventing proximal and distal DVT and PE events in hip arthroplasty patients, but resulted in a much lower bleeding risk (1.3% IPCD vs 4.3% LMWH) [28]. This adds to the argument that patients with a decreased risk of VTE should not undergo chemoprophylaxis but use only mechanical prophylaxis, thereby sparing them the adverse risk of bleeding. However, it is still unclear whether combined modalities of chemical and mechanical prophylaxis are better than either chemoprophylaxis or mechanical prophylaxis alone in overall functional outcomes. A study in 2013 found that there were no significant differences in the patient-reported quality of life outcomes and therapist-reported knee range of motion between patients who had developed DVT and those who had not [17]. Our study showed that the type

Table 5 Multivariate analysis using demographics, comorbidities and surgical factors found to be significant on univariate analysis

Statement	Odds Ratio (95% Confidence interval)	P-value
Ethnicity		0.089
Chinese	0.184	
Malay	0.400	
Indian	0.275	
Others	0.354	
Length of Stay	1.134 (1.101–1.168)	0.00
Previous Lower Limb VTE	3.963 (1.327–11.831)	0.014

Table 6 Multivariate Analysis Using Postoperative Outcome Scores Found to be Significant on Univariate Analysis

Statement	Odds Ratio (95% Confidence interval)	p-value
post op 6 months SF36 (MCS)	1.182 (0.566–1.571)	0.032
post op 12 months SF36 (MCS)	0.971 (0.569–1.574)	0.132
post op 24 months SF36 (MCS)	1.063 (0.573–1.578)	0.014
post op 12 months WOMAC	1.342 (0.888–1.900)	0.21

of thromboprophylaxis was independently associated with post op 6 months SF36 (PCS) and post op 24 months SF36 (MCS). Anticoagulation has been associated with decreased risk of acute myocardial infarction and stroke [29]. Given our patient demographics, it is possible this could have played a role in higher patient outcome scores despite no significant difference in VTE incidence. Further studies will have to be done to explore this finding.

Our incidence of VTE is low compared to that of Caucasian populations. In a review of the literature, there is only a single study on a Caucasian population which revealed similar a similar incidence of DVT -Gelfer et al. showed an incidence of DVT of 6.6% in a THA and TKA population that was treated only by mechanical prophylaxis therapy coupled with aspirin [30]. An explanation for this difference between the Asian and Western populations is most likely due to the prevalence of prothrombotic factors in Caucasians which cause them to have a higher risk of developing VTEs as compared to Asians, regardless of the type of surgery performed [31]. In fact, the low probability of Asian populations having postoperative DVT and PE as compared to Western populations was first highlighted by Tinckler et al. in 1964 [32]. There are some data that support genetic differences as a partial cause of a lower risk of VTE in Asians. The most common of the known genetic mutations is a gene known as factor V Leiden [33] which increases DVT risk by about 7 times in heterozygotes, and about 80 times in homozygotes. It has been shown to be found in approximately 5% of Caucasians, but is less common in Africans and rare in Asians [34]. Another genetic trait that predisposes to DVT and PE is the prothrombin promoter G20210A mutation. This is found in 4 to 6% of Caucasians and enhances transcription of the prothrombin gene, yielding higher prothrombin levels and consequently easier generation of thrombin, the key enzyme in blood clotting [35].

Last but not least, our study noted an apparent correlation between proximal DVT as well as bilateral DVT and the development of PE. All the PEs that had an accompanying DVT in the study had proximal DVT. Li et al. had identified a similar relationship in her study which showed the risk of developing a silent PE in patients with proximal DVT [36]. Larger scale studies would be beneficial in further investigating this possible relationship. Strengths of our study are that we have a large cohort of patients in a 10 year follow up period with no loss to follow up in the public sector. This is due to our National Electronic Healthcare Registry in Singapore which combines patient information in all our public hospitals. However as it does not include the private hospitals, there could have been loss to follow up to private institutions during the study period. Care was also standardized across the study as the methods were part of the hospital protocol. It is also one of the first

studies to show a difference in functional outcomes scores (SF-36) between the type of thromboprophylaxis for total knee arthroplasty. A limitation of our study is that we employed the usage of Doppler Ultrasound, which is operator dependent. Thus we could have missed out on certain DVTs that could have been picked up by venograms.

In Asian patients on thromboprophylaxis post-TKA, there is no significant difference in incidence of DVT between patients on chemoprophylaxis to those without. Mechanical postoperative thromboprophylaxis may be adequate in post-TKA DVT prevention, in our local context. A randomized controlled trial in Asians should be done to assess if the addition of chemoprophylaxis on top of mechanical thromboprophylaxis might lead to more harm than good.

Conclusion
In one of the largest Asian studies specifically investigating the incidence of DVT after TKA, we found that the incidence is low at 4.5%. The study institution's policy for VTE prevention included routine mechanical thromboprophylaxis and duplex ultrasound. With this policy, VTE rates that are clinically relevant were very low.

This is in contrast to recent studies that showed higher post-operative VTE rates similar to Western populations.. In addition, patients who were administered chemoprophylaxis did not have a statistically significant difference in incidence of VTE although it did show a correlation with higher post-operative outcome scores indicating better function.

Abbreviations
BMI: Body Mass Index; CI: Confidence Interval; DVT: Deep Venous Thrombosis; OR: Odd Ratio; PE: Pulmonary Embolism; SF-36: Short Form-36; TKA: Total Knee Arthroplasty; VTE: Venous Thromboembolism; WOMAC: Western Ontario and McMaster Universities Osteoarthritis Index

Acknowledgements
Not applicable.

Author details
[1]Department of Orthopaedic Surgery, Singapore General Hospital, 20 College Road, Academia, Level 4, Singapore 169865, Singapore. [2]Department of Haematology, Tan Tock Seng Hospital, Singapore, Singapore. [3]Department of Orthopaedic Surgery, Sengkang General Hospital, Singapore, Singapore. [4]Department of Hematology-Oncology, National University Cancer Institute, National University Hospital, Singapore, Singapore.

References

1. Steiner C, Andrews R, Barrett M, Weiss A. HCUP projections: mobility/orthopedic procedures 2003 to 2012. HCUP projections report# 2012–03 2012. US Agency for Healthcare Research and Quality.
2. Geerts WH, Bergqvist D, Pineo GF, Heit JA, Samama CM, Lassen MR, Colwell CW. Prevention of venous thromboembolism: American College of Chest Physicians evidence-based clinical practice guidelines. Chest. 2008;133(6):381–453.
3. Cohen AT. Asia-Pacific thrombosis advisory board consensus paper on prevention of venous thromboembolism after major orthopaedic surgery. Thromb Haemost. 2010;104(05):919–30.
4. Atichartakarn V, Pathepchotiwong K, Keorochana S, Eurvilaichit C. Deep vein thrombosis after hip surgery among Thai. Arch Intern Med. 1988;148(6):1349–53.
5. Kim YH, Suh JS. Low incidence of deep-vein thrombosis after cementless total hip. J Bone Joint Surg Am. 1988;70:878–82.
6. Mok CK, Hoaglund FT, Rogoff SM, Chow SP, Yau AC. The pattern of deep-vein thrombosis and clinical course of a group of Hong Kong Chinese patients following hip surgery for fracture of the proximal femur. Clin Orthop Relat Res. 1980;(147):115–20.
7. Lee LH. Clinical update on deep vein thrombosis in Singapore. Ann Acad Med Singap. 2002;31(2):248–52.
8. Mont MA, Jacobs JJ, Boggio LN, Bozic KJ, Della Valle CJ, Goodman SB, Lewis CG, Yates AJ Jr, Watters WC III, Turkelson CM, Wies JL. Preventing venous thromboembolic disease in patients undergoing elective hip and knee arthroplasty. J Am Acad Orthop Surg. 2011;19(12):768–76.
9. Falck-Ytter Y, Francis CW, Johanson NA, Curley C, Dahl OE, Schulman S, Ortel TL, Pauker SG, Colwell CW Jr. Prevention of VTE in orthopedic surgery patients: antithrombotic therapy and prevention of thrombosis: American College of Chest Physicians evidence-based clinical practice guidelines. Chest. 2012;141(2):e278S–325S.
10. Dhillon KS, Askander A, Doraisamy S. Postoperative deep-vein thrombosis in Asian patients is not a rarity: a prospective study of 88 patients with no prophylaxis. J Bone Joint Surg Br. 1996;78(3):427–30.
11. Patel VP, Walsh M, Sehgal B, Preston C, DeWal H, Di Cesare PE. Factors associated with prolonged wound drainage after primary total hip and knee arthroplasty. JBJS. 2007;89(1):33–8.
12. Lyder CH. Pressure ulcer prevention and management. Jama. 2003;289(2):223–6.
13. Fuji T, Nakamura M, Takeuchi M. Darexaban for the prevention of venous thromboembolism in Asian patients undergoing orthopedic surgery: results from 2 randomized, placebo-controlled, double-blind studies. Clin Appl Thromb Hemost. 2014;20(2):199–211.
14. Kanchanabat B, Stapanavatr W, Meknavin S, Soorapanth C, Sumanasrethakul C, Kanchanasuttirak P. Systematic review and meta-analysis on the rate of postoperative venous thromboembolism in orthopaedic surgery in Asian patients without thromboprophylaxis. Br J Surg. 2011;98(10):1356–64.
15. Bellamy N. WOMAC Osteoarthritis index: a user's guide. London, Ontario: University of Western Ontario; 1996.
16. Gandek B, Ware JE Jr, Aaronson NK, Alonso J, Apolone G, Bjorner J, Brazier J, Bullinger M, Fukuhara S, Kaasa S, Leplège A. Tests of data quality, scaling assumptions, and reliability of the SF-36 in eleven countries: results from the IQOLA Project. J. Clin. Epidemiol. 1998;51(11):1149–58.
17. Zhou Z, Yew AK, Chin PL, Lo NN, Yeo SJ, Chia SL. Total knee arthroplasty complicated by distal deep venous thromboembolism: does it affect the functional outcome? Proceedings of Singapore Healthcare. 2013;22(4):262–6.
18. Hill J, Treasure T. Reducing the risk of venous thromboembolism (deep vein thrombosis and pulmonary embolism) in patients admitted to hospital: summary of the NICE guideline. Heart. 2010;96(11):879–82.
19. Kearon C, Akl EA, Comerota AJ, Prandoni P, Bounameaux H, Goldhaber SZ, Nelson ME, Wells PS, Gould MK, Dentali F, Crowther M. Antithrombotic therapy for VTE disease: antithrombotic therapy and prevention of thrombosis: American College of Chest Physicians evidence-based clinical practice guidelines. Chest. 2012 1;141(2):e419S–96S.
20. Eikelboom JW, Karthikeyan G, Fagel N, Hirsh J. American Association of Orthopedic Surgeons and American College of Chest Physicians guidelines for venous thromboembolism prevention in hip and knee arthroplasty differ: what are the implications for clinicians and patients? Chest. 2009;135(2):513–20.
21. Sharfman ZT, Campbell JC, Mirocha JM, Spitzer AI. Balancing thromboprophylaxis and bleeding in total joint arthroplasty: impact of eliminating enoxaparin and predonation and implementing pneumatic compression and tranexamic acid. J arthroplasty. 2016;31(6):1307–12.
22. Cusick LA, Beverland DE. The incidence of fatal pulmonary embolism after primary hip and knee replacement in a consecutive series of 4253 patients. J Bone Joint Surg Br. 2009;91(5):645–8.
23. Sharrock NE, Della Valle AG, Go G, Lyman S, Salvati EA. Potent anticoagulants are associated with a higher all-cause mortality rate after hip and knee arthroplasty. Clin Orthop Relat Res. 2008;466(3):714–21.
24. Wong KL, Daguman R, Lim KH, Shen L, Lingaraj K. Incidence of deep vein thrombosis following total knee arthroplasty: a Doppler ultrasonographic study. J Orthop Surg. 2011;19(1):50–3.
25. Wang CJ, Wang JW, Chen LM, Chen HS, Yang BY, Cheng SM. Deep vein thrombosis after total knee arthroplasty. J Formos Med Assoc. 2000;99(11):848–53.
26. Ko PS, Chan WF, Siu TH, Khoo J, Wu WC, Lam JJ. Deep venous thrombosis after total hip or knee arthroplasty in a "low-risk" Chinese population. J Arthroplast. 2003;18(2):174–9.
27. Piovella F, Wang CJ, Lu H, Lee K, Lee LH, Lee WC, Turpie AG, Gallus AS, Planès A, Passera R, Rouillon A. Deep-vein thrombosis rates after major orthopedic surgery in Asia. An epidemiological study based on postoperative screening with centrally adjudicated bilateral venography. J Thromb Haemost. 2005;3(12):2664–70.
28. Colwell CW Jr, Froimson MI, Mont MA, Ritter MA, Trousdale RT, Buehler KC, Spitzer A, Donaldson TK, Padgett DE. Thrombosis prevention after total hip arthroplasty: a prospective, randomized trial comparing a mobile compression device with low-molecular-weight heparin. JBJS. 2010;92(3):527–35.
29. Clayville LR, Anderson KV, Miller SA, Onge EL. New options in anticoagulation for the prevention of venous thromboembolism and stroke. Pharmacy and Therapeutics. 2011;36(2):86.
30. Gelfer Y, Tavor H, Oron A, Peer A, Halperin N, Robinson D. Deep vein thrombosis prevention in joint arthroplasties: continuous enhanced circulation therapy vs low molecular weight heparin. J arthroplasty. 2006;21(2):206–14.
31. White RH, Keenan CR. Effects of race and ethnicity on the incidence of venous thromboembolism. Thromb Res. 2009;123:S11–7.
32. Tinckler LF. Absence of pulmonary embolism in asians? Br Med J. 1964;1(5381):502.
33. Klatsky AL, Armstrong MA, Poggi J. Risk of pulmonary embolism and/or deep venous thrombosis in Asian-Americans. Am J Cardiol. 2000;85(11):1334–7.
34. De Stefano V, Martinelli I, Mannucci PM, Paciaroni K, Chiusolo P, Casorelli I, Rossi E, Leone G. The risk of recurrent deep venous thrombosis among heterozygous carriers of both factor V Leiden and the G20210A prothrombin mutation. N Engl J Med. 1999;341(11):801–6.
35. Hessner MJ, Luhm RA, Pearson SL, Endean DJ, Friedman KD, Montgomery RR. Prevalence of prothrombin G20210A, factor V G1691A (Leiden), and methylenetetrahydrofolate reductase (MTHFR) C677T in seven different populations determined by multiplex allele-specific PCR. Thromb Haemost. 1999;81(05):733–8.
36. Li F, Wang X, Huang W, Ren W, Cheng J, Zhang M, Zhao Y. Risk factors associated with the occurrence of silent pulmonary embolism in patients with deep venous thrombosis of the lower limb. Phlebology. 2014;29(7):442–6.

4

Evaluation of unmet clinical needs in prophylaxis and treatment of venous thromboembolism in at-risk patient groups: Pregnancy, elderly and obese patients

Benjamin Brenner[1,2]*, Roopen Arya[3], Jan Beyer-Westendorf[4,5], James Douketis[6,7], Russell Hull[8], Ismail Elalamy[2,9], Davide Imberti[10] and Zhenguo Zhai[11]

Abstract

Background: Venous thromboembolism (VTE) accounts for an estimated 900,000 cases per year in the US alone and constitutes a considerable burden on healthcare systems across the globe.

Objective: To understand why the burden is so high, qualitative and quantitative research was carried out to gain insights from experts, guidelines and published studies on the unmet clinical needs and therapeutic strategies in VTE prevention and treatment in three populations identified as being at increased risk of VTE and in whom VTE prevention and treatment were regarded as suboptimal: pregnant women, the elderly and obese patients.

Methodology: A gap analysis methodology was created to highlight unmet needs in VTE management and to discover the patient populations considered most at risk. A questionnaire was devised to guide qualitative interviews with 44 thrombosis and haemostasis experts, and a review of the literature on VTE in the specific patient groups from 2015 to 2017 was completed. This was followed by a Think Tank meeting where the results from the research were discussed.

Results: This review highlights the insights gained and examines in detail the unmet needs with regard to VTE risk-assessment tools, biomarkers, patient stratification methods, and anticoagulant and dosing regimens in pregnant women, the elderly and obese patients.

Conclusions: Specifically, in pregnant women at high risk of VTE, low-molecular-weight heparin (LMWH) is the therapy of choice, but it remains unclear how to use anticoagulants when VTE risk is intermediate. In elderly patients, evaluation of the benefit of VTE prophylaxis against the bleeding risk is particularly important, and a head-to-head comparison of efficacy and safety of LMWH versus direct oral anticoagulants is needed. Finally, in obese patients, lack of guidance on anticoagulant dose adjustment to body weight has emerged as a major obstacle in effective prophylaxis and treatment of VTE.

Keywords: Venous thromboembolism, Elderly, Pregnant, Pregnancy, Obese, Obesity, Anticoagulants, Low-molecular-weight heparin

* Correspondence: b_brenner@rambam.health.gov.il
[1]Department of Hematology and Bone Marrow Transplantation, Rambam Health Care Campus, Haifa, Israel
[2]Department of Obstetrics and Gynaecology, The First I.M. Sechenov Moscow State Medical University, Moscow, Russia
Full list of author information is available at the end of the article

Background

Venous thromboembolism (VTE), comprising deep vein thrombosis (DVT) and pulmonary embolism (PE), remains a major concern for healthcare systems globally. Despite improved prophylaxis and treatment options, and current risk-assessment tools, morbidity and mortality related to VTE remains high in patient populations such as pregnant women, the elderly and obese patients [1].

VTE is the main cause of mortality in women during the post-partum period [2]. Acute VTE is linked to substantial long-term mortality in the elderly (21% of 991 patients in a Swiss cohort study with a median follow-up time of 30 months) [3]. Patients with VTE who are morbidly obese are more likely to have extended hospital and intensive care unit stays [4]. Thus, the suboptimal use of anticoagulants in these patients and the increased cost burden related to longer hospital stays needs to be addressed.

A lack of adequate population-specific risk-assessment tools, along with uncertainties around correct dosing regimens and concern over increased bleeding risk, may be linked to these elevated mortality and morbidity rates [5, 6]. In addition, although guidelines exist on prophylaxis and treatment of these patients, discrepancies occur between recommendations, leading to low adherence by physicians to such guidance [7–9]. Moreover, there is a paucity of evidence on these patient populations due to problems of recruiting individuals to randomised controlled trials (RCT), which may be linked to patients' comorbidities, frailty and concern over foetal development and maternal well-being [10, 11].

Considering the above, it is important to examine the evidence presented in guidelines, published studies and reviews, and through expert opinion, in order to highlight unmet needs and inconsistencies in clinical practice, with a view to homogenising VTE prevention and treatment strategies.

Methodology

Quantitative mapping was performed to identify key opinion leaders who were active online and in publications, patient advocacy groups, scientific associations, editorial boards, guidelines, clinical trials and congress activities in the thrombosis and haemostasis field. From this list, experts were selected from a range of countries dependent on their availability to attend a telephone interview. Forty-four key opinion leaders were contacted between February and August 2017 from 12 different countries or regions: Canada, Brazil, five European countries, Middle East, Africa, Russia, China and Japan. The interviews followed a pre-determined questionnaire [see Additional file 1] and a gap analysis was carried out on the information received. The data revealed areas of

unmet need with regard to VTE management with cancer, the critically ill, pregnant women, the elderly and obese patients. Of these five patient groups, the first two were discussed in a previous paper and the latter three were chosen for discussion in this paper [12] additional file 2. A comprehensive literature search was conducted in PubMed, Cochrane Library and current guidelines (January 2015 to December 2018) using the terms: pregnant, pregnancy, obese, obesity, elderly and venous thromboembolism. Further insights were gained during a Thrombosis Think Tank meeting in Paris in February 2018, during which the authors discussed the findings from the qualitative and quantitative research in order to establish unmet clinical needs and examine therapeutic approaches to bridging the gaps in VTE management in these three patient groups.

Prophylaxis and treatment of VTE during pregnancy and post-partum

Despite a relatively low absolute risk of VTE of 1.2 per 1000 pregnancies, VTE remains a leading cause of maternal mortality in developed countries [2, 13, 14]. VTE can occur at any time during pregnancy, but increases 20-fold during the post-partum period [13]. Timely diagnosis depends on awareness of the condition and recognition of risk factors, including a family history of or previous thrombophilia (heritable: antithrombin deficiency, protein C deficiency, protein S deficiency, factor V Leiden, prothrombin gene mutation; acquired: antiphospholipid antibodies, persistent lupus anticoagulant and/or persistent moderate/high titre anticardiolipin antibodies and/or β2-glycoprotein 1 antibodies) or VTE, obesity, increased maternal age, reduced mobility and hospitalisation, and is critical to avoid VTE-induced mortality [13].

Guideline recommendations for pregnant and post-natal women at risk of VTE

Various guidelines on prevention and treatment of VTE in ante- and post-partum women and women with recurrent pregnancy loss exist, and of the experts interviewed, the American College of Chest Physicians (ACCP) and the Royal College of Obstetricians and Gynaecologists (RCOG) were indicated as the main guidelines being followed (Table 1).

However, due to a lack of evidence-based data in this population, the recommendations provided by national and international guidelines often vary and have not recently been updated, apart from the American Society of Hematology (ASH) guidelines on VTE in pregnancy published in 2018 [10, 14]. For example, the guidelines on prophylaxis of VTE in women after a caesarean section show divergent recommendations. A study by Palmerola, et al., comparing guideline recommendations for

Table 1 Guidelines followed by experts interviewed

Question	Expert opinion
What guidelines and clinical protocols do you use for prevention and treatment of VTE, including guidance on dose and duration, in ante- or post-partum pregnant women and in women with recurrent pregnancy loss?	• ACCP/CHEST
	• ISTH
	• Italian Society of Thrombosis and Haemostasis
	• RCOG
	• National guidelines
	• Involved in the generation of national guidelines
	• Follow own experience
	• No guidelines are being followed

ACCP/CHEST, American College of Chest Physicians; ISTH, International Society of Thrombosis and Haemostasis; RCOG, Royal College of Obstetricians and Gynaecologists; VTE, venous thromboembolism

thromboprophylaxis after a caesarean section from RCOG, the American College of Obstetricians and Gynecologists, and ACCP found that 85, 1 and 35% of patients, respectively, would receive pharmacologic prophylaxis if the guidance were followed, thus highlighting significant gaps in consistency between recommendations [15].

The underlying cause is the lack of RCTs in this patient population and over-reliance on observational data, especially case–control studies that provide a lower level of evidence [16]. Many studies on prevention and management of VTE in pregnancy are performed on a small patient population due to patient enrolment difficulties, as women are reluctant to take additional medication, particularly when it is administered through injections. For example, the TIPPS study aimed to examine the effects of dalteparin in pregnancy and recruited only 292 pregnant women with thrombophilia over 12 years [17]. Thrombophilia was defined in this study as two abnormal tests and no normal tests for protein S, protein C or antithrombin; two positive tests for anticardiolipin immunoglobulin M (IgM) (> 30 U/ml), anticardiolipin immunoglobulin G (IgG) (> 30 U/ml), anti-β2 glycoprotein IgG (> 20 U/ml), anti-β2 glycoprotein IgM (> 20 U/ml), or lupus anticoagulant; and one positive test for factor V Leiden (heterozygous or homozygous) or prothrombin gene defect (heterozygous or homozygous) [17]. Most of the studies involving pregnant women provide outcomes without achieving statistical significance and, due to an absence of high-level evidence, prophylaxis is often not provided [16]. Insights from the qualitative research carried out for this paper noted that in China, country-level guidelines have not yet been developed and there is an inconsistent approach to prophylaxis.

VTE risk-assessment models and biomarkers

A history of VTE or heritable thrombophilia (factor V Leiden mutation, prothrombin gene mutation, antithrombin deficiency, protein C deficiency, protein S deficiency) are established risk factors of VTE in pregnant women [18]; however, the data from the qualitative interviews underlined the need to develop new tools to identify additional risk factors for pregnant women. The STRATHEGE score study by Chauleur, et al., involving pregnant women with at least one VTE risk factor, established a simple scoring system to evaluate VTE risk, but the low event rate meant the discriminatory power of the score could not be assessed [19]. However, a subsequent study, aimed at evaluating the effectiveness of the STRATHEGE score following its implementation in 21 French maternity units, demonstrated a significantly reduced risk of VTE and placental vascular complications of 50 and 30%, respectively [20]. Another VTE risk score, which was developed through a logistic regression model and based on 14 risk factors, including comorbidities and VTE history in the first 6 weeks post-partum, offers a benefit of predicting VTE events in the early post-partum period more accurately than current models provided by UK and Swedish national guidelines, but further validation is needed [21]. Alternatively, the EThIG trial assessed a risk evaluation strategy and effectiveness of heparin prophylaxis in low-risk and high/very high-risk pregnant women groups. Risk-stratified dalteparin prophylaxis was associated with a low incidence of symptomatic VTE and few adverse events [22].

In terms of biomarkers, it is known that D-dimer levels, an exclusion criterion for VTE, increase during pregnancy and peak in the third trimester at levels above the conventional cut-off, making them of little use [23]. Several studies have looked at recording D-dimer reference intervals during the three trimesters in healthy pregnancy and suggested pregnancy-associated cut-off levels that may assist clinical decision-making on VTE prophylaxis [23, 24]. Soluble fibrin monomer forms a complex with fibrinogen in the bloodstream early in coagulation, and measuring levels of the complex has also been proposed as a marker to screen for VTE [25]. However, recent studies have questioned the predictive utility of all conventional and candidate VTE biomarkers for use during pregnancy and the puerperium [26, 27].

In summary, further research is needed to develop more precise risk-assessment tools and improve the diagnostic value of biomarkers in order to tailor thromboprophylaxis for this patient population.

Prophylaxis and treatment of VTE in ante- and post-partum periods

Thromboprophylaxis is recommended in all pregnant women with an estimated VTE risk above 5% but is advised against for a risk below 1%. However, the approach to the management of pregnant women with an estimated risk between 1 and 5% remains debatable (Table 2) [2, 14, 30].

The 2015 RCOG guidelines state that prophylaxis should be used from the start of pregnancy in women with four VTE risk factors, from week 28 in those with three risk factors, and women with two risk factors should receive 10 days of post-partum prophylaxis [13]. This implies that nearly half of pregnant women are eligible for post-partum prophylaxis [31]. The ACCP guidelines suggest that the presence of one of the major

risk factors or two minor risk factors, or one following emergency caesarean section indicates a post-partum VTE risk > 3% [28].

In the post-partum period, the risk of VTE is high in the first 2 weeks after giving birth. Guidelines [13, 28] suggest that prophylaxis should continue for 6 weeks post-partum, although experts noted that, considering the increase in risk is greatest in the first 2–3 weeks only, this recommendation may be contested, unless a history of VTE is present in a patient. Since VTE risk is high in the first week following a caesarean section, thromboprophylaxis is given post-partum for 10 days in the UK following all non-elective caesarean sections and for elective caesarean-section patients with one other VTE risk according to RCOG guidance [13]. This may account for the observed decrease in maternal deaths from 1985 to 2014 [32]. In Germany, post-partum prophylaxis depends on the type of caesarean section, i.e., prophylaxis after elective caesarean section lasts for 10–14 days and after an emergency caesarean section is extended for up to 3 months.

Direct oral anticoagulants (DOAC) should not be used in pregnancy, or when breastfeeding, as their effects on the foetus or the new-born child are currently unknown [14, 33, 34]. However, despite guideline recommendations,

Table 2 Subpopulations of pregnant women recommended for LMWH prophylaxis or treatment

Question	Expert opinion	Guideline recommendations
Which subpopulation(s) of pregnant women, ante- or post-partum, or those with recurrent pregnancy loss, should be treated with LMWHs such as enoxaparin?	• Women with recurrent pregnancy loss • No evidence to support use of LMWH to prevent recurrent pregnancy loss • Women with antiphospholipid syndrome or with heterozygosity of factor V Leiden mutation • Those undergoing IVF • Those with previous unprovoked or provoked VTE • LMWH is recommended in the case of a severe event such as placenta abruption, intrauterine foetus death or VTE	• ACCP/CHEST [28]: For women requiring long-term VKA treatment who are attempting pregnancy, a switch to LMWH is recommended. In women with no VTE risk factors, prophylaxis is not recommended following a caesarean section. No routine prophylaxis for patients following assisted reproduction • ASH [14]: Prophylaxis is only advised for women undergoing assisted reproductive therapy with severe ovarian hyperstimulation syndrome. For women with previous unprovoked or provoked VTE, ante-partum prophylaxis is advised. For women with antithrombin deficiency who are homozygous for the factor V Leiden regardless of family history, ante-partum and post-partum prophylaxis is recommended. In those with protein S or C deficiency, post-partum prophylaxis is advised • Italian Society of Thrombosis and Haemostasis [29]: Ante- and post-partum prophylaxis is recommended for women with thrombophilic defects. LMWH is recommended in women with prior VTE. Ante- and post-partum LMWH prophylaxis is suggested for women with prior obstetric complications and one thrombophilic defect • RCOG [13]: LMWH is the preferred anticoagulant to treat acute VTE and for antenatal and post-natal prophylaxis. 10 days prophylaxis with LMWH is recommended after an emergency caesarean section and after a planned caesarean section if there are additional risk factors

ACCP/CHEST, American College of Chest Physicians; ASH, American Society of Hematology; IVF, in-vitro fertilisation; LMWH, low-molecular-weight heparin; RCOG, Royal College of Obstetricians and Gynaecologists; VKA, vitamin K antagonists; VTE, venous thromboembolism clinical experience in Germany (as documented subjectively by local opinion leaders) and a recent review of 137 pregnant women with DOAC exposure suggest that administration of DOACs during early pregnancy does not indicate a high risk of embryopathy, and pregnancy termination for these women may not be necessary [35].

In summary, low-molecular-weight heparin (LMWH) is the preferred anticoagulant for both prophylaxis and treatment during pregnancy. However, guidelines and opinions differ on how to stratify risk, the most effective duration of prophylaxis and the safety of DOACs during pregnancy.

LMWH dose adjustment

In pregnant women at very high risk of thromboembolic complications and especially in those with acute VTE, monitoring of anti-Xa activity is often recommended (and performed), aiming to ensure adequate dosing of LMWH, which can be challenging in pregnant women. However, there is considerable uncertainty about the strategy (peak or trough anti-Xa levels) and the target ranges, the impact of these target ranges on clinical outcomes, and the accuracy and reproducibility of the assays [36]. Taken together, the experts agreed that anti-Xa monitoring in pregnant women at very high risk for thromboembolism is widely used and likely beneficial, but also agreed that many details of this strategy are still under debate, indicating a large unmet need for better evidence in this setting (Table 3).

Clinical practice in the UK recommends dose adjustment as per body weight in pregnant women for both treatment and prophylaxis, and, as a result, only a few breakthrough clots occur, although generous dosage given as recommended by RCOG guidelines may be a reason for these outcomes [13]. In Israel, anti-Xa levels are measured for both treatment and prophylaxis, although usually approximately 60% of women on a therapeutic dose and 20% of women on a prophylactic dose need

these doses to be adjusted at around 20–25 weeks. In Italy, the experts interviewed used a fixed dose of LMWH for prophylaxis in pregnant women with a history of thrombosis.

Some of the experts have questioned the ideal dose of LMWH for thromboprophylaxis and treatment in pregnancy. The ongoing Highlow study, an RCT of intermediate-dose LMWH adjusted to actual body weight versus fixed low-dose nadroparin, may inform this clinical question for thromboprophylaxis [37].

Challenges in the management of VTE in elderly patients

With life expectancy increasing in the developed world, a new definition of 'the elderly' should be considered, which should include significant comorbidities such as coronary, hepatic, renal and cognitive functions, as well as frailty, rather than focusing on age alone (Table 4).

The interviewed experts noted that impaired renal and cognitive functions, but not age per se, may be the major factors influencing the decision for or against antithrombotic therapy, as well as treatment outcome. However, 26 of the interviewees acknowledged that such patients are usually excluded from clinical trials, which limits evidence and guideline recommendations [40]. Evidence shows that the risk of venous thrombosis, which associates with illnesses characteristic to advanced age, increases exponentially with age, but thromboprophylaxis remains suboptimal in this patient group due to fear of bleeding since thrombotic and bleeding risk profiles usually overlap in this population [41, 42].

VTE risk-assessment models and biomarkers in the elderly

The experts agreed that VTE risk assessment in elderly patients should include comorbidities, concomitant medications and frailty to identify those at high risk of VTE. Furthermore, biomarkers may help to increase the predictive performance of VTE risk-assessment strategies. In the setting of primary VTE prophylaxis in acutely ill medical

Table 3 Methods of identifying optimal anticoagulant dose in thrombophilic pregnant women and those with pregnancy loss

Question	Expert opinion	Guideline recommendations
What method do you use to identify optimal dose of anticoagulants in thrombophilic pregnant women and those with pregnancy loss, e.g., PK/PD modelling or other methods?	• Anti-Xa monitoring • Factor Xa activity in prophylaxis is not measured • Routine monitoring of the dose is not recommended, the clinical picture of each patients is more important • PK/PD data is not usually used • The PK/PD profile is required • LMWH dose adjusted to weight • Fixed dose • Full-dose enoxaparin for high-risk patients	• ACCP/CHEST [28]: Anti-Xa measuring is not advised. Intermediate-dose LMWH dose is recommended in pregnant women with a history of VTE, with thrombophilia or with a risk of pregnancy loss • ASH [14]: Routine anti-Xa monitoring to guide dosing is not advised • Italian Society of Thrombosis and Haemostasis [29]: Monitoring platelet count during prophylaxis with LMWH is advised. No evidence to suggest use of anti-Xa monitoring to adjust LMWH dose • RCOG [13]: Titration of LMWH dose against the woman's booking or early pregnancy weight is advised. Routine measurement of anti-Xa is not recommended except in women < 50 kg or > 90 kg

ACCP/CHEST, American College of Chest Physicians; ASH, American Society of Hematology; LMWH, low-molecular-weight heparin; PK/PD, pharmacokinetic/pharmacodynamic; RCOG, Royal College of Obstetricians and Gynaecologists; VTE, venous thromboembolism

Table 4 Practical considerations for treating elderly patients with high risk of VTE

Question	Expert opinion	Guideline recommendations
Are there any practical considerations when treating elderly patients with high risk of VTE, such as specific risk factors, contra-indications, comorbidities or practicalities of administration?	• Higher bleeding risk • Traditional regimens increase the risk of bleeding • The risk of internal bleeding • Need to evaluate the risk of stroke through bleeding • Renal function may be compromised • Dosage due to the reduction in kidney function • Dosage taking into consideration contra-indications • Co-medications • Lack of clinical trials • Affordability is an issue	All recommendations are non-age specific. ACCP/CHEST [28]: • Hepatic failure, severe renal failure, rheumatic disease, current cancer and age ≥ 80 are all independent risk factors for bleeding NICE [38]: • Balance the patient's risk of VTE against their bleeding risk SIGN [39]: • Patients undergoing total hip replacement with increased risk of bleeding should be given mechanical prophylaxis alone

ACCP/CHEST, American College of Chest Physicians; NICE, The National Institute for Health and Care Excellence; SIGN, Scottish Intercollegiate Guidelines Network; VTE, venous thromboembolism

patients, the MAGELLAN study found that in patients with an average age of 71.4 years, high concentrations of D-dimer ($> 2\ \mu g\ mL^{-1}$ mean) at day 10 were a predictor of increased VTE risk for up to 35 days [43]. Subsequently, this informed the selection criteria for the APEX study, which used a D-dimer level of ≥2x the upper limit of normal to examine primary VTE prevention for acutely ill medical patients aged 60–74 [44]. The ADJUST-PE study demonstrated that an age-adjusted D-dimer cut-off of age × 10 in patients > 50 years was successful in ruling out patients at risk of VTE [45]. However, using this biomarker to drive primary VTE prophylaxis decisions may not be effective in elderly patients due to an increase of circulating D-dimer in this patient population, which may not necessarily be linked to increased VTE risk [42, 46]. Consequently, further studies need to establish a more accurate threshold for biomarkers such as D-dimer before they can be routinely used for risk stratification and treatment decisions.

At the same time, elderly fragile patients are at an increased risk of falls and bleeding, but bleeding scores are unreliable in this population and their use is limited [47]. Moreover, elderly women seem to be at 20–25% higher risk of bleeding than men [11, 48, 49].

The experts noted that VTE risk-assessment guidance differs across countries. Further work is needed to develop a simple-to-use risk-assessment score for elderly patients that incorporates age, gender, comorbidities and bleeding risk.

Consideration of anticoagulants for prophylaxis in the elderly

There is little evidence regarding ideal anticoagulants for prophylaxis of the elderly largely due to the under-representation of this group of patients in clinical studies, owing to several comorbidities which increase the chance of exclusion from a trial [40]. Therefore, certain guideline recommendations may have been extrapolated from studies with younger cohorts and may not necessarily extend to this patient population [42]. Patients > 75 years of age have an increased risk of VTE [42] and, according to the ACCP, hospitalised medical patients > 70 years should be offered pharmacological VTE prophylaxis with fondaparinux, LMWH or unfractionated heparin (UFH) [29]. Yet, a systematic review and meta-analysis comparing efficacy and safety of LMWH versus UFH reported an overall increase in the rate of major haemorrhage with heparin prophylaxis compared to no prophylaxis [50]. However, the LMWH group showed a statistically significant bleeding risk reduction over the UFH group and LMWH demonstrated a better efficacy profile than UFH in terms of reducing DVT risk (Table 5) [50].

The experts agreed that thromboprophylaxis should only be prescribed following careful benefit–risk assessments, but it is essential to consider drug compliance, major and non-major bleeding risks, and comorbidities, including renal function, hypertension, infections and coronary artery disease. Evidence from expert interviews demonstrates disparities in thromboprophylaxis practice from country to country. In general, elderly patients are underprophylaxed due to the perceived increased risk of bleeding in this population [51]. In Germany, evidence from a VTE registry shows that patients > 65 years of age are often underprophylaxed out of hospital and increasing public awareness on VTE risk situations has been suggested as a possible solution [52]. In France, according to national experts, elderly patients often receive

Table 5 Subgroups of elderly patients for whom LMWH may be the optimal choice

Question	Expert opinion	Guideline recommendations
In which subgroups of elderly patients would you consider LMWHs, such as enoxaparin, the optimal choice?	• Only if the patient has a specific condition • In patients with cancer and VTE • In patients with ACS • Used in percutaneous coronary interventions, ACS and thrombolytic therapy • Those with a history of internal bleeding • LMWH preferred due to the ability to change dosage based on kidney function and age • Intermediate risk PE • Patients with acute PE who do not use DOACs • Patients with comorbidities, GI problems and chronic inflammatory disease • Patients with provoked VTE post-operatively • LMWH used with inpatients but not used with outpatients	All recommendations are non-age specific. ACCP/CHEST [28]: • Acutely ill hospitalised patients at increased risk of thrombosis • Critically ill patients • Outpatients with solid tumours who have additional risk factors for VTE and low bleeding risk NICE [38]: • Patients with renal impairment needing pharmacological VTE prophylaxis • People with myeloma or pancreatic cancer receiving chemotherapy • People receiving palliative care • Those admitted to the critical care unit • 1 month of VTE prophylaxis for patients with fragility fractures of the pelvis, hip or proximal femur • 10 days of LMWH for people undergoing elective hip replacement surgery • 7 days minimum VTE prophylaxis with LMWH for patient undergoing open vascular surgery or major endovascular procedures, lower limb amputation SIGN [39]: • Patients undergoing total hip replacement should receive prophylaxis with LMWH • Patients with cancer and cancer surgery • In patients with non-haemorrhagic stroke at high risk of VTE • Patients with suspected PE or DVT should receive therapeutic doses

ACCP/CHEST, American College of Chest Physicians; ACS, acute coronary syndrome; DOAC, direct oral anticoagulant; DVT, deep vein thrombosis; GI, gastrointestinal; LMWH, low-molecular-weight heparin; NICE, The National Institute for Health and Care Excellence; PE, pulmonary embolism; SIGN, Scottish Intercollegiate Guidelines Network; VTE, venous thromboembolism

prophylaxis but many of these patients are prophylaxed with either the incorrect type of anticoagulant or a sub-optimal dose, therefore increasing the bleeding risk without achieving antithrombotic effect [53]. In China, in-hospital prophylaxis is insufficient and a lack of VTE knowledge and understanding of the guidelines is leading to non-standard approaches to thromboprophylaxis

[54]. Published data from Italian national registries have shown that in contrast to widely used extended prophylaxis following a surgical procedure, medical prophylaxis is rare [55].

Expert opinion suggests that extended prophylaxis of 35 days should be given for patients at high risk of VTE, such as post-surgery or cancer patients (Table 6).

Table 6 Extended prophylaxis in elderly patients

Question	Expert opinion	Guideline recommendations
Should extended prophylaxis be used in elderly patients, e.g., for hip fractures?	• In patients with cancer • In patients undergoing surgery • Hip/knee replacements • In patients with multiple fractures at risk of recurrent VTE • Injections can only be used for 2 weeks, oral is the preferred treatment • Generally given for 10–14 days but can be extended to 30–35 days • Primary prophylaxis is currently recommended for 35 days • Recommended for 1 month but often extended for 3 months • This should only be for very high-risk patients but we don't know how to identify them • Yes, but length of time is not well defined	All recommendations are non-age specific. ACCP/CHEST [28]: • Extended-duration thromboprophylaxis up to 35 days reduces VTE in hip replacement, hip fracture and abdominal malignancy surgery NICE [38]: • There is a recommendation for research by the NICE guideline committee regarding extended-duration prophylaxis for patients undergoing elective total hip replacement surgery SIGN [39]: • Following total hip replacement, particularly those with previous VTE

ACCP/CHEST, American College of Chest Physicians; NICE, The National Institute for Health and Care Excellence; SIGN, Scottish Intercollegiate Guidelines Network; VTE, venous thromboembolism.

This statement was supported by Dentali, et al., 2016, who conducted a pooled analysis that suggested a potential benefit of extended antithrombotic prophylaxis in acutely ill patients [56]. Indeed, the EXCLAIM trial showed reduced rates of VTE in medically ill patients > 75 years of age when LMWH was administered for up to 38 days following hospital discharge; however, this was counterbalanced by an increase in major bleeding [57]. Therefore, extended prophylaxis should be assessed on an individual basis [58].

VTE treatment and secondary prevention after VTE in elderly patients

Elderly patients receiving therapeutic anticoagulation for VTE are at increased risk of long-term mortality with comorbid burden, polypharmacy and a low level of physical activity as predictors of major bleeding, one of the most common causes of death [3]. Thus, selection of the optimal antithrombotic agent, its dose and duration of treatment, and whether this should continue beyond hospitalisation is particularly important. Although LMWH remains an option for hospitalised, elderly patients with different comorbidities such as chronic inflammatory conditions, gastrointestinal system problems, poor renal function, active cancer, acute or chronic lung or heart conditions, and acute infections, extended-duration treatment with LMWH is rare, mainly due to its inconvenience and cost [59, 60]. As a consequence, short courses of initial LMWH therapy are followed by oral anticoagulation with a vitamin K antagonists (VKA) such as warfarin. During the last decade, DOACs have taken the place of LMWH/VKAs in acute and long-term VTE treatment due to the convenience of administration and an excellent dose-response relationship without the need for monitoring or frequent dose adjustments [61]. Indeed, several reviews examining study evidence on DOACs compared to VKAs for VTE treatment in patients ≥75 years of age have demonstrated better efficacy and safety of DOACs over VKAs, with no increase in the risk of bleeding [62, 63]. However, when the different DOACs are examined individually, varying profiles are revealed. The AMPLIFY trial noted improved efficacy and safety of apixaban (10 mg twice daily for 7 days followed by 5 mg twice daily for 6 months) compared to standard therapy (enoxaparin followed by warfarin) in patients ≥75 years [64], whereas the RE-COVER II trial, which compared dabigatran to warfarin, found that efficacy and risk of bleeding increased exponentially with age with dabigatran and decreased with warfarin [65]. The Hokusai-VTE study, comparing edoxaban to warfarin, observed an increased bleeding risk linked to age regardless of treatment, but noted a reduction in recurrent VTE for patients > 80 years of age on the DOAC regimen [66]. In the EINSTEIN-DVT and PE trials, there was a 1.4% reduction in recurrent VTE events and a 3.3% reduction in major bleeding in patients

≥75 years of age receiving rivaroxaban compared to standard enoxaparin/VKA treatment [67].

The elderly subpopulations of patients ≥75 years of age in these trials, however, consist of small sample sizes from 13 to 43% of the total study populations [63]. In addition, the majority of these trials compared DOACs to VKAs, and clinical trials are now needed to directly compare extended treatment with LMWHs to treatment with DOACs in elderly patients ≥75 years of age, along with a need for real-life evidence in elderly patients with a high risk of DOAC accumulation [62].

In summary, more studies need to be carried out to establish the most effective and safe antithrombotic treatment for elderly patients outside the hospital setting. Although DOACs are considered convenient in these situations, studies on their safety have produced varying results.

Thromboprophylaxis and treatment of VTE in obese patients

Obesity is increasing rapidly around the world, and it presents a significant health burden [68]. Adult obesity is classified into three categories: class I obesity is defined by a body mass index (BMI) of 30.0–34.9 kg/m^2; class II obesity by a BMI of 35.0–39.9 kg/m^2; and class III obesity, or severe obesity, by a BMI ≥40.0 kg/m^2 [69]. Weight is a VTE risk factor when a BMI exceeds 30 kg/m^2 [68], and BMI has a strong linear relationship with the incidence of VTE [4]. The inflammatory and metabolic perturbations associated with obesity are thought to provoke a hypercoagulability state in these patients, and central obesity plus high fibrinogen levels may be considered as clinical markers [70]. Genetically pre-determined elevated BMI is associated with a 57% higher risk of VTE (odds ratio 1.57; 95% confidence interval 1.08–1.97; $p = 0.003$), as shown by Mendelian randomisation analysis between BMI- and VTE-associated genetic variants [71]. Presence of other risk factors of VTE, including hospitalisation, pregnancy and use of combined oestrogen–progestin hormonal contraceptives, increases VTE risk in obese patients and exacerbates the severity of VTE [72–74]. An association between elevated BMI and VTE risk has also been recently identified in paediatric patients [75]. Despite greater understanding, a number of questions remain unanswered concerning a definition of high-risk subpopulations who are obese and who may benefit from thromboprophylaxis, the choice of anticoagulants and selection of optimal regimens for thromboprophylaxis, and treatment of VTE in obese patients.

Guideline recommendations for obese patients

Clinical practice guidelines such as, National Institute for Health and Care Excellence (NICE), ASH and International Society of Thrombosis and Haemostasis highlight the need for further research regarding dosing regimens for obese patients [14, 76, 77]. Indeed, the experts interviewed considered that prophylaxis and treatment for obese patients should be stratified into subgroups but this is not fully reflected in current guidelines (Table 7).

In certain specific patient subpopulations, such as pregnant women with a BMI ≥40, guidelines suggest prophylactic LMWH dosage appropriate to a patient's weight should be considered [13], whereas bariatric surgery patients should be given a higher dose of LMWH in combination with graduated elastic compression stockings or intermittent pneumatic compression devices [79]. It is also suggested to avoid dose capping of LMWH, especially in patients with cancer, and to administer LMWH as a twice-daily regimen to allow an adequate total dose to be administered [78, 80].

Due to limited published data on the safety of DOACs, guidelines do not recommend DOACs in patients with a BMI > 40 kg/m^2 or > 120 kg, and pharmacokinetic/pharmacodynamic data suggest that drug exposure, the peak concentration and half-life of DOACs can be compromised by obesity, leading to underexposure in severely obese patients [76].

Anticoagulants, doses and regimens in prophylaxis

The evidence for using anticoagulant thromboprophylaxis in obese patients is scarce according to the experts, as obese (BMI > 30 kg/m^2) and severely obese (BMI > 40 kg/m^2) patients are under-represented in clinical studies. Despite this, the physicians interviewed prefer LMWHs over DOACs for thromboprophylaxis of obese patients. A recent pooled data analysis from 11 out of 14 primary studies highlighted the advantages of weight-based or higher-than-fixed dosing of enoxaparin, which increased the probability of achieving desired anti-Xa levels [81]. However, due to insufficient evidence and quality of studies on LMWH dose adjustment, caution should be taken in patients with a weight > 120–125 kg [81]. Indeed, in the UK, NICE have highlighted the need for further research regarding dose strategies for obese patients before recommendations can be made [56]. In Israel, the experts indicated that weight-adjusted regimens are mostly used for thromboprophylaxis in obese patients, and the Canadian experts noted that empiric LMWH dose regimens based on a patient's weight have been introduced in some hospitals in Canada: patients < 40 kg are given a reduced dose of LMWH (e.g., enoxaparin 30 mg daily) whereas patients > 100 kg receive a higher dose of LMWH, typically increased by 50% (e.g., enoxaparin 60 mg daily or dalteparin 7500 international units [IU] daily). With the latter option, however, they suggest a dose limit should be introduced to avoid overtreatment. The type of LMWH is important, as clearance of different LMWH varies in obese patients. Qualitative interviews revealed divergence of country-specific clinical practices and clinicians' opinions regarding adjustment

Table 7 High-risk obese patient subgroups that may require variations of VTE treatment

Question	Expert opinion	Guideline recommendations
Do considerations for treatment of obese patients at high risk of VTE vary between patient subgroups?	• Subgroups in obese patients are poorly studied • Treatments vary between different patient weight groups: obese, morbidly obese • The subgroup of obese patients > 120 kg is problematic • Different weight groups require different anticoagulant treatments • Standardised treatment regimens with enoxaparin exist in some hospitals • Medical and surgical obese patients need to be considered as two separate groups • Bariatric surgery or non-bariatric surgery patients and medical patients should be considered separately • Surgical obese patients should be differentiated into those undergoing bariatric surgery or any other surgery • There are differences in how these patients are defined as high risk	ACCP [28]: • Graduated compression stockings are recommended for severely obese patients considering long distance travel ISTH [76]: • Standard dosing of DOACs is recommended for obese patients with a weight < 120 kg • DOACs should not be used in obese patients with a weight > 120 kg but if they are then drug-specific peak and trough levels should be checked NICE [38]: • Further research is needed regarding dose strategies of LMWH for very obese people (BMI > 35) who are admitted to hospital or receiving day procedures • Mechanical prophylaxis is recommended for patients undergoing bariatric surgery RCOG [13]: • Risk of VTE during pregnancy increases with a BMI > 25 and ante-partum immobilisation SOGC [30]: • Recommended dose increases for UFH, enoxaparin, dalteparin and tinzaparin are indicated for obese pregnant women Thrombosis Canada [78]: • Obese patients between 40–100 kg are recommended higher doses of dalteparin, enoxaparin and tinzaparin than patients < 40 kg to be taken once daily. This dose is increased to twice daily for those weighing 101–120 kg

ACCP, American College of Chest Physicians; BMI, body mass index; DOAC, direct oral anticoagulant; ISTH, International Society of Thrombosis and Haemostasis; LMWH, low-molecular-weight heparin; NICE, National Institute for Health and Care Excellence; RCOG, Royal College of Obstetricians and Gynaecologists; SOGC, Society of Obstetricians and Gynaecologists of Canada; UFH, unfractionated heparin; VTE, venous thromboembolism of prophylactic LMWH doses to a patient's weight or BMI (Fig. 1).

Several recent studies have demonstrated advantages of adjusting prophylactic dosage to a patient's weight to achieve adequate VTE control. High-dose UFH, 7500 IU three-times daily, or enoxaparin, 40 mg twice daily, were more effective in reducing the risk for VTE from 1.48 to 0.77% in patients > 100 kg and discharged from hospital than low-dose UFH (5000 IU twice/three-times daily) or enoxaparin (40 mg once daily), with no increase in bleeding being reported [82]. Similarly, the comparative ITOHENOX study, which evaluated two enoxaparin regimens (60 mg versus 40 mg) in acutely ill obese patients with a BMI ≥30 kg/m², found normal anti-Xa levels in 69 and 31% of patients receiving 60 mg and 40 mg daily, respectively, with no significant difference in bleeding rates between the two groups [83]. Patients with an average BMI of 62.1 kg/m² achieved adequate goal peak anti-Xa levels more frequently when weight-based higher-dose enoxaparin (0.5 mg/kg) was administered compared with a weight-adjusted lower-dose (0.4 mg/kg) or fixed-dose (40 mg daily) regimen [84].

Weight-based enoxaparin dosage for prophylaxis appears more effective than BMI-stratified dosing in achieving anti-Xa levels that are presumed adequate for VTE prophylaxis in severely obese women (BMI ≥40 kg/m²) after caesarean delivery [80]. Similarly, another study has shown that post-caesarean weight-based thromboprophylaxis with enoxaparin at 0.5 mg/kg twice daily in women with a BMI ≥35 kg/m² is more effective than fixed dosage of 40 mg daily in achieving prophylactic anti-Xa levels [85].

Efficacy and safety of DOACs in thromboprophylaxis of obese patients has not been adequately investigated. Various Phase III studies of DOACs have a subpopulation of obese patients, but many of those studies are inconsistent in their design, and stratification based on BMI or weight is not always available [79]. Fixed-dose DOACs are generally thought to be inappropriate for patients with a high BMI, specifically a BMI in the range of 30–40 kg/m² and in severely obese with a BMI > 40 kg/m² [80].

In summary, due to conflicting data from a small amount of research-based studies in this population, it is uncertain whether dose adjustment should be based on weight, BMI or a fixed-dose regimen (Fig. 2).

Treatment of VTE in obese patients

The majority of experts from the qualitative interviews agree on adjusting LMWH dose to a patient's weight for treatment of VTE (Fig. 1).

In obese patients with a weight > 100 kg and acute VTE, twice-daily dosing with LMWH is suggested. In selected patients, measurement of peak anti-factor Xa levels may be appropriate to ensure that an adequate anticoagulant effect is attained. Therapeutic levels of anticoagulant effect are not established with LMWH therapy and do not appear to correlate with treatment efficacy (VTE recurrence risk) or safety (bleeding risk) [86]. Nonetheless, target peak therapeutic levels have been suggested to be 0.6–1.0 IU/mL for obese patients receiving a twice-daily treatment dose of LMWH and > 1.0 IU/mL for patients receiving once-daily LMWH [86–88].

Recent studies on DOACs showed similar efficacy and safety to that of VKAs in patients with high, normal and low body weight and acute VTE, with similar rates of bleeding episodes recorded [89]. A study by Ihaddadene, et al., and the experts' personal clinical experience suggest that DOACs, such as rivaroxaban, at a fixed dose is effective in patients with a weight range of 50–150 kg [90]. Moreover, analysis of prospectively collected non-

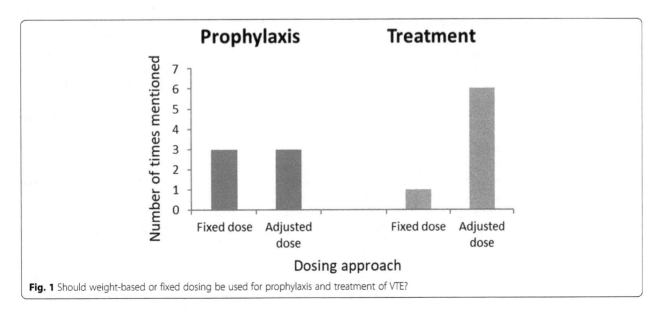

Fig. 1 Should weight-based or fixed dosing be used for prophylaxis and treatment of VTE?

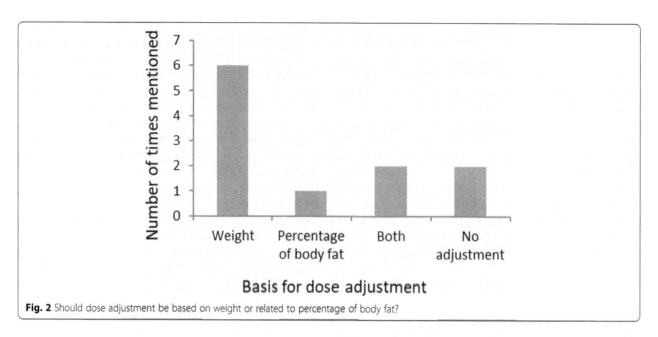

Fig. 2 Should dose adjustment be based on weight or related to percentage of body fat?

interventional data in stroke prevention in patients with a BMI range of 13.7–57.2 kg/m^2 and atrial fibrillation or VTE revealed that obese patients treated with a standard dose of DOACs had the lowest rate of cardiovascular events, major bleeding events and all-cause mortality than the normal-weight patients, suggesting that fixed-dose DOACs may provide a safe option in obese patients [91]. Creatinine clearance is greater in obese patients; therefore, it may be suggested to use DOACs with less dependence on renal clearance, such as apixaban or rivaroxaban, in these patients [92]. However, the experts interviewed agreed that further evidence needs to be generated to recommend DOACs for obese patients in a routine clinical setting.

Anticoagulants and dose regimens in bariatric surgery
The number of patients undergoing bariatric surgery procedures is increasing, and VTE prevention research in this area warrants more attention to define best practices. Patients undergoing bariatric surgery are considered at high VTE risk due, in part, to such patients having multiple non-surgical factors that increase risk, and VTE is also likely one of the most common causes of death in this population [93, 94]. In the US, bariatric surgery is the most common surgery [95]. However, studies carried out on patients undergoing bariatric surgery do not necessarily reflect up-to-date practices according to the experts, as patients are currently discharged from hospital 1–2 days post-surgery and therefore thromboprophylaxis should be considered in an out-of-hospital setting. Evidence-based guidance is sparse, but it suggests that the LMWH dose should be increased for prophylaxis, with a weight-based or staggered dose, after bariatric surgery [39]. Indeed, a systematic review, which sought to

discover if weight-adjusted thromboprophylaxis is safe and effective in the post-operative period, showed that prophylactic doses of heparin, adjusted to a patient's weight, achieved a significantly better reduction in the in-hospital VTE rate when compared with non-adjusted prophylactic dose (0.54% versus 2.0%) [94]. A risk-assessment tool was designed to predict the risk of post-discharge VTE, which was 0.29% in a 30-day post-bariatric surgery period with a 28-fold increase in mortality in those with VTE ($p < 0.001$) [94]. More than 80% of VTE events occur in a post-hospitalisation period, and this proportion is likely to become larger as bariatric surgery is increasingly done as a day procedure or with a minimal hospital stay [94]. In a prophylactic setting following bariatric surgery, anti-Xa measurements (trough levels if intent is to identify over-dosing and peak levels if intent is to identify under-dosing) should be considered 3–5 days after starting prophylaxis, but patients typically are sent home 1–2 days post-operatively and are in the acute-phase setting, so routinely measuring anti-Xa levels may be impractical. The experts considered that the determination of VTE is typically made pre-procedure, so anti-Xa levels appear uninformative in stratifying patients for prophylaxis.

Conclusions
The findings from the interviews with experts, the Thrombosis Think Tank meeting and the desktop research highlight the inconsistency of guideline recommendations and the heterogeneous views of physicians on effective primary and secondary VTE prophylaxis and VTE prevention in these high-risk medical patients. There is a paucity of user-friendly, population-adapted VTE risk-assessment models to provide reliable stratification of medical patients

for anticoagulant therapy, and current biomarkers show promise when investigated in research studies, but many have little value in the routine clinical setting [43].

LMWH remains the anticoagulant of choice in pregnant women and obese patients, where DOACs are not currently recommended. Similarly, in the elderly, LMWH demonstrates a better safety and efficacy profile than UFH for thromboprophylaxis. LMWH dose adjustment remains a significant problem in obese patients and pregnant women, with conflicting views on adjustment of prophylactic dose related to weight or BMI. Simple guidance needs to be generated for clinicians, as many are not familiar with the use of pharmacokinetic data to adjust dosing regimens.

Although further clinical studies are needed to address the VTE prophylaxis gaps, ultimately, global communication on best-practice strategies and homogeneity of guideline recommendations through increasing research data would help join up the gaps in clinical practice and improve the outcomes of medical patients.

Abbreviations
ACCP: American College of Chest Physicians; ASH: American Society of Hematology; BMI: Body mass index; DOAC: Direct oral anticoagulants; DVT: Deep vein thrombosis; IU: International unit; LMWH: Low-molecular-weight heparin; NICE: The National Institute for Health and Care Excellence; PE: Pulmonary embolism; RCOG: Royal College of Gynaecologists; RCT: Randomised controlled trial; UFH: Unfractionated heparin; VKA: Vitamin K antagonists; VTE: Venous thromboembolism

Acknowledgements
Editorial support, in the form of medical writing, assembling tables based on authors' detailed directions, collating author comments, copyediting and referencing was provided by Dr. Egle McDonald and Jane Juif, HealthCare21 Communications Ltd., Macclesfield, Cheshire, SK10 2XA, UK, and was funded by Sanofi.

Authors' contributions
All authors analysed and discussed the gap analysis data and results from the interviews. RA edited the section on pregnancy, JB-W edited the section on the elderly and JD edited the section on obese patients. All authors read and approved the final manuscript.

Author details
[1]Department of Hematology and Bone Marrow Transplantation, Rambam Health Care Campus, Haifa, Israel. [2]Department of Obstetrics and Gynaecology, The First I.M. Sechenov Moscow State Medical University, Moscow, Russia. [3]King's Thrombosis Centre, Department of Haematological Medicine, King's College Hospital Foundation NHS Trust, London, UK. [4]Thrombosis Research Unit, Department of Medicine I, Division Hematology, University Hospital 'Carl Gustav Carus' Dresden, Dresden, Germany. [5]King's Thrombosis Service, Department of Haematology, King's College London, London, UK. [6]Department of Medicine, McMaster University, Hamilton, Ontario, Canada. [7]Thrombosis and Atherosclerosis Research Institute, Hamilton, Ontario, Canada. [8]Foothills Medical Centre and Thrombosis Research Unit, University of Calgary, Calgary, Canada. [9]Hematology and Thrombosis Center, Tenon University Hospital, Sorbonne University, INSERM U938, Sorbonne University, Paris, France. [10]Hospital of Piacenza, Piacenza, Italy. [11]Department of Pulmonary and Critical Care Medicine, Center of Respiratory Medicine, China-Japan Friendship Hospital, National Clinical Research Center for Respiratory Diseases, Beijing, China.

References
1. Heit JA, Spencer FA, White RH. The epidemiology of venous thromboembolism. J Thromb Thrombolysis. 2016;41(1):3–14.
2. Chan WS, Rey E, Kent NE, Group VTEiPGW, Chan WS, Kent NE, et al. Venous thromboembolism and antithrombotic therapy in pregnancy. J Obstet Gynaecol Can. 2014;36(6):527–53.
3. Faller N, Limacher A, Mean M, Righini M, Aschwanden M, Beer JH, et al. Predictors and causes of long-term mortality in elderly patients with acute venous thromboembolism: a prospective cohort study. Am J Med. 2017; 130(2):198–206.
4. Lee YR, Blanco DD. Efficacy of standard dose unfractionated heparin for venous thromboembolism prophylaxis in morbidly obese and non-morbidly obese critically ill patients. J Thromb Thrombolysis. 2017;44(3):386–91.
5. Patil S, Ayad M, Maithili S, Patel B. Preventable vs non-preventable VTE in hospitalized patients. Chest. 2016;150(4):598A.
6. Spencer FA, Gurwitz JH, Schulman S, Linkins LA, Crowther MA, Ginsberg JS, et al. Venous thromboembolism in older adults: a community-based study. Am J Med. 2014;127(6):530–7.
7. Suh J, Desai A, Desai A, Cruz JD, Mariampillai A, Hindenburg A. Adherence to thromboprophylaxis guidelines in elderly patients with hospital acquired venous thromboembolism: a case control study. J Thromb Thrombolysis. 2017;43(2):172–8.
8. Thériault T, Touchette M, Goupil V, Echenberg D, Lanthier L. Thromboprophylaxis adherence to the ninth edition of American college of chest physicians antithrombotic guidelines in a tertiary care Centre: a cross-sectional study. J Eval Clin Pract. 2016 Dec;22(6):952–7.
9. Arcelus JI, Felicissimo P. DEIMOS investigators. Venous thromboprophylaxis duration and adherence to international guidelines in patients undergoing major orthopaedic surgery: results of the international, longitudinal, observational DEIMOS registry. Thromb Res. 2013 Jun;131(6):e240–6.
10. Bates SM, Middeldorp S, Rodger M, James AH, Greer I. Guidance for the treatment and prevention of obstetric-associated venous thromboembolism. J Thromb Thrombolysis. 2016;41(1):92–128.
11. Engbers MJ, van Hylckama VA, Rosendaal FR. Venous thrombosis in the elderly: incidence, risk factors and risk groups. J Thromb Haemost. 2010;8(10):2105–12.
12. Brenner B, Hull R, Arya R, Beyer-Westendorf J, Douketis J, Elelamy I, et al. Evaluation of unmet clinical needs in prophylaxis and treatment of venous thromboembolism in high-risk patient groups: cancer and critically ill. Thromb J. 2019;17:6.
13. Royal College of Obstetricians & Gynaecologists. Thrombosis and Embolism during Pregnancy and the Puerperium, Reducing the Risk. 2015. Available at: https://www.rcog.org.uk/en/guidelines-research-services/guidelines/gtg3 7a/. Accessed Dec 2018.
14. Bates SM, Rajasekhar A, Middeldorp S, McLintock C, Rodger MA, James AH, et al. American Society of Hematology 2018 guidelines for management of venous thromboembolism: venous thromboembolism in the context of pregnancy. Blood Adv. 2018;2(22):3317–59.
15. Palmerola KL, D'Alton ME, Brock CO, Friedman AM. A comparison of recommendations for pharmacologic thromboembolism prophylaxis after caesarean delivery from three major guidelines. BJOG. 2016;123(13):2157–62.
16. Bain E, Wilson A, Tooher R, Gates S, Davis LJ, Middleton P. Prophylaxis for venous thromboembolic disease in pregnancy and the early postnatal period. Cochrane Database Syst Rev. 2014;2:CD001689.
17. Rodger MA, Hague WM, Kingdom J, Kahn SR, Karovitch A, Sermer M, et al. Antepartum dalteparin versus no antepartum dalteparin for the prevention

of pregnancy complications in pregnant women with thrombophilia (TIPPS): a multinational open-label randomised trial. Lancet. 2014;384(9955):1673–83.

18. Gerhardt A, Scharf RE, Greer IA, Zotz RB. Hereditary risk factors for thrombophilia and probability of venous thromboembolism during pregnancy and the puerperium. Blood. 2016;128(19):2343–9.

19. Chauleur C, Quenet S, Varlet MN, Seffert P, Laporte S, Decousus H, et al. Feasibility of an easy-to-use risk score in the prevention of venous thromboembolism and placental vascular complications in pregnant women: a prospective cohort of 2736 women. Thromb Res. 2008;122(4):478–84.

20. Chaleur C, Gris JC, Laporte S, Chapelle C, Bertoletti L, Eguy V, et al. Benefit of risk score-guided prophylaxis in pregnant women at risk of thrombotic events: a controlled before-and-after implementation study. Thromb Haemost. 2018;118(9):1564–71.

21. Sultan AA, West J, Grainge MJ, Riley RD, Tata LJ, Stephansson O, et al. Development and validation of risk prediction model for venous thromboembolism in postpartum women: multinational cohort study. BMJ. 2016;355:i6253.

22. Bauersachs RM, Dudenhausen J, Faridi A, Fischer T, Fung S, Geisen U, et al. Risk stratification and heparin prophylaxis to prevent venous thromboembolism in pregnant women. Thromb Haemost. 2007;98(6):1237–45.

23. Gutiérrez García I, Pérez Cañadas P, Martínez Uriarte J, García Izquierdo O, Angeles Jódar Pérez M, García de Guadiana Romualdo L. D-dimer during pregnancy: establishing trimester-specific reference intervals. Scand J Clin Lab Invest. 2018;78(6):439–42.

24. Ercan Ş, Özkan S, Yücel N, Orçun A. Establishing reference intervals for D-dimer to trimesters. J Matern Fetal Neonatal Med. 2015;28(8):983–7.

25. Kawamura M, Fukuda N, Suzuki A, Kobayashi Y, Matsuda M, Kanda R, Kiseki H, Tsukahara Y, Hashimura N. Use of fibrin monomer complex for screening for venous thromboembolism in the late pregnancy and post-partum period. J Obstet Gynaecol Res. 2014;40(3):700–4.

26. Refaai MA, Riley P, Mardovina T, Bell PD. The clinical significance of fibrin monomers. Thromb Haemost. 2018;118(11):1856–66.

27. Hunt BJ, Parmar K, Horspool K, Shephard N, Nelson-Piercy C, Goodacre S. DiPEP research group. The DiPEP (diagnosis of PE in pregnancy) biomarker study: an observational cohort study augmented with additional cases to determine the diagnostic utility of biomarkers for suspected venous thromboembolism during pregnancy and puerperium. Br J Haematol. 2018; 180(5):694–704.

28. Kahn SR, Lim W, Dunn AS, Cushman M, Dentali F, Akl EA, et al. Prevention of VTE in nonsurgical patients: antithrombotic therapy and prevention of thrombosis, 9th ed: American College of Chest Physicians evidence-based clinical practice guidelines. Chest. 2012;141(2 Suppl):e195S–e226S.

29. Lussana F, Dentali F, Abbate R, d'Aloja E, D'Angelo A, De Stefano V, et al. Screening for thrombophilia and antithrombotic prophylaxis in pregnancy: Guidelines of the Italian Society for Haemostasis and Thrombosis (SISET). Thromb Res. 2009;124(5):e19–25.

30. Society of Obstetricians and Gynaecologists of Canada (2014) Venous Thromboembolism and Antithrombotic Therapy in Pregnancy. Available at: http://www.jogc.com/article/S1701-2163(15)30569-7/pdf. Accessed May 2019.

31. Omunakwe HE, Roberts LN, Patel JP, Subramanian D, Arya R. Impact on thromboprophylaxis rates of implementing Royal College of Obstetricians and Gynaecologists' guidance for reducing the risk of ante- and postnatal venous thromboembolism. BJOG Exchange. 2017. In response to: Palmerola KL, D'Alton ME, Brock CO, Friedman AM. A comparison of recommendations for pharmacologic thromboembolism prophylaxis after caesarean delivery from three major guidelines. BJOG. 2016;123(13):2157–2162.

32. MBRACE-UK: saving lives, improving mothers' care. https://www.npeu.ox.ac.uk/downloads/files/mbrrace-uk/reports/MBRRACE-UK%20Maternal%20Report%202017%20-%20Web.pdf Accessed May 2019.

33. Cohen H, Arachchillage DR, Middeldorp S, Beyer-Westendorf J, Abdul-Kadir R. Management of direct oral anticoagulants in women of childbearing potential: guidance from the SSC of the ISTH. J Thromb Haemost. 2016; 14(8):1673–6.

34. Thrombosis Canada. Pregnancy: Venous Thromboembolism Treatment. 2018. Available at: http://thrombosiscanada.ca/wp-content/uploads/2018/06/Pregnancy-VTE-Treatment-11May2018.pdf Accessed Feb 2019.

35. Beyer-Westendorf J, Michalski F, Tittl L, Middeldorp S, Cohen H, Kadir

36. Goland S, Schwartzenberg S, Fan J, Kozak N, Khatri N, Elkayam U. Monitoring of anti-Xa in pregnant patients with mechanical prosthetic valves receiving low-molecular-weight heparin: peak or trough levels? J Cardiovasc Pharmacol Ther. 2014;19(5):451–6.

37. Bleker SM, Buchmüller A, Chauleur C, Ní Áinle F, Donnelly J, Verhamme P, et al. Low-molecular-weight heparin to prevent recurrent venous thromboembolism in pregnancy: rationale and design of the Highlow study, a randomised trial of two doses. Thromb Res. 2016;144:62–8.

38. National Institute for Health and Care Excellence (2018) Venous thromboembolism in over 16s: reducing the risk of hospital-acquired deep vein thrombosis or pulmonary embolism: recommendations for research. Available at: https://www.nice.org.uk/guidance/ng89/chapter/Recommendations-for-research#2-dose-strategies-for-people-who-are-obese Accessed June 2019.

39. Scottish Intercollegiate Guidelines Network. Prevention and management of venous thromboembolism: a national clinical guideline. 2014. Available at: http://www.sign.ac.uk/assets/sign122.pdf. Accessed Dec 2018.

40. Crome P, Cherubini A, Oristrell J. The PREDICT (increasing participation of the elderly in clinical trials) study: the charter and beyond. Expert Rev Clin Pharmacol. 2014;7(4):457–68.

41. Silverstein RL, Bauer KA, Cushman M, Esmon CT, Ershler WB, Tracy RP. Venous thrombosis in the elderly: more questions than answers. Blood. 2007;110(9):3097–101.

42. Tritschler T, Aujesky D. Venous thromboembolism in the elderly: a narrative review. Thromb Res. 2017;155:140–7.

43. Cohen AT, Spiro TE, Spyropoulos AC, Desanctis YH, Homering M, Buller HR, et al. D-dimer as a predictor of venous thromboembolism in acutely ill, hospitalized patients: a subanalysis of the randomized controlled MAGELLAN trial. J Thromb Haemost. 2014;12(4):479–87.

44. Cohen AT, Harrington R, Goldhaber SZ, Hull R, Gibson CM, Hernandez AF, et al. The design and rationale for the acutely medically ill venous thromboembolism prevention with extended duration Betrixaban (APEX) study. AHJ. 2014;167(3):335–41.

45. Righini M, Van Es J, Den Exter PL, Roy PM, Verschuren F, Ghuysen A, et al. Age-adjusted D-dimer cutoff levels to rule out pulmonary embolism: the ADJUST-PE study. JAMA. 2014;311(11):1117–24.

46. Tita-Nwa F, Bos A, Adjei A, Ershler WB, Longo DL, Ferrucci L. Correlates of D-dimer in older persons. Aging Clin Exp Res. 2010;22(1):20–3.

47. Scherz N, Méan M, Limacher A, Righini M, Jaeger K, Beer HJ, et al. Prospective, multicenter validation of prediction scores for major bleeding in elderly patients with venous thromboembolism. J Thromb Haemost. 2013;11(3):435–43.

48. Lapner S, Cohen N, Kearon C. Influence of sex on risk of bleeding in anticoagulated patients: a systematic review and meta-analysis. J Thromb Haemost. 2014;12(5):595–605.

49. Blanco-Molina A, Enea I, Gadelha T, Tufano A, Bura-Riviere A, Di Micco P, et al. Sex differences in patients receiving anticoagulant therapy for venous thromboembolism. Medicine (Baltimore). 2014;93(17):309–17.

50. Alikhan R, Bedenis R, Cohen AT. Heparin for the prevention of venous thromboembolism in acutely ill medical patients (excluding stroke and myocardial infarction). Cochrane Database Syst Rev. 2014;5:CD003747.

51. Lacut K, Le Gal G, Mottier D. Primary prevention of venous thromboembolism in elderly medical patients. Clin Interv Aging. 2008;3(3):399–411.

52. Kröger K, Moerchel C, Bus C, Serban M. Venous thromboembolism in Germany: results of the GermAn VTE registry (GATE-registry). Int J Clin Pract. 2014;68(12):1467–72.

53. Bergmann JF, Mouly S. Thromboprophylaxis in medical patients: focus on France. Semin Thromb Hemost. 2002;3:51–5.

54. Tang X, Sun B, Yang Y, Tong Z. A survey of the knowledge of venous thromboembolism prophylaxis among the medical staff of intensive care units in North China. PLoS One. 2015;10(9):e0139162.

55. Di Micco P, Bura-Riviere A, Poggio R, Tiraferri E, Quintavalla R, Visonà A, et al. Clinical characteristics of Italian patients with venous thromboembolism enrolled in the RIETE registry. Italian J Med. 2011;5(4):255–60.

56. Dentali F, Mumoli N, Fontanella A, et al. Efficacy and safety of extended antithrombotic prophylaxis in elderly medically ill patients. Eur Respir J. 2017;49:1601887.

57. Yusen RD, Hull RD, Schellong SM, Tapson VF, Monreal M, Samama MM, et al. Impact of age on the efficacy and safety of extended-duration thromboprophylaxis in medical patients. Subgroups analysis from the EXCLAIM randomised trial. Thromb Haemost. 2013;110(6):1152–63.

58. Hull RD, Merali T, Mills A, Stevenson AL, Liang J. Venous thromboembolism in elderly high-risk medical patients: time course of events and influence of risk factors. Clin Appl Thromb Hemost. 2013;19(4):357–62.

59. Connell NT, Abel GA, Connors JM. Cost-effectiveness analysis of warfarin versus low-molecular weight heparin for the treatment of malignancy-associated venous thromboembolism. Blood. 2015;126:746.

60. Schulman S. Advantages and limitations of the new anticoagulants. J Intern Med. 2014;275(1):1–11.

61. Kearon C, Akl EA, Ornelas J, Blaivas A, Jimenez D, Bounameaux H, et al. Antithrombotic therapy for VTE disease: CHEST guideline and expert panel report. Chest. 2016;149(2):315–52.

62. Geldhof V, Vandenbriele C, Verhamme P, Vanassche T. Venous thromboembolism in the elderly: efficacy and safety of non-VKA oral anticoagulants. Thromb J. 2014;12:21.

63. Sadlon AH, Tsakiris DA. Direct oral anticoagulants in the elderly: systematic review and meta-analysis of evidence, current and future directions. Swiss Med Wkly. 2016;146:w14356.

64. Agnelli G, Buller HR, Cohen A, Curto M, Gallus AS, Johnson M, et al. Apixaban for extended treatment of venous thromboembolism. N Engl J Med. 2013;368(8):699–708.

65. Schulman S, Kakkar AK, Goldhaber SZ, Schellong S, Eriksson H, Mismetti P, et al. Treatment of acute venous thromboembolism with dabigatran or warfarin and pooled analysis. Circulation. 2014;129(7):764–72.

66. Vanassche T, Verhamme P, Wells PS, Segers A, Ageno W, Brekelmans MPA, et al. Impact of age, comorbidity, and polypharmacy on the efficacy and safety of edoxaban for the treatment of venous thromboembolism: an analysis of the randomized, double-blind Hokusai-VTE trial. Thromb Res. 2018;162:7–14.

67. Prins MH, Lensing AWA, Bauersachs R, van Bellen B, Bounameaux H, Brighton TA, et al. Oral rivaroxaban versus standard therapy for the treatment of symptomatic venous thromboembolism: a pooled analysis of the EINSTEIN-DVT and PE randomized studies. Thromb J. 2013;11(1):21.

68. Nejat EJ, Polotsky AJ, Pal L. Predictors of chronic disease at midlife and beyond--the health risks of obesity. Maturitas. 2010;65(2):106–11.

69. World Health Organization Europe: body mass index. Available at: http://www.euro.who.int/en/health-topics/disease-prevention/nutrition/a-healthy-lifestyle/body-mass-index-bmi. Accessed Dec 2018.

70. Taura P, Rivas E, Martinez-Palli G, Blasi A, Holguera JC, Balust J. Clinical markers of the hypercoagulable state by rotational thrombelastometry in obese patients submitted to bariatric surgery. Surg Endosc. 2014;28(2):543–51.78.

71. Klarin D, Emdin CA, Natarajan P, Conrad MF. INVENT Consortium, Kathiresan S. Genetic analysis of venous thromboembolism in UK biobank identifies the ZFPM2 locus and implicates obesity as a causal risk factor. Circ Cardiovasc Genet. 2017;10(2):e001643.

72. Fausett MB, Vogtlander M, Lee RM, Esplin MS, Branch DW, Rodgers GM, et al. Heparin-induced thrombocytopenia is rare in pregnancy. Am J Obstet Gynecol. 2001;185(1):148–52.

73. Yang G, De Staercke C, Hooper WC. The effects of obesity on venous thromboembolism: a review. Open J Prev Med. 2012;2(4):499–509.

74. Horton LG, Simmons KB, Curtis KM. Combined hormonal contraceptive use among obese women and risk for cardiovascular events: a systematic review. Contraception. 2016;94(6):590–604.

75. Halvorson EE, Ervin SE, Russell TB, Skelton JA, Davis S, Spangler J. Association of obesity and pediatric venous thromboembolism. Hosp Pediatr. 2016;6(1):22–6.

76. Martin K, Beyer-Westendorf J, Davidson BL, Huisman MV, Sandset PM, Moll S. Use of the direct oral anticoagulants in obese patients: guidance from the SSC of the ISTH. J Thromb Haemost. 2016;14(6):1308–13.

77. National Institute for Health and Care Excellence (2015) Venous thromboembolism: reducing the risk for patients in hospital. Available at: https://www.nice.org.uk/guidance/CG92/chapter/introduction. Accessed Dec 2018.

78. Thrombosis Canada 2017: Thrombosis Canada (2017) Thromboprophylaxis: Hospitalized Medical Patients. Available at: http://thrombosiscanada.ca/wp-content/uploads/2017/06/10.-Thromboprophylaxis-Medical-Patients-2017May17.pdf Accessed May 2019.

79. Nicolaides AN, Fareed J, Kakkar AK, Comerota AJ, Goldhaber SZ, Hull R, et al. Prevention and treatment of venous thromboembolism--international consensus statement. Int Angiol. 2013;32(2):111–260.

80. Easaw JC, Shea-Budgell MA, Wu CM, Czaykowski PM, Kassis J, Kuehl B, et al. Canadian consensus recommendations on the management of venous thromboembolism in patients with cancer. Part 2: treatment. Curr Oncol. 2015;22(2):144–55.

81. He Z, Morrissey H, Ball P. Review of current evidence available for guiding optimal enoxaparin prophylactic dosing strategies in obese patients-actual weight-based vs fixed. Crit Rev Oncol Hematol. 2017;113:191–4.

82. Wang TF, Milligan PE, Wong CA, Deal EN, Thoelke MS, Gage BF. Efficacy and safety of high-dose thromboprophylaxis in morbidly obese inpatients. Thromb Haemost. 2014;111(1):88–93.

83. Miranda S, Le Cam-Duchez V, Benichou J, Donnadieu N, Barbay V, Le Besnerais M, et al. Adjusted value of thromboprophylaxis in hospitalized obese patients: a comparative study of two regimens of enoxaparin: the ITOHENOX study. Thromb Res. 2017;155:1–5.

84. Freeman A, Horner T, Pendleton RC, Rondina MT. Prospective comparison of three enoxaparin dosing regimens to achieve target anti-factor Xa levels in hospitalized, medically ill patients with extreme obesity. Am J Hematol. 2012;87(7):740–3.

85. Stephenson ML, Serra AE, Neeper JM, Caballero DC, McNulty J. A randomized controlled trial of differing doses of postcesarean enoxaparin thromboprophylaxis in obese women. J Perinatol. 2016;36(2):95–9.

86. Boneu B, de Moerloose P. How and when to monitor a patient treated with low molecular weight heparin. Semin Thromb Hemost. 2001;27(5):519–22.

87. Egan G, Ensom MH. Measuring anti-factor Xa activity to monitor low-molecular-weight heparin in obesity: a critical review. Can J Hosp Pharm. 2015;68(1):33–47.

88. Samama MM, Poller L. Contemporary laboratory monitoring of low molecular weight heparins. Clin Lab Med. 1995;15(1):119–23.

89. Di Minno MN, Lupoli R, Di Minno A, Ambrosino P, Scalera A, Dentali F. Effect of body weight on efficacy and safety of direct oral anticoagulants in the treatment of patients with acute venous thromboembolism: a meta-analysis of randomized controlled trials. Ann Med. 2015;47(1):61–8.

90. Ihaddadene R, Carrier M. The use of anticoagulants for the treatment and prevention of venous thromboembolism in obese patients: implications for safety. Expert Opin Drug Saf. 2016;15(1):65–74.

91. Tittl L, Endig S, Marten S, Reitter A, Beyer-Westendorf I, Beyer-Westendorf J. Impact of BMI on clinical outcomes of NOAC therapy in daily care - results of the prospective Dresden NOAC registry (NCT01588119). Int J Cardiol. 2018;262:85–91.

92. Güler E, Babur Güler G, Demir GG, Hatipoğlu S. A review of the fixed dose use of new oral anticoagulants in obese patients: is it really enough? Anatol J Cardiol. 2015;15(12):1020–9.

93. Ikesaka R, Delluc A, Le Gal G, Carrier M. Efficacy and safety of weight-adjusted heparin prophylaxis for the prevention of acute venous thromboembolism among obese patients undergoing bariatric surgery: a systematic review and meta-analysis. Thromb Res. 2014;133(4):682–7.

94. Aminian A, Andalib A, Khorgami Z, Cetin D, Burguera B, Bartholomew J, et al. Who should get extended thromboprophylaxis after bariatric surgery? A risk assessment tool to guide indications for post-discharge pharmacoprophylaxis. Ann Surg. 2017;265(1):143–50.

95. Pierce J, Galante J, Scherer LA, Chang EJ, Wisner D, Ali M. PL-202: bariatric surgery in the balance: a paradigm shift in general surgery. Surg Obes Relat Dis. 2010;6(3):S10.

5

Rivaroxaban versus warfarin for treatment and prevention of recurrence of venous thromboembolism in African American patients

Olivia S. Costa[1,2], Stanley Thompson[3], Veronica Ashton[4], Michael Palladino[5], Thomas J. Bunz[6] and Craig I. Coleman[1,2]*

Abstract

Background: African Americans are under-represented in trials evaluating oral anticoagulants for the treatment of acute venous thromboembolism (VTE). The aim of this study was to evaluate the effectiveness and safety of rivaroxaban versus warfarin for the treatment of VTE in African Americans.

Methods: We utilized Optum® De-Identified Electronic Health Record data from 11/1/2012–9/30/2018. We included African Americans experiencing an acute VTE during a hospital or emergency department visit, who received rivaroxaban or warfarin as their first oral anticoagulant within 7-days of the acute VTE event and had ≥1 provider visit in the prior 12-months. Differences in baseline characteristics between cohorts were adjusted using inverse probability-of-treatment weighting based on propensity scores (standard differences < 0.10 were achieved for all covariates). Our primary endpoint was the composite of recurrent VTE or major bleeding at 6-months. Three- and 12-month timepoints were also assessed. Secondary endpoints included recurrent VTE and major bleeding as individual endpoints. Cohort risk was compared using Cox regression and reported as hazard ratios (HRs) with 95% confidence intervals (CIs).

Results: We identified 2097 rivaroxaban and 2842 warfarin users with incident VTE. At 6-months, no significant differences in the composite endpoint (HR = 0.96, 95%CI = 0.75–1.24), recurrent VTE (HR = 1.02, 95%CI = 0.76–1.36) or major bleeding alone (HR = 0.93, 95%CI = 0.59–1.47) were observed between cohorts. Analysis at 3- and 12-months provided consistent findings for these endpoints.

Conclusions: In African Americans experiencing an acute VTE, no significant difference in the incidence of recurrent VTE or major bleeding was observed between patients receiving rivaroxaban or warfarin.

Keywords: African Americans, Anticoagulants, Rivaroxaban, Venous thromboembolism, Warfarin

* Correspondence: craig.coleman@hhchealth.org
[1]Department of Pharmacy Practice, University of Connecticut School of Pharmacy, 69 North Eagleville Road, Unit 3092, Storrs, CT 06269, USA
[2]Evidence-Based Practice Center, Hartford Hospital, Hartford, CT, USA
Full list of author information is available at the end of the article

Background

There is ample evidence suggesting African Americans have an increased incidence of venous thromboembolism (VTE) and poorer disease outcomes compared to other racial groups [1–5]. Despite race-based differences in VTE incidence and prognosis, African Americans have been under-represented in randomized controlled trials (RCTs) evaluating non-vitamin K oral anticoagulants (NOACs) for the management of VTE [6–10]. As a result, there is a scarcity of data evaluating NOACs for the treatment and secondary prevention of VTE.

The objective of this study was to evaluate the effectiveness and safety of rivaroxaban versus warfarin in the treatment and prevention of recurrent VTE in African Americans managed in routine practice.

Methods

We performed a retrospective cohort analysis using United States (US) Optum® De-Identified Electronic Health Record (EHR) data from November 1, 2012 to September 30, 2018 [11]. The Optum EHR database includes longitudinal patient-level medical record data for 97 million patients seen at 700 hospitals and 7000 clinics across the United States. The database includes records of prescriptions as prescribed and administered, lab results, vital signs, body measurements, diagnoses, procedures, and information derived from clinical notes using natural language processing. This database contains data on insured and uninsured patients of all ages and races to provide a representative sample of all African American patients with acute VTE in the US.

To be included in this study patients had to be African American, admitted to the hospital, emergency department or observation unit for acute deep vein thrombosis (DVT) or pulmonary embolism (PE), have received rivaroxaban or warfarin as their first oral anticoagulant (OAC) within 7-days of the acute VTE event (index date) and had at least one provider visit in the 12-months prior to the acute VTE event (baseline period). We excluded patients with another indication for OAC use (i.e. atrial fibrillation, prophylaxis after hip/knee replacement, valvular heart disease).

Our primary endpoint for this analysis was the composite of recurrent VTE or major bleeding at 3-, 6- and 12-months [12, 13]. Recurrent VTE was defined as a subsequent hospitalization with a primary International Classification of Diseases-10th Revision (or cross-walked ICD-9 to ICD-10) diagnosis code for DVT (ICD-10 = 180–182) or PE (ICD-10 = 126) [12]. Major bleeding was defined as a subsequent hospitalization for a bleeding event using the validated Cunningham algorithm [13]. This algorithm defines a hospitalization as bleeding-related based on the presence of an ICD-10 bleeding code in the primary position or the presence of select non-primary diagnosis ICD-10 codes accompanied by a billing code indicating a blood transfusion or processing of blood products for transfusion. Secondary endpoints included recurrent VTE and major bleeding as separate endpoints, as well as, intracranial hemorrhage (ICH), gastrointestinal bleeding (GIB) and genitourinary bleeding (GUB). Patients were followed for up to 12-months or until endpoint occurrence, end-of-EHR activity or through September 30, 2018 (an intent-to-treat approach).

Differences in baseline characteristics between the rivaroxaban and warfarin cohorts were adjusted for using inverse probability-of-treatment weighting (IPTW) based on propensity scores [14]. For the IPTW analysis, propensity scores (and subsequent patient weights) were estimated using generalized boosted models on the basis of 10,000 regression trees using the 'TWANG' package (version 1.5) and R statistical software version 3.4.3 (The R Project for Statistical Computing) which implements an automated, nonparametric machine learning method. The weights were derived to obtain estimates of the population average treatment effect. Variables entered in the generalized boosted modeling procedure (including demographics, comorbidities and concurrent non-anticoagulant medications) are depicted in Table 1 and were identified during the 12-month baseline period. The presence of residual differences in measured covariates following cohort weighting was assessed by calculating absolute standardized differences (< 0.1 was considered well-balanced for each variable) [14].

Baseline categorical data were reported as percentages and continuous data as medians with 25, 75% ranges. Endpoint incidence were reported as proportions (the number experiencing an event divided by total number of patients in the cohort). Weighted Cox proportional hazards regression analysis were performed using the 'SURVEY' package version 3.36 in R. Patients assigned weights at the extremes (<1st or > 99th percentile) were recalibrated to the corresponding threshold values prior to weighted regression analyses [14]. The proportional hazard assumption was tested based on Schoenfeld residuals and was found valid for all endpoints.

We performed sensitivity analyses in which an on-treatment approach (i.e., patients followed for up to 12-months or until endpoint occurrence, index OAC discontinuation [30-day permissible gap] or switch, end-of-EHR activity or through September 30, 2018) was utilized and differences in baseline characteristics between the rivaroxaban and warfarin cohorts were adjusted using IPTW based on propensity scores. An additional sensitivity analysis was performed in which differences in baseline characteristics between the rivaroxaban and warfarin cohorts were adjusted by propensity score matching calculated via multivariable logistic regression using 'MatchIT' in R.

Table 1 Characteristics of the Rivaroxaban and Warfarin Intent-To-Treat Cohorts After IPTW

	Rivaroxaban N = 2097 %	Warfarin N = 2842 %	Absolute Standardized Difference
Demographics			
Age, median (25, 75% range)	50 (39, 62)	51 (40, 64)	–
Age 18–49 years	45.5	43.6	0.04
Age 50–64 years	29.6	29.2	0.01
Age 65–74 years	13.1	13.7	0.02
Age 75–79 years	4.3	4.7	0.02
Age ≥ 80 years	7.5	8.9	0.05
Female sex	56.4	56.4	0.00
Pulmonary embolism (±deep vein thrombosis)	18.6	19.1	0.01
Comorbidities			
Chronic obstructive pulmonary disease	8.6	9.6	0.04
Asthma	13.1	13.6	0.02
Heart Failure	5.1	5.4	0.01
Hypertension	53.5	55.2	0.03
Ischemic stroke	3.6	4.3	0.04
Diabetes	22.3	23.0	0.02
Dementia	2.6	3.3	0.04
Coronary artery disease	0.8	0.7	0.01
Carotid stenosis	0.6	0.8	0.03
Peripheral vascular disease	5.5	5.8	0.01
Myocardial infarction	5.2	5.9	0.03
Percutaneous coronary intervention	3.5	4.1	0.03
Coronary artery bypass grafting	2.4	2.8	0.02
Gastrointestinal bleed	0.3	0.5	0.02
Intracranial hemorrhage	0.0	0.3	0.07
Acute kidney injury	11.0	12.5	0.05
Other kidney injury	0.3	0.5	0.04
Inflammatory bowel disease	1.2	1.6	0.04
eGFR > 90 mL/minute	53.6	51.7	0.04
eGFR 60–89 mL/minute	30.9	30.8	0.00
eGFR 30-59 mL/minute	11.1	11.3	0.01
eGFR 15–29 mL/minute	1.9	2.7	0.06
eGFR < 15 mL/minute	1.7	2.6	0.06
eGFR unknown	0.7	0.7	0.01
Liver disease	1.6	1.6	0.00
Coagulopathy	3.1	3.5	0.02
Gastroesophageal reflux disease	18.9	18.8	0.00
Anemia	25.5	27.7	0.05

Table 1 Characteristics of the Rivaroxaban and Warfarin Intent-To-Treat Cohorts After IPTW (Continued)

	Rivaroxaban N = 2097 %	Warfarin N = 2842 %	Absolute Standardized Difference
Sleep apnea	10.4	10.2	0.01
Smoking	27.4	27.4	0.00
Hemorrhoids	2.3	2.6	0.02
Alcohol abuse	0.4	0.3	0.02
Anxiety	12.6	12.2	0.01
Depression	1.6	1.8	0.02
Psychosis	1.5	1.5	0.00
BMI < 18.5 kg/m^2	1.9	1.9	0.00
BMI 18.5–24.9 kg/m^2	15.8	16.5	0.02
BMI 25.0–29.9 kg/m^2	24.8	24.6	0.01
BMI 30.0–34.9 kg/m^2	23.0	23.0	0.00
BMI 35.0–39.9 kg/m^2	14.7	14.3	0.01
BMI ≥40 kg/m^2	18.4	18.4	0.00
BMI < 18.5 kg/m^2	1.3	1.2	0.01
Rheumatoid arthritis	6.2	5.8	0.02
Osteoarthritis	18.9	19.9	0.03
Headache	10.7	11.1	0.01
Diverticulitis	3.8	3.8	0.00
H. pylori treatment	0.4	0.6	0.02
Hypothyroidism	0.8	0.9	0.00
Solid tumor	9.5	10.2	0.02
Metastatic cancer	3.5	3.8	0.01
Major surgery	9.8	9.7	0.01
Varicose veins	1.4	1.3	0.01
Comedications			
Aspirin	22.7	24.0	0.03
P2Y12 platelet inhibitor	3.1	4.0	0.05
Nonsteroidal anti-inflammatory drug	31.8	30.8	0.02
Celecoxib	1.1	1.0	0.01
Angiotensin-converting enzyme inhibitor or receptor blocker	31.1	32.2	0.02
Beta-blocker	23.5	25.3	0.04
Diltiazem	1.8	2.0	0.01
Verapamil	0.9	1.1	0.02
Dihydropyridine calcium channel blocker	21.2	21.8	0.01
Loop diuretic	11.0	11.9	0.03
Thiazide	21.2	21.4	0.00
Digoxin	0.5	0.8	0.04
Statin	23.7	24.5	0.02
Other cholesterol medication	2.0	2.1	0.01
Metformin	11.7	11.5	0.01

Table 1 Characteristics of the Rivaroxaban and Warfarin Intent-To-Treat Cohorts After IPTW *(Continued)*

	Rivaroxaban N = 2097 %	Warfarin N = 2842 %	Absolute Standardized Difference
Sulfonylurea or glinides	5.1	6.0	0.04
Thiazolidinediones	0.5	0.6	0.02
Dipeptidyl peptidase 4 inhibitors	1.5	1.4	0.01
Glucagon-like peptide-1 agonist	0.5	0.3	0.03
Insulin	7.8	8.9	0.04
Selective serotonin reuptake or serotonin-norepinephrine reuptake inhibitor	10.6	11.3	0.02
Other antidepressants	9.0	9.7	0.03
Proton pump inhibitors	21.4	22.6	0.03
Histamin-2 receptor antagonist	8.4	9.0	0.02
Systemic corticosteroids	17.8	18.8	0.03
Alpha-glucosidase inhibitor	0.1	0.0	0.04
Hypnotic medication	3.7	3.6	0.00
Sodium-glucose cotransporter-2 inhibitor	0.3	0.2	0.02

Each eligible rivaroxaban user was 1:1 propensity score matched using greedy nearest neighbor matching without replacement and a caliper = 0.25 standard deviations of the propensity score. For sensitivity analysis, Cox proportional hazards regression analysis was performed using IBM SPSS version 25.0 (IBM Corp, Armonk, NY).

The report for this analysis was written to comply with the Reporting of Studies Conducted using Observational Routinely-Collected Health Data (RECORD) statement [15].

Results

In total, we identified 48,429 patients with a primary diagnosis for VTE with ≥1 provider visit in the 12-months prior to the index VTE event. Of these, 6158 were African Americans and 4939 were initiated on OAC with either rivaroxaban or warfarin within 7-days of the index event. The median age of included patients was 51 years, 56.4% o were female, 18.4% were morbidly obese (body mass index ≥40 kg/m^2), 9.7% had a history of prior major surgery, 3.7 and 9.9% and had a history of/active metastatic cancer or a solid tumor, respectively, and nearly 1 in 5 patients had a PE ± DVT.

Following IPTW, patients were deemed well-balanced on all independent variables entered into the propensity-score model as demonstrated by absolute standardized differences between the rivaroxaban and warfarin users < 0.1. Upon Cox regression, rivaroxaban use (N = 2097) was not associated with a statistically significant difference in the incidence of

the composite endpoint of recurrent VTE or major bleeding at 3-months (4.57% versus 4.58%, HR = 1.08, 95%CI = 0.82–1.42), 6-months (5.01% versus 5.84%, HR = 0.96, 95%CI = 0.75–1.24) or 12-months (5.82% versus 7.32%, HR = 0.93, 95%CI = 0.74–1.16) of follow-up (Table 2) compared to warfarin (N = 2842). No significant differences were observed between the cohorts for either of the components when evaluated separately at these same time points, nor were there significant differences in the incidence of ICH (HR = 0.66, 95%CI = 0.12–3.59 at 3-months; HR = 0.50, 95%CI = 0.10–2.50 at 6-months and HR = 0.76, 95%CI = 0.27–2.19 at 12-months), GI (HR = 1.16, 95%CI = 0.61–2.21 at 3-months; HR = 0.84, 95%CI = 0.47–1.51 at 6-months and HR = 0.80, 95%CI = 0.47–1.37 at 12-months) and GU bleeding (HR = 1.08, 95%CI = 0.30–3.93 at 3-months; HR = 0.80, 95%CI = 0.24–2.63 at 6-months and HR = 0.88, 95%CI = 0.29–2.63 at 12-months). Sensitivity analyses 1) employing propensity score matching (N = 2068 users of rivaroxaban or warfarin per group) and 2) based upon an on-treatment analysis approach both provided similar results to the base-case analysis for the composite endpoint, recurrent VTE and major bleeding alone at each timepoint (Tables 3 and 4).

Discussion

This EHR-based study evaluated African American patients experiencing a VTE treated with rivaroxaban or warfarin in routine practice. Our analysis suggested there was no significant difference in the incidence of the composite endpoint of recurrent VTE or major bleeding between the treatment groups after 3-, 6- or 12-months of follow up. No significant differences were observed between the cohorts for either of the components when evaluated separately at these same time points, nor were there significant differences in the incidence of ICH, GI or GU bleeding. Our conclusions were also similar when an on-treatment approach and propensity score matching were utilized.

African American patients have been under-enrolled in RCTs evaluating NOACs for the treatment of VTE [7–10]. Moreover, no sub-analyses of an RCT has reported on the efficacy and/or safety of NOACs in a cohort of African American patients. Consequently, our present analysis provides important new data to aid in clinical decision-making. The findings of our study were generally consistent with those of the pooled EINSTEIN trial analysis which included a small portion (2.6%) of black patients and the prospective, nonrandomized XALIA registry study [5, 9, 16]. In the pooled EINSTEIN trial analysis, rivaroxaban (n = 4151) was found to be non-inferior to enoxaparin/vitamin K antagonist (VKA) (n = 4131) for the endpoint of recurrent VTE with a 2.1 and 2.3% incidence, respectively (HR = 0.89; 95%CI = 0.66–1.19). These results were echoed in XALIA which found no significant difference in recurrent VTE risk

Table 2 Event Incidence and Hazard Ratios with 95% Confidence Intervals for IPTW Analysis of the Rivaroxaban and Warfarin Cohorts Using an Intent-To-Treat Approach

	Rivaroxaban N = 2097 n (%)	Warfarin N = 2842 n (%)	HR (95%CI)
3-Month			
Composite of recurrent venous thromboembolism or major bleeding	96 (4.58)	130 (4.57)	1.08 (0.82–1.42)
Recurrent venous thromboembolism	74 (3.53)	96 (3.38)	1.07 (0.78–1.46)
Major bleeding	27 (1.29)	40 (1.41)	1.19 (0.72–1.97)
Intracranial hemorrhage	2 (0.10)	5 (0.18)	0.66 (0.12–3.59)
Gastrointestinal bleeding	17 (0.81)	24 (0.84)	1.16 (0.61–2.21)
Genitourinary bleeding	4 (0.19)	6 (0.21)	1.08 (0.30–3.93)
6-Month			
Composite of recurrent venous thromboembolism or major bleeding	105 (5.01)	166 (5.84)	0.96 (0.75–1.24)
Recurrent venous thromboembolism	81 (3.86)	115 (4.05)	1.01 (0.76–1.36)
Major bleeding	30 (1.43)	59 (2.08)	0.93 (0.59–1.47)
Intracranial hemorrhage	2 (0.10)	7 (0.25)	0.50 (0.10–2.50)
Gastrointestinal bleeding	18 (0.86)	37 (1.30)	0.84 (0.47–1.51)
Genitourinary bleeding	4 (0.19)	9 (0.32)	0.80 (0.24–2.63)
12-Month			
Composite of recurrent venous thromboembolism or major bleeding	122 (5.82)	208 (7.32)	0.93 (0.74–1.16)
Recurrent venous thromboembolism	89 (4.24)	140 (4.93)	0.95 (0.72–1.2)
Major bleeding	39 (1.86)	80 (2.81)	0.92 (0.62–1.36)
Intracranial hemorrhage	5 (0.24)	13 (0.46)	0.76 (0.27–2.19)
Gastrointestinal bleeding	21 (1.00)	47 (1.65)	0.80 (0.47–1.37)
Genitourinary bleeding	5 (0.24)	10 (0.35)	0.88 (0.29–2.63)

CI Confidence interval, HR Hazard ratio, N Number

between rivaroxaban (n = 2619) (1.4%) and standard-of-care management (typically parenteral bridging to a VKA) (n = 2149) (2.3%) of acute DVT (±PE) in routine practice (propensity score-adjusted HR = 0.91; 95%CI = 0·54–1·54). While reductions in the risk of major bleeding was observed with rivaroxaban (1.0%) compared to enoxaparin/VKA (1.7%) in the EINSTEIN clinical trial program (HR = 0.54; 95%CI = 0.37–0.79), no significant difference was observed in XALIA for rivaroxaban (0.8%) versus standard-of-care (2.1%) management (propensity score-adjusted HR = 0.77; 95%CI = 0.40–1.50).

This study has limitations worthy of discussion. First, multiple biases including misclassification, sampling and confounding bias are always important limitations in non-randomized, retrospective studies that may impact their internal validity [17]. We attempted to reduce the probability of misclassification bias by using validated coding schema to identify comorbidities and endpoints (when possible). Our methodology appeared to be effective given we reported recurrent VTE rates just slightly above previously published studies [9, 16,

18] (which was anticipated as black patients have been hypothesized to be at a higher risk of thrombosis compared to other races [1–5]) as well as a similar incidence of major bleeding (range in prior studies: 0.77–2.1%) [9, 16, 18]. Second, we used EHR data for US patients [11]; and therefore, our results are most generalizable to a US population. Third, we did not calculate time in therapeutic international normalized ratio (INR) range for warfarin patients. While INR control is somewhat predictive of the effectiveness and safety of vitamin K antagonists, it is well known that VTE patients treated with warfarin in routine US clinical practice spend only ~ 56% of their time during the first 3 months of treatment (when recurrent VTE is most likely) in the therapeutic INR range [19, 20] and African American patients may have among the poorest INR control [21]. Given the Optum EHR data used for this study covers patients throughout the US regardless of insurer (or no insurance), it is likely patients included in this study experienced at least similar suboptimal INR control. Fourth, results of the on-treatment analysis which was performed to supplement

Table 3 Characteristics of the 1:1 Propensity Score Matched (Sensitivity Analysis) Rivaroxaban and Warfarin Cohorts

	Rivaroxaban N = 2068 %	Warfarin N = 2068 %	Absolute Standardized Difference
Demographics			
Age, median (25, 75% range)	50 (39, 62)	51 (40, 64)	–
Age 18–49 years	46.32	48.21	0.04
Age 50–64 years	30.03	30.32	0.01
Age 65–74 years	13.10	12.28	0.03
Age 75–79 years	4.59	3.77	0.04
Age ≥ 80 years	5.95	5.42	0.02
Female sex	56.19	55.66	0.01
Pulmonary embolism (±deep vein thrombosis)	18.09	17.89	0.01
Comorbidities			
Chronic obstructive pulmonary disease	8.37	7.98	0.01
Asthma	13.25	13.10	0.00
Heart Failure	4.84	4.93	0.00
Hypertension	52.80	51.45	0.27
Ischemic stroke or transient ischemic attack	2.95	2.85	0.01
Diabetes	21.13	21.03	0.00
Dementia	2.18	2.03	0.01
Coronary artery disease	0.68	0.87	0.02
Carotid stenosis	0.63	0.53	0.01
Peripheral vascular disease	5.51	5.42	0.00
Myocardial infarction	5.08	4.59	0.02
Percutaneous coronary intervention	3.34	3.13	0.01
Coronary artery bypass grafting	1.93	2.18	0.02
Gastrointestinal bleed	0.24	0.29	0.01
Intracranial hemorrhage	0.00	0.00	NA
Acute kidney injury	10.06	9.38	0.02
Other kidney injury	0.24	0.24	0.00
Inflammatory bowel disease	0.77	0.82	0.01
eGFR > 90 mL/minute	55.42	58.32	0.06
eGFR 60–89 mL/minute	0.48	0.73	0.03
eGFR 30-59 mL/minute	31.09	28.97	0.05
eGFR 15–29 mL/minute	10.88	10.06	0.03
eGFR < 15 mL/minute	1.21	1.11	0.01
eGFR unknown	0.77	0.68	0.01
Liver disease	1.50	1.93	0.03
Coagulopathy	3.00	3.00	0.00
Gastroesophageal reflux disease	18.76	18.96	0.00
Anemia	24.13	23.55	0.01
Sleep apnea	10.20	10.64	0.01
Smoking	28.77	28.19	0.01
Hemorrhoids	2.22	2.37	0.01
Alcohol abuse	0.34	0.34	0.00
Anxiety	12.28	14.02	0.05

Table 3 Characteristics of the 1:1 Propensity Score Matched (Sensitivity Analysis) Rivaroxaban and Warfarin Cohorts *(Continued)*

	Rivaroxaban N = 2068 %	Warfarin N = 2068 %	Absolute Standardized Difference
Depression	1.69	1.60	0.01
Psychosis	1.50	1.16	0.03
BMI < 18.5 kg/m^2	1.60	1.74	0.01
BMI 18.5–24.9 kg/m^2	15.43	14.46	0.03
BMI 25.0–29.9 kg/m^2	24.71	25.29	0.01
BMI 30.0–34.9 kg/m^2	23.26	23.79	0.01
BMI 35.0–39.9 kg/m^2	14.70	15.47	0.02
BMI ≥40 kg/m^2	19.15	17.65	0.04
BMI unknown	1.16	1.60	0.03
Rheumatoid arthritis	5.80	6.53	0.03
Osteoarthritis	18.86	18.23	0.02
Headache	10.15	10.59	0.01
Diverticulitis	3.72	3.77	0.00
H. pylori treatment	0.39	0.34	0.01
Hypothyroidism	0.87	0.87	0.00
Solid tumor	9.72	8.90	0.03
Metastatic cancer	3.72	3.29	0.02
Major surgery	10.11	10.01	0.00
Varicose veins	1.26	1.35	0.01
Comedications			
Aspirin	22.10	21.47	0.02
P2Y12 platelet inhibitor	2.90	2.80	0.01
Nonsteroidal anti-inflammatory drug	31.33	33.95	0.05
Celecoxib	1.02	1.35	0.03
Angiotensin-converting enzyme inhibitor or receptor blocker	30.66	29.21	0.03
Beta-blocker	22.44	21.52	0.02
Diltiazem	1.55	1.69	0.01
Verapamil	0.87	0.87	0.00
Dihydropyridine calcium channel blocker	20.31	19.44	0.02
Loop diuretic	10.69	9.91	0.03
Thiazide	21.08	20.45	0.02
Digoxin	0.44	0.39	0.01
Statin	23.02	21.66	0.03
Other cholesterol medication	2.13	1.98	0.01
Metformin	11.41	11.17	0.01
Sulfonylurea or glinides	4.64	4.30	0.02
Thiazolidinediones	0.34	0.53	0.03
Dipeptidyl peptidase 4 inhibitors	1.35	1.64	0.02
Glucagon-like peptide-1 agonist	0.29	0.44	0.02
Insulin	7.54	7.06	0.02
Selective serotonin reuptake or serotonin-norepinephrine reuptake inhibitor	10.88	10.74	0.00
Other antidepressants	8.95	8.80	0.01
Proton pump inhibitors	21.23	21.03	0.00

Table 3 Characteristics of the 1:1 Propensity Score Matched (Sensitivity Analysis) Rivaroxaban and Warfarin Cohorts *(Continued)*

	Rivaroxaban N = 2068 %	Warfarin N = 2068 %	Absolute Standardized Difference
Histamin-2 receptor antagonist	9.14	8.46	0.02
Systemic corticosteroids	18.13	18.09	0.00
Alpha-glucosidase inhibitor	0.00	0.00	0.00
Hypnotic medication	3.68	4.01	0.02
Sodium-glucose cotransporter-2 inhibitor	0.15	0.19	0.01

our intention-to-treat analysis should be interpreted with caution as it is unclear how accurately EHRs maintain up-to-date patient medication profiles. Moreover, an EHR entry to initiate an OAC does neither guarantee a patient took the medication nor (as in claim data sets) assures patients even picked up their prescription at the pharmacy. Finally, absent randomization in a study, residual confounding cannot be fully excluded due to the possibility of confounding from unobserved or unmeasured covariates [11].

Conclusions

In conclusion, our EHR-based study suggests rivaroxaban is no worse than warfarin at preventing recurrent VTE with no increased risk of major bleeds in African Americans. Our findings are similar to those found in the EINSTEIN clinical trials and consistent with the results from the XALIA study. Additional real-world analyses with an increased sample size to evaluate the effectiveness and safety of rivaroxaban for treatment and prevention of VTE in African Americans are warranted.

Table 4 Results of Sensitivity Analyses

	1:1 Propensity Score Matching	On-Treatment Approach
3-Month		
Composite of recurrent venous thromboembolism or major bleeding	1.10 (0.82–1.46)	1.10 (0.83–1.45)
Recurrent venous thromboembolism	1.08 (0.78–1.50)	1.11 (0.81–1.52)
Major bleeding	1.28 (0.73–2.25)	1.17 (0.69–1.98)
Intracranial hemorrhage	1.04 (0.15–7.37)	0.65 (0.12–3.47)
Gastrointestinal bleeding	1.11 (0.56–2.19)	1.08 (0.55–2.13)
Genitourinary bleeding	1.39 (0.31–6.21)	1.05 (0.29–3.75)
6-Month		
Composite of recurrent venous thromboembolism or major bleeding	1.00 (0.767–1.31)	1.05 (0.81–1.37)
Recurrent venous thromboembolism	1.04 (0.76–1.41)	1.12 (0.83–1.53)
Major bleeding	1.02 (0.62–1.69)	1.01 (0.62–1.66)
Intracranial hemorrhage	0.70 (0.12–4.20)	0.65 (0.12–3.47)
Gastrointestinal bleeding	0.80 (0.43–1.47)	0.94 (0.50–1.78)
Genitourinary bleeding	1.39 (0.31–6.21)	0.85 (0.25–2.84)
12-Month		
Composite of recurrent venous thromboembolism or major bleeding	0.98 (0.76–1.25)	1.04 (0.80–1.34)
Recurrent venous thromboembolism	1.00 (0.75–1.34)	1.10 (0.82–1.47)
Major bleeding	0.99 (0.64–1.5)	0.98 (0.61–1.57)
Intracranial hemorrhage	0.94 (0.29–3.10)	0.82 (0.21–3.30)
Gastrointestinal bleeding	0.84 (0.47–1.48)	0.88 (0.47–1.65)
Genitourinary bleeding	1.34 (0.36–5.00)	1.03 (0.33–3.24)

Abbreviations

CI: Confidence intervals; DVT: Deep vein thrombosis; EHR: Electronic health record; HR: Hazard ratio; ICH: Intracranial hemorrhage; IPTW: Inverse probability-of-treatment weighting; GI: Gastrointestinal; GU: Genitourinary; NOACs: Non-vitamin K oral anticoagulants; OAC: Oral anticoagulant; PE: Pulmonary embolism; RCTs: Randomized controlled trials; RECORD: Reporting of studies conducting using observational routinely-collected health data; US: United States; VTE: Venous thromboembolism

Acknowledgements

Data used in this study were obtained from the Optum Inc. under a license to Janssen Scientific Affairs LLC (and provided to Dr. Coleman under a third-party agreement) and are not publicly available.

Authors' contributions

C. I. Coleman, V. Ashton, and M. Palladino conceptualized and designed the study. O. S. Costa, C. I. Coleman and T. J. Bunz analyzed the data. O. S. Costa, C. I. Coleman, S. Thompson, V. Ashton, M. Palladino, T. J. Bunz interpreted the data. The manuscript was written primarily by O. S. Costa and C. I. Coleman; all remaining authors aided and/or contributed to revisions. All authors substantially contributed to this project, read and approved the manuscript and assume responsibility for the contents of the manuscript.

Author details

[1]Department of Pharmacy Practice, University of Connecticut School of Pharmacy, 69 North Eagleville Road, Unit 3092, Storrs, CT 06269, USA. [2]Evidence-Based Practice Center, Hartford Hospital, Hartford, CT, USA. [3]TeamHealth LifePoint Group, Southaven, MS, USA. [4]Real World Value and Evidence, Janssen Scientific Affairs LLC, Titusville, NJ, USA. [5]Medical Affairs, Janssen Pharmaceuticals Inc., Titusville, NJ, USA. [6]Department of Pharmacoepidemiology, New England Health Analytics LLC, Granby, CT, USA.

References

1. White RH, Zhou H, Romano PS. Incidence of idiopathic deep venous thrombosis and secondary thromboembolism among ethnic groups in California. Ann Intern Med. 1998;128:737–40.
2. White RH, Zhou H, Murin S, Harvey D. Effect of ethnicity and gender on the incidence of venous thromboembolism in a diverse population in California in 1996. Thromb Haemost. 2005;93:298–305.
3. Schneider D, Lilienfeld DE, Im W. The epidemiology of pulmonary embolism: racial contrasts in incidence and in-hospital case fatality. J Natl Med Assoc. 2006;98:1967–72.
4. Dowling NF, Austin H, Dilley A, Whitsett C, Evatt BL, Hooper WC. The epidemiology of venous thromboembolism in Caucasians and African-Americans: the GATE study. J Thromb Haemost. 2003;1:80–7.
5. Jackson LR 2nd, Peterson ED, Okeagu E, Thomas K. Review of race/ethnicity in non vitamin K antagonist oral anticoagulants clinical trials. J Thromb Thrombolysis. 2015;39:222–7.
6. Di Nisio M, Ageno W, Rutjes AW, Pap AF, Büller HR. Risk of major bleeding in patients with venous thromboembolism treated with rivaroxaban or with heparin and vitamin K antagonists. Thromb Haemost. 2016;115:424–32.
7. Agnelli G, Buller HR, Cohen A, et al. Oral apixaban for the treatment of acute venous thromboembolism. N Engl J Med. 2013;369:799–808.
8. Buller HR, Decousus H, Grosso MA, et al. Edoxaban versus warfarin for the treatment of symptomatic venous thromboembolism. N Engl J Med. 2014; 369:1406–15.
9. Prins MH, Lensing AW, Bauersachs R, et al. Oral rivaroxaban versus standard therapy for the treatment of symptomatic venous thromboembolism: a pooled analysis of the EINSTEIN-DVT and PE randomized studies. Thromb J. 2013;11:21.
10. Schulman S, Kearson C, Kakkar AK, et al. Dabigatran versus warfarin in the treatment of acute venous thromboembolism. N Engl J Med. 2009;361: 2342–52.
11. Optum. Optum EHR Offering. Optum Inc, 2018. Available at: https://www.optum.com/campaign/ls/data-new-era-of-visibility/download.html (Last accessed on July 28, 2019).
12. White RH, Garcia M, Sadeghi B, et al. Evaluation of the predictive value of ICD-9-CM coded administrative data for venous thromboembolism in the United States. Thromb Res. 2010;126:61–7.
13. Cunningham A, Stein CM, Chung CP, Daugherty JR, Smalley WE, Ray WA. An automated database case definition for serious bleeding related to oral anticoagulant use. Pharmacoepidemiol Drug Saf. 2011;20:560–6.
14. Austin PC. An introduction to propensity score methods for reducing the effects of confounding in observational studies. Multivariate Behav Res. 2011;46:399–424.
15. Benchimol EI, Smeeth L, Guttmann A, Harron K, Moher D, Petersen I, Sørensen HT, von Elm E, Langan SM. RECORD Working Committee. The REporting of studies Conducted using Observational Routinely-collected health Data (RECORD) statement. PLoS Med. 2015;12:e1001885.
16. Ageno W, Mantovani LG, Haas S. Safety and effectiveness of oral rivaroxaban versus standard anticoagulation for the treatment of symptomatic deep-vein thrombosis (XALIA): an international prospective, non-interventional study. Lancet Haematol. 2016;3:e12–21.
17. Gandhi SK, Salmon W, Kong SX, Zhao SZ. Administrative databases and outcomes assessment: an overview of issues and potential utility. J Manag Care Spec Pharm. 1999;5:215–22.
18. Coleman CI, Turpie AG, Bunz TJ, Beyer-Westendorf J. Effectiveness and safety of rivaroxaban versus warfarin in patients with provoked venous thromboembolism. J Thromb Thrombolysis. 2018;46:339–45.
19. Erkens PM, ten Cate H, Büller HR, Prins MH. Benchmark for time in therapeutic range in venous thromboembolism: a systematic review and meta-analysis. PLoS One. 2012;7:e42269. https://doi.org/10.1371/journal.pone.0042269.
20. Limone BL, Hernandez AV, Michalak D, Bookhart BK, Coleman CI. Timing of recurrent venous thromboembolism early after the index event: a meta-analysis of randomized controlled trials. Thromb Res. 2013;132:420–6.
21. Yong C, Xu X, Than C, Ullal A, Schmitt S, Azarbal F, Heidenreich P, Turakhia M. Racial disparities in warfarin time in INR therapeutic range in patients with atrial fibrillation: findings from the TREAT-AF study. Circulation. 2013; 128:A14134.

6

Comparative analysis of enoxaparin versus rivaroxaban in the treatment of cancer associated venous thromboembolism: Experience from a tertiary care cancer centre

Anadil Faqah[1]*[ID], Hassan Sheikh[2], Muhammad Abu Bakar[3], Fatima Tayyaab[1] and Sahrish Khawaja[1]

Abstract

Background: Venous Thromboembolism (VTE) in cancer patients is associated with increased mortality and morbidity. While newer data on use of direct oral anticoagulants (DOACs) in treating cancer associated thrombosis (CAT) is promising; its data is still few and inconsistent across literature. We designed the study to assess if rivaroxaban would be an appealing alternate choice to treat CAT.

Methods: We conducted a retrospective study to evaluate the efficacy and safety profile of rivaroxaban versus enoxaparin in cancer patients after developing a symptomatic deep vein thrombosis (DVT) or pulmonary embolism (PE). Baseline patient characteristics and laboratory values were assessed in each arm. Primary efficacy outcome was measured by radiographically confirmed VTE recurrence at different intervals. Primary safety outcome was measured by presence of major and minor bleeding using the ISTH scale.

Results: Our study recruited 150 cancer patients with radiologically confirmed DVT and PE; 80 patients were evaluated in enoxaparin arm and 70 patients in rivaroxaban arm. Our results showed that there was no statistically significant difference between the incidence of VTE recurrence at 6 months between the enoxaparin and rivaroxaban arm (10% vs 14.2%, $p = 0.42$). Historically significant risk factors for VTE in cancer patients such as high platelet count, high leukocyte count, low hemoglobin level, high risk gastrointestinal, genitourinary and lung cancers were not found to be significantly associated with the risk of VTE recurrence. Primary safety outcome analysis also showed no statistically significant difference in major (11.2% vs 11.4%) and minor (15% vs 10%) bleeding between enoxaparin versus rivaroxaban arm respectively ($p = 0.65$).

Conclusion: We conclude that there was no significant difference seen between the efficacy and safety profile of enoxaparin and rivaroxaban in our cancer patient population.

Keywords: Anticoagulants, Rivaroxaban, Factor Xa inhibitor, Thrombosis, Low-molecular-weight-heparin, Cancer-associated-thrombosis

* Correspondence: anadilfaqah@skm.org.pk
Presented as a poster presentation at International Academy for Clinical Hematology. Paris, France (19-21 Sept,2019)
[1]Department of Internal Medicine, Shaukat Khanam Memorial Cancer Hospital & Research Centre, Lahore, Pakistan
Full list of author information is available at the end of the article

Introduction

Venous Thromboembolism (VTE) which broadly consists of deep vein thrombosis (DVT) and pulmonary embolism (PE) is associated with a poor prognosis in patients with cancer and remains a leading cause of mortality and morbidity [1]. Cancer patients are at 6 to 7 fold increased risk of venous thromboembolism (VTE) compared with age-matched controls corresponding to an annual incidence of about one thrombotic event per 200 active cancer patients [2]. Therefore adequate management of VTE is of utmost importance for clinicians involved in the care of cancer patients.

There has been substantial advances in the management of cancer associated thrombosis (CAT) in the last few decades. Low molecular weight heparin (LMWH) which was once considered the gold standard is no more the only treatment option available [3–5]. Direct oral anticoagulants (DOACs) i.e. rivaroxaban, apixaban, and edoxaban which are taken orally and do not require laboratory monitoring have become an appealing alternate choice as oppose to LMWH which require daily subcutaneous injections. The initial literature on use of DOACs was drawn from meta-analysis evaluating randomized controlled trials (RCTs) with cancer subgroups i.e. RECOVER, AMPLIFY, Hokusai-VTE, EINSTEIN-PE & DVT. They drew conclusion that DOACs were non-inferior to LMWH in preventing recurrent VTE and are associated with similar bleeding rates [6–11]. On the contrary its key criticism stems from the fact that only less than 7% of the study population in these RCTs had cancer.

More recently two randomized control trials (SELECT D & Hokusai VTE- Cancer) have emerged involving the use of DOACs versus LMWH in preventing cancer associated thrombosis [12, 13].These studies showed that DOACs were noninferior to LMWH in preventing recurrent VTE; however this is with increased risk of bleeding. In the randomized SELECT D trial, 203 patients were compared with dalteparin versus rivaroxban. The VTE recurrence rate for dalteparin versus rivaroxban was 11% versus 4% respectively [HR 0.43 (0.19–0.9)]. However major bleeding risk for dalterparin versus rivaroxaban was 4% versus 6% respectively [HR 1.83 (068–4.96)]. In the randomized Hokusai VTE trial, 1050 patients were compared with LMWH for 5 days followed by oral edoxaban versus dalteparin. The VTE recurrence rate for dalteparin versus edoxaban was 11.3% versus 7.9% respectively. However major bleeding risk for dalterparin versus edoxaban was 4% versus 6.9% respectively.

Following these recent trials, American Society of Clinical Oncology (ASCO) and National Comprehensive Cancer Network (NCCN) have revised their recommendations and have added the use of rivaroxaban and edoxaban for cancer associated thrombosis treatment [14, 15]. Although the recommendations for the use of DOACs have recently become popular in guidelines, they are still few and inconsistent across the current literature. In the absence of multiple large randomized controlled trials and dearth of literature in cancer population we designed a retrospective single center study to investigate the efficacy and safety profile of rivaroxaban over enoxaparin in preventing recurrent cancer associated thrombosis.

Patients and methods
Design
This study was a single center retrospective chart review study utilizing data from the Shaukat Khanum Cancer Memorial Hospital and Research Centre (SKMCH) cancer registry between January 1, 2012 to Dec 31,2017 following the approval by the Institutional Review Board. Patients who received anticoagulation therapy with enoxaparin or rivaroxaban from January 1, 2012 to Dec 31,2017 were identified using a report generated from pharmacy charge codes.

Patient population
Patients were included if they were at least 18 years of age, had a diagnosis of cancer and concurrent radiological diagnosis of DVT and/or PE, and were prescribed treatment with either rivaroxaban or enoxaparin during the study period. Patients were excluded if the length of anticoagulation therapy was less than 30 days, if therapy with enoxaparin or rivaroxaban was initiated more than 6 months after DVT or PE diagnosis, or if they did not receive therapeutic doses of the therapy. Patients with DVT of upper extremity were also excluded.

Outcome
The primary efficacy outcome was the incidence of radiologically confirmed new or recurrent DVT or PE in 30 days, 3 months and 6 months using fisher exact test. The secondary endpoint of the study was to compare the safety of enoxaparin vs rivaroxaban in cancer patients for the treatment of DVT or PE.

The primary safety outcome was determined by the incidence and severity of bleeding, based on the International Society of Thrombosis and Hemostasis (ISTH) definition. Major bleeding was defined as clinically overt if it was associated with a drop in hemoglobin of 2 g/dL, required transfusions of 2 units of packed red blood cells, involved critical site bleeding (intracranial, intraspinal, intraocular, retroperitoneal, or pericardial area), or if it contributed to death. Minor bleeding was defined as overt bleeding not meeting the criteria for major bleeding but associated with medical intervention, unscheduled contact with a physician, interruption or discontinuation of anticoagulation treatment, or associated with any discomfort or impairment of activities of daily life.

Study procedure

The following information was extracted from the medical records for each eligible patient: age, gender, demographics, Body-Mass Index, laboratory results at time of VTE diagnosis, cancer type, presence of active cancer, chemotherapy history, metastatic malignancy, comorbidities (coronary artery disease, hypertension, diabetes, renal insufficiency) prior history of VTE, surgery within 30 days or central venous catheter.

Patients who received therapeutic doses of Enoxaparin were matched with a similar population of patients who were treated with therapeutic doses of Rivaroxaban in a 1:1 ratio. Wilcox in rank sum test was performed to compare continuous variables. The Fisher exact test was performed to compare categorical variables. All data were analyzed using SAS 9.4 with a significance level of a = 0.05.

Results

Patient population

Between January 12,012 to December 31, 2017, a total of 245 patients were screened and 150 eligible patients were included in the study; 95 patients excluded from the study consisted of those who had treatment for less than 6 months, administered non-therapeutic doses, absconded and treatment overlap with both rivaroxaban and enoxaparin (Fig. 1). Of the total 150 patients, 80 patients were treated with enoxaparin and 70 patients were treated with rivaroxaban.

The baseline characteristics, comorbidities were reasonably comparable between treatment arms. (Table 1) except for average leukocyte count 9.67+/– 4.96 in the enoxaparin arm compared to 8.16 +/– 3.79 in rivaroxaban arm; also average albumin level was 3.46+/– 0.78 in enoxaparin arm compared to 3.75+/– 0.56 in rivaroxaban arm. Indication for anticoagulation for our population included DVT only 70, PE only 76 and DVT/PE both 4. Interestingly enough baseline comorbidities which included coronary heart disease, diabetes, hypertension and renal insufficiency were similar in both arms and mostly absent. However most of our cohort had active malignancy at the time of VTE diagnosis 90.1%, including 48.05% patients with metastatic disease and 63.4% receiving chemotherapy. GI malignancy was the primary in enoxaparin arm whereas GU malignancy was the primary in rivaroxaban arm. Risk factors for thrombosis such as central line and immobilization/ major surgery were similar in both groups.

Recurrent VTE

Table 2 shows a comparison of the incidence of VTE recurrence and bleeding events. Overall, rivaroxaban had a similar rate of VTE recurrence at 6 months with 10 (14.3%) events versus 8 (10.1%) events with Enoxaparin (*p* = 0.42). The incidence of recurrent DVT at 6 months in patients treated with enoxaparin (3.75%) was lower compared to rivaroxaban (8.75%) at 6 months, however there was no statistical significance (*p* = 0.11). The incidence of recurrent PE in patients treated with enoxaparin (6.25%) was higher compared to rivaroxaban with

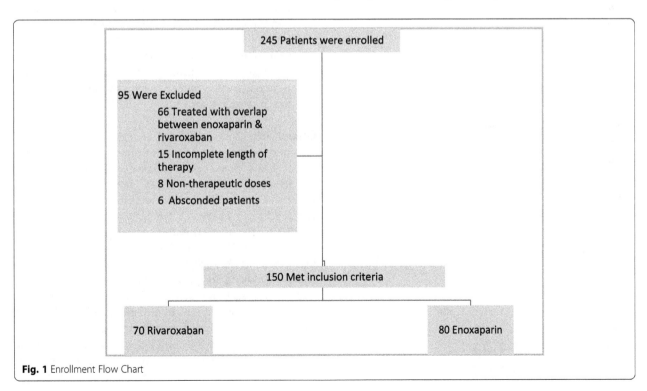

Fig. 1 Enrollment Flow Chart

Table 1 Demographic Table: This will include all the following information in both Enoxaparin and Rivaroxaban Arm

Variables	Enoxaparin 80 (53.3%)	Rivaroxaban 70 (46.7%)	p-value
Baseline Demographics			
Age in years	48.67 ± 14.45	51.84 ± 13.49	0.17
Gender			0.25
Male	37 (46.2%)	39 (55.7%)	
Female	43 (53.8%)	31 (44.3%)	
BMI	23.63 ± 4.64	25.20 ± 5.43	0.05
Baseline Co-Morbids			
Coronary Artery Disease			1.00
No	79 (98.8%)	69 (98.6%)	
Yes	1 (1.2%)	1 (1.4%)	
Hypertension			0.30
No	70 (87.5%)	57 (81.4%)	
Yes	10 (12.5%)	13 (18.6%)	
Diabetes Mellitus			0.49
No	64 (80.0%)	59 (84.3%)	
Yes	16 (20.0%)	11 (15.7%)	
Creatinine Clearance			0.78
Less than 60	8 (10.0%)	8 (11.4%)	
Equal or above 60	72 (90.0%)	62 (88.6%)	
Baseline Malignancy History			
Active Cancer			0.58
No	9 (11.2%)	6 (8.6%)	
Yes	71 (88.8%)	64 (91.4%)	
Cancer Type			0.07
GI	23 (28.8%)	18 (26.1%)	
Breast	9 (11.2%)	17 (24.6%)	
GU	21 (26.2%)	22 (31.9%)	
Lungs	4 (5.0%)	3 (4.3%)	
Misc.	23 (28.8%)	9 (13.0%)	
Disease status			0.89
Non-metastatic	42 (52.5%)	36 (51.4%)	
Metastatic	38 (47.5%)	34 (48.6%)	
Chemotherapy			0.82
No	30 (37.5%)	25 (35.7%)	
Yes	50 (62.5%)	45 (64.3%)	
Baseline Laboratory Findings			
Hemoglobin Level	10.65 ± 2.19	13.12 ± 14.21	0.13
Platelet Level	274.93 ± 140.70	302.60 ± 153.84	0.25
Leukocyte Count	9.67 ± 4.96	8.16 ± 3.79	0.04
Albumin	3.46 ± 0.78	3.75 ± 0.56	0.01
Creatinine	0.81 ± 0.64	0.73 ± 0.27	0.34
Creatinine clearance	128.02 ± 82.76	114.30 ± 45.65	0.22

Table 2 Efficacy and Safety Outcome

Variables	Enoxaparin 80 (53.3%)	Rivaroxaban 70 (46.7%)	p-value
Primary Efficacy Outcomes			
VTE Recurrence			0.42
No	72 (90.0%)	60 (85.7%)	
Yes	8 (10.0%)	10 (14.3%)	
• DVT recurrence			0.11
Proximal	3 (100.0%)	6 (100.0%)	
Distal	0 (0.0%)	0 (0.0%)	
• PE recurrence			0.07
Central	5 (100.0%)	2 (50.0%)	
Sub segmental	0 (0.0%)	2 (50.0%)	
Primary Safety Outcomes			
Safety outcome			0.65
No bleeding	59 (73.8%)	55 (78.6%)	
Minor bleeding	12 (15.0%)	7 (10.0%)	
Major bleeding	9 (11.2%)	8 (11.4%)	

(5.71%) at 6 months, however there was no statistical significance ($p = 0.08$).

Bleeding

Nine patients receiving enoxaparin had major bleeds, compared with eight patients in the rivaroxaban arm. (Table 2). The cumulative major bleed rate at 6 months was comparable with no significant difference between 11.2% for enoxaparin arm and 11.4% for rivaroxaban arm. An additional twelve patients receiving enoxaparin had minor bleeds, compared with seven patients in the rivaroxaban arm. (Table 2). The cumulative minor bleed rate at 6 months was again comparable with no significant difference between 15% for enoxaparin arm and 10% for rivaroxaban arm.

Discussion

One of the population based study from Walker European Journal has shown a steady increase in the absolute rate of venous thrombosis from 10 VTE (per 1000 person-years) to 20 VTE (per 1000 person-years) from 1997 to 2007 in cancer patients; where as it has remained steady i.e. 4 VTE (per 1000 person-years) in non-cancer group [1]. This rise in cancer associated thrombosis poses a serious problem that diminishes the patient's life span and quality of life. Hence identifying adequate management of cancer associated thrombosis is imperative especially when use of anticoagulation is complicated by a delicate balance between risk of recurrent VTE and major bleeding.

Our study showed the cumulative VTE recurrence risk in enoxaparin and rivaroxaban at 6 months is consistent with the current literature. However there was a non-significant increase in VTE recurrence in rivaroxaban as compared to enoxaparin. It was noted that while recurrent VTE estimate in enoxaparin arm was comparable with previous RCTs (HOKUSAI-VTE, HOKUSAI-VTE CANCER and SELECT D); there was higher recurrent VTE estimate in rivaroxaban arm when compared to current data. On analyzing our data we found out that 50.6% of our population indication for anticoagulation was PE while it was only 29.7% in Chaudhury et al. and 39% in Young et al.; explaining that our patient population was more at risk at baseline [16]. We also noted that our study had larger percentage of gastric (7.3% Vs 3%) and cervical cancer (6.6% Vs 3%); which studies have shown to also cause a higher rate of VTE recurrence [17]. We also separately analyzed the demographic details of each one of the 6 recurrent DVT patients in rivaroxaban arm and found that 4 of 6 had gastric or pancreatic cancer, low albumin, BMI less than 22 and shared co-morbid (Diabetes, Hypertension and Coronary Artery Disease). All of which explains low nutritional reserve resulting in poor gut absorption for oral anticoagulant and inconversely higher adverse outcomes. We also analyzed historically significant risk factors for VTE in cancer patients such as high platelet count, high leukocyte count, low hemoglobin level, high risk gastrointestinal, genitourinary and lung cancers. They were not found to be independently significantly associated with the risk of VTE recurrence [18].

Another important objective of our study was to evaluate the safety outcome i.e. to access rates of major bleeding and clinically relevant non-major bleeding (CRNMB). Our study showed comparable major bleeding and CRNMB rates in rivaroxaban and enoxaparin arm as shown in RECOVER/RECOVER-2. It is worth mentioning that the trends in bleeding rate are not consistent across trials [6, 19]. The bleeding rates in our study were strikingly higher (11% Vs 4–7%) when compared with previously observed rates and were mainly related to GI bleed. Although bleeding rates as high as 16% in enoxaparin plus warfarin arm in CANT HANOX 2002 study and 9% in enoxaparin in ONCENOX 2006 study were seen in prior studies; however, no study has shown bleeding rates higher than 7% (HOKUSAI-VTE Cancer) with DOACs.

Rivaroxaban is a factor Xa inhibitor which directly and reversibly binds to factor Xa and competitively inhibits factor Xa. It is 10,000 fold more selective for factor Xa and it does not require co-factors to exert its anticoagulant effect [20, 21]. It is plausible that the enhanced antithrombotic effects of rivaroxaban as opposed to LMWH which acts on factor X indirectly, is associated with a greater perturbation of coagulation and predisposing to more bleeding. We take this as a learning opportunity to consider modifying DOAC doses to best suit your patient's needs depending on their demographic and disease specific details. When we individually analyzed 8 episodes of major bleeding with rivaroxaban in our study population we found out they were mainly in older population i.e. aged 65 years or higher with poor nutritional reserve i.e. low albumin, BMI less than 22 and had an advanced metastatic breast or prostate cancer.

Our study despite being a retrospective study and having limited number of participants provides solutions for real world situations. It is felt that despite availability of results from SELECT D & Hokusai VTE-Cancer trial our study still manages to highlight that "one size fits all" cannot be applied to all patients and physicians will need to use their best clinical judgement. We believe NOACs have a promising future in cancer associated VTE due to its ease in utilization and comparable results with LMWH in preventing recurrent VTE. However we are still concerned about its safety profile. Especially as our study showed higher rates of major bleeding with Rivaroxaban when compared to SELECT D & Hokusai VTE-Cancer trial. This is particularly true for complex cancer patients due to rivaroxaban's unpredictable higher risk of GI bleeding, inability to measure anticoagulant activity by using standard essays, potential interaction with medicines and altered metabolism in renal dysfunction, hepatic metastasis and lack of antidote. In addition patients with gastric and pancreatic cancer who have undergone surgical resection will have altered gut absorption hence making rivaroxaban pharmacodynamics even more unpredictable.

Conclusion

We conclude that there was no significant difference seen between the efficacy and safety profile of enoxaparin and rivaroxaban in our cancer patient population. While rivaroxaban has recently become popular in cancer associated VTE due to its ease in utilization and comparable results with LMWH in preventing recurrent VTE. Attention also needs to be paid on patient's disease specific details and demographics before favoring DOACs over LMWH.

Abbreviations
VTE: Venous Thromboembolism; CAT: Cancer Associated Venous Thrombosis; ISTH: International Society of Thrombosis and Hemostasis; LMWH: Low Molecular Weight Heparin; NCCN: National Comprehensive Cancer Network; ASCO: American Society of Clinical Oncology; DOACs: Direct oral anticoagulants; CRNMB: Clinically relevant non-major bleeding; FDA: Food and Drug Association; PE: Pulmonary Embolism; DVT: Deep Vein Thrombosis

Authors' contributions
Dr. Anadil Faqah and Dr. Hassan Sheikh designed, conducted and wrote the paper; Mr. Abu Bakr analyzed the results and made the figures; Dr. Fatima Tayyaab and Dr. Sahrish Khawaja performed data extraction and assisted in writing paper. The author(s) read and approved the final manuscript.

Author details
[1]Department of Internal Medicine, Shaukat Khanam Memorial Cancer Hospital & Research Centre, Lahore, Pakistan. [2]Department of Hematology and Oncology, Shaukat Khanam Memorial Cancer Hospital & Research Centre, Lahore, Pakistan. [3]Department of Cancer Registry, Shaukat Khanam Memorial Cancer Hospital & Research Centre, Lahore, Pakistan.

References

1. Timp JF, Braekkan SK, Versteeg HH, et al. Epidemiology of cancer-associated venous thrombosis. Blood. 2013;122(10):1712–23.

2. Martinez BK, Sheth J, Patel N, et al. Systematic review and meta-analysis of real-world studies evaluating rivaroxaban for Cancer-associated venous thrombosis. Pharmacotherapy. 2018;38(6):610–8.

3. Lee AYY, Levine MN, Baker RI, et al. Low-molecular-weight heparin versus a coumarin for the prevention of recurrent venous thromboembolism in patients with cancer. N Engl J Med. 2003;349(2):146–53.

4. Kuderer NM, Lyman GH. Guidelines for treatment and prevention of venous thromboembolism among patients with cancer. Thromb Res. 2014; 133(Suppl 2(0 2)):S122–7.

5. Streiff MB. An overview of the NCCN and ASCO guidelines on cancer-associated venous thromboembolism. Cancer Investig. 2009;27(Suppl 1):41–52.

6. Schulman S, Kearon C, Kakkar AK, et al. Dabigatran versus warfarin in the treatment of acute venous thromboembolism. N Engl J Med. 2009;361(24): 2342–52.

7. Agnelli G, Buller HR, Cohen A, et al. Oral apixaban for the treatment of acute venous thromboembolism. N Engl J Med. 2013;369(9):799–808.

8. Büller HR, Décousus H, Grosso MA, et al. Edoxaban versus warfarin for the treatment of symptomatic venous thromboembolism. N Engl J Med. 2013; 369(15):1406–15.

9. Landman GW, Gans ROB. Oral rivaroxaban for symptomatic venous thromboembolism. N Engl J Med. 2011;364(12):1178.

10. Büller HR, Prins MH, Lensing AWA, et al. Oral rivaroxaban for the treatment of symptomatic pulmonary embolism. N Engl J Med. 2012;366(14):1287–97.

11. Posch F, Königsbrügge O, Zielinski C, et al. Treatment of venous thromboembolism in patients with cancer: a network meta-analysis comparing efficacy and safety of anticoagulants. Thromb Res. 2015;136(3): 582–9.

12. van Es N, Di Nisio M, Bleker SM, et al. Edoxaban for treatment of venous thromboembolism in patients with cancer: rationale and design of the hokusai VTE-cancer study. Thromb Haemost. 2015;114(6):1268–76.

13. Young AM, Marshall A, Thirlwall J, et al. Comparison of an oral factor xa inhibitor with low molecular weight heparin in patients with cancer with venous thromboembolism: results of a randomized trial (SELECT-D). J Clin Oncol. 2018;36(20):2017–23.

14. Streiff MB, Holmstrom B, Angelini D, et al. NCCN Guidelines® insights cancer-associated venous thromboembolic disease, version 2.2018 featured updates to the NCCN guidelines. J Natl Compr Cancer Netw. 2018;16(11): 1289–303.

15. Key NS, Khorana AA, Kuderer NM, et al. Venous thromboembolism prophylaxis and treatment in patients with Cancer: ASCO clinical practice guideline update. J Clin Oncol. 2019;38(5):496–520.

16. Chaudhury A, Balakrishnan A, Thai C, et al: The efficacy and safety of rivaroxaban and Dalteparin in the treatment of Cancer associated venous thrombosis. Indian J Hematol Blood Transfus , 2018.

17. Horsted F, West J, Grainge MJ. Risk of venous thromboembolism in patients with cancer: a systematic review and meta-analysis. PLoS Med. 2012;9(7): e1001275.

18. Lee EC, Cameron SJ: Cancer and thrombotic risk: the platelet paradigm. Front Cardiovasc Med , 2017.

19. Schulman S, Kakkar AK, Goldhaber SZ, et al. Treatment of acute venous thromboembolism with dabigatran or warfarin and pooled analysis. Circulation. 2014;129(7):764–72.

20. DeHaas KA: The direct Oral anticoagulants Apixaban, rivaroxaban, and edoxaban. Am Soc Clin Lab Sci , 2017.

21. Eriksson BI, Quinlan DJ, Eikelboom JW. Novel Oral Factor Xa and Thrombin Inhibitors in the Management of Thromboembolism. Annu Rev Med. 2011; 62:41–57.

7

Prevalence of venous obstructions in (recurrent) venous thromboembolism

Pascale Notten[1,2†] (iD), Rob H. W. Strijkers[3†], Irwin Toonder[3], Hugo ten Cate[2,3,4] and Arina J. ten Cate-Hoek[2,3,4,5*]

Abstract

Background: The role of venous obstructions as a risk factor for recurrent venous thromboembolism has never been evaluated. This study aimed to determine whether there is a difference in prevalence of venous obstructions between patients with and without recurrent venous thromboembolism. Furthermore, its influence on the development of post-thrombotic syndrome and patient-reported quality of life was assessed.

Methods: This matched nested case-control study included 32 patients with recurrent venous thromboembolism (26 recurrent deep-vein thrombosis and 6 pulmonary embolism) from an existing prospective cohort of deep-vein thrombosis patients and compared them to 24 age and sex matched deep-vein thrombosis patients without recurrent venous thromboembolism. All participants received standard post-thrombotic management and underwent an additional extensive duplex ultrasonography. Post-thrombotic syndrome was assessed by the Villalta-scale and quality of life was measured using the SF36v2 and VEINES-QOL/Sym-questionnaires.

Results: Venous obstruction was found in 6 patients (18.8%) with recurrent venous thromboembolism compared to 5 patients (20.8%) without recurrent venous thromboembolism (Odds ratio 0.88, 95%CI 0.23–3.30, $p = 1.000$). After a median follow-up of 60.0 months (IQR 41.3–103.5) the mean Villalta-score was 5.55 ± 3.02 versus 5.26 ± 2.63 ($p = 0.909$) and post-thrombotic syndrome developed in 20 (62.5%) versus 14 (58.3%) patients, respectively (Odds ratio 1.19, 95%CI 0.40–3.51, $p = 0.752$). If venous obstruction was present, it was mainly located in the common iliac vein ($n = 7$, 63.6%). In patients with an objectified venous obstruction the mean Villalta-score was 5.11 ± 2.80 versus 5.49 ± 2.87 in patients without venous obstruction ($p = 0.639$). Post-thrombotic syndrome developed in 6 (54.5%) versus 28 (62.2%) patients, respectively (Odds ratio 1.37, 95%CI 0.36–5.20, $p = 0.736$). No significant differences were seen regarding patient-reported quality of life between either groups.

(Continued on next page)

* Correspondence: arina.tencate@maastrichtuniversity.nl
†Pascale Notten and Rob H. W. Strijkers contributed equally to this work.
[2]CARIM, Cardiovascular Research Institute Maastricht, School for Cardiovascular Diseases, Maastricht University Medical Centre, P.O. Box 616, Maastricht 6200 MD, the Netherlands
[3]Laboratory for Clinical Thrombosis and Hemostasis, Maastricht University, P.O. Box 616, Maastricht 6200 MD, The Netherlands
Full list of author information is available at the end of the article

(Continued from previous page)

Conclusions: In this exploratory case-control study patients with recurrent venous thromboembolism did not have a higher prevalence of venous obstruction compared to patients without recurrent venous thromboembolism. The presence of recurrent venous thromboembolism or venous obstruction had no impact on the development of post-thrombotic syndrome or the patient-reported quality of life.

Keywords: Venous thromboembolism, Deep vein thrombosis, Recurrence, Postthrombotic syndrome, Quality of life

Background

Following the acute phase, a substantial number of deep-vein thrombosis (DVT) patients face long-term post-thrombotic consequences. Despite optimal conservative treatment comprising of anticoagulation therapy, early mobilisation, and the use of therapeutic compression stockings, a recurrent venous thromboembolism (reVTE) will occur in about one-third of the patients within 10 years following a first DVT [1, 2] with even higher risks in case of an unprovoked event [3, 4].

Subsequently, there is an increased risk of post-thrombotic syndrome (PTS) [5]. PTS is a chronic condition characterised by a painful, swollen limb with paraesthesia, skin changes, venous claudication, and ultimately venous ulceration. It develops in 20–50% of all DVT patients [6–8] and is associated with a negative impact on the quality of life (QoL) [9] and increased health care costs [10].

According to Virchow's triad a disturbed or turbulent blood flow is one of the factors increasing the risk of thrombus formation. Obstruction of the venous tract, which can either be due to an anatomical anomaly, or an intraluminal or extraluminal obstruction [11], induces impairment of the venous outflow [12]. This may lead to an increased risk of thrombosis due to stasis. However, it remains unknown if the presence of pre-existent venous obstruction (VO, meaning the presence of central venous obstructions and/or additional anatomic anomalies) is increased in patients with reVTE compared to patients without recurrence.

Since visualisation of the venous tract in the lower abdomen and pelvis with assessment of the inferior caval vein (ICV), common iliac vein (CIV), external iliac vein (EIV), and common femoral vein (CFV) is not incorporated into the standard diagnostic work-up for DVT, detection of VO through additional imaging is usually limited to patients presenting with more severe symptomatology in the acute phase and clinically suspect of having an iliofemoral DVT. Consequently, little is known regarding the presence of VO in relation to reVTE.

The risk of reVTE in case of venous outflow obstructions may be lowered by using (long-term) anticoagulant therapy. Additionally, new treatment modalities such as venous stenting make it possible to overcome (asymptomatic) central obstructions and restore venous flow

[13]. Therefore, if the presence of VO increases the risk for recurrent thrombosis, the preferred treatment strategy in these patients might switch from conservative into a more invasive treatment also influencing the duration of anticoagulant therapy.

This exploratory case-control study had the aim to assess the prevalence of VO in patients with reVTE (i.e. recurrent DVT or pulmonary embolism (PE)) compared to patients without reVTE. In addition, the association of reVTE and VO with PTS and the experienced QoL was analysed. The underlying hypothesis was that the presence of VO increases the risk of both reVTE and PTS and is associated with a reduced QoL as well.

Methods

Study design

This matched nested case-control study was based on a selection of patients from an existing prospective cohort of patients with a venous thromboembolism (VTE) who received treatment according to international guidelines at the department of Internal Medicine in the Maastricht University Medical Centre, the Netherlands [14]. All patients with a first-time DVT of the femoropopliteal tract or more cranial vein segments were eligible for participation. Because the assessment for the diagnosis in the acute phase was not based on an extended duplex ultrasonography (DUS), the more cranial vein segments were not routinely identified/specified in the cohort database. Patients were excluded if they were younger than 18 years of age, pregnant, known to have an active malignancy, or if the patient refused unexpected medical findings to be communicated to the patient as well as to their general practitioner. Patients who had experienced a reVTE during follow-up were invited to participate in the current study by mail. When willing, they were requested to return a signed informed consent. Subsequently, an equal number of patients without reVTE (controls) who were matched by age and sex, were selected and approached. Informed consent had to be obtained before participation.

This study has been approved by the Medical Ethical Committee of the Maastricht University Medical Centre. All authors had full access to all the data in this study.

Clinical assessment

All participants were invited for a single study visit at the outpatient clinic during which study assessments were performed. All study visits and assessments were performed by the same physician (RS) and registered vascular technologist (IT).

Data collection

A standardised case record form was used to gather all study data. This form included demographics, patient characteristics, disease-specific details (dates of primary and recurrent VTEs, provoked or unprovoked cause, risk factors), current post-thrombotic treatment (use of anti-coagulant therapy, type of anticoagulant therapy, duration of treatment, adherence to compression therapy), clinical scores (Villalta-scale [15]) as well as results of an extended duplex ultrasonography assessment (presence of trabeculations or compression per vein segment, reflux, anatomic anomalies, and collaterals) of the affected leg.

Patient characteristics

The cohort database ascertained by medical records were used to obtain patient characteristics such as demographics, medical history concerning VTE, and details on the reVTE. Risk factors considered to be associated with reVTE were recent surgery, trauma or immobilization, long-term travelling, inflammation, the use of oral contraceptives, pregnancy and puerperium, obesity, a family history of VTE, and thrombophilia (factor V Leiden, antithrombin deficiency, prothrombin mutation, protein C deficiency, protein S deficiency, persistently elevated factor VIII, and/or antiphospholipid antibodies). The current use of anticoagulant medication and compression therapy as well as current risk enhancing factors for reVTE were assessed during the study visit.

Duplex

A standardised extended DUS was performed by one dedicated registered venous technologist (IT) assessing the inferior caval vein (ICV), common iliac vein (CIV), external iliac vein (EIV), common femoral vein (CFV), femoral vein (FV), deep femoral vein (DFV), and popliteal vein (PV) of the affected leg(s) in supine position. Venous outflow obstruction through the presence of anatomical anomalies, intraluminal post-thrombotic trabeculations and/or extraluminal compression was recorded for each vein segment separately. Reflux of the CFV and PV was assessed in upright position and based on a prolonged retrograde flow [16]. All DUS assessments were performed using an Esaote Spa© 2019 type MyLabAlpha with a broadband 1–8 MHz curved array probe (AC2541).

Post-thrombotic morbidity and quality of life

The Villalta-scale [15] was recorded to assess post-thrombotic morbidity at the time of the study visit. PTS was diagnosed according to the definition by the International Society on Thrombosis and Haemostasis (ISTH) which requires a single Villalta-score of 5 or higher or the presence of a venous ulcer obtained at 6 months or more after the initial thrombotic event [17]. PTS severity was categorised into none (Villalta score 0–4), mild (5–9), moderate (10–14), or severe (≥15 or the presence of a venous ulcer). Patient reported quality of life was assessed using the generic SF36v2 [18] and disease-specific VEINES QOL/Sym [19–21] questionnaires.

Study outcomes

The primary study outcome was the prevalence of VO in patients with reVTE compared to patients who had not developed reVTE. Secondary study outcomes regarded duplex findings, the development of PTS, and patient-reported QoL.

A reVTE comprised a recurrent DVT (reDVT) in the legs and/or PE. ReDVT was defined as an objectified DVT of the limb involving a new venous segment or a previously involved venous segment for which earlier symptomatic and imaging improvement had been obtained in a patient with at least one prior episode of DVT [22]. Results of imaging assessments were to be compared with previous assessments and reDVT was diagnosed in case of a) a new non-compressible, previously unaffected, or normalized vein segment (popliteal, femoral, iliac, or caval), b) extension of the thrombus margin, or c) an increased thrombus size [23–25]. PE was defined as the presence of complete or partial occlusion of the lung arteries in CT-pulmonary angiogram [22]. VO was defined as presence of either extraluminal compression of the CFV and/or more cranial vein segments (e.g. due to May Thurner Syndrome, adjacent anatomical structures, or a tumour), or any anatomical anomalies (e.g. agenesis, hypoplasia, aneurysms, anatomical variances and duplicates). In this study, post-thrombotic sequelae were registered separately and were defined as the presence of intraluminal trabeculations and/or synechiae.

Statistical analysis

Analyses were performed for the primary and secondary study outcomes by comparing the group of patients with reVTE versus those without reVTE. The study was matched on age and sex; stratified analyses on these matching factors was performed. In addition, subgroup analyses were performed for the baseline characteristics as well as secondary outcomes using the comparisons: provoked versus unprovoked VTE and VO versus no VO. Descriptive statistics were performed on patient characteristics and study outcomes using Student t-tests or Mann-Whitney U-tests for continuous variables and the Chi-squared or Fisher Exact test for categorical variables. Continuous data was presented as mean ± standard deviation, categorical data was presented with absolute number and percentages or Odds ratio (OR) and their associated 95% confidence interval (95%CI). The Jonckheere-Terpstra test was performed on the Villalta scores (total score, subjective score, and objective score) for trends. A significance level of 0.05 (two-sided) or less was considered statistically significant. All analyses were performed using SPSS, version 24.

Results
Patient characteristics
Forty patients with reVTE that were alive and whose contact data were available were identified from the cohort database of DVT patients treated at the outpatient clinic of the Maastricht University Medical Centre [14]. Twenty-nine patients responded to our invitation to participate in this exploratory case-control study and signed the informed consent form.

These 29 patients were then age and sex matched to 29 controls who had not experienced reVTE according to the data available in the database. Therefore, in total 58 patients signed informed consent and were included in the study. Information obtained during data ascertainment of the patients' medical records and at the study visit showed that in two out of the 29 patients the recurrent event concerned an upper extremity thrombosis. Furthermore, five of the 29 matched controls for whom no reVTE was recorded in the database actually had experienced a reVTE. Hence the final study sample includes 56 patients of which 32 patients with reVTE (26 reDVT and 6 PE) and 24 patients who had not experienced a recurrent event (Table 1). Patients had a median age of 67.0 (Inter Quartile Range 57.0–71.0) years and were predominantly male (82.1%). An unprovoked cause of the first DVT was significantly more common in patients with reVTE: 23 out of 32 patients (71.9%) versus ten out of 24 patients (41.7%), ($P = 0.03$). In seven patients (six (18.8%) versus one (4.2%); $p = 0.219$) thrombophilia was known; the prevalence of elevated factor VIII (defined as > 213%

Table 1 Baseline characteristics

	Recurrent VTE N = 32	No recurrent VTE N = 24	P-value
Age, years	68.0 (61.3–72.0)	65.0 (45.3–70.8)	0.223
Sex			0.298
- Male	28 (87.5)	18 (75.0)	0.298
- Female	4 (12.5)	6 (25.0)	0.298
Unprovoked DVT	23 (71.9)	10 (41.7)	0.030
Affected side initial event			0.697
- Left	13 (40.6)	11 (45.8)	0.697
- Right	19 (59.4)	13 (54.2)	0.697
Affected side recurrent event			
- Ipsilateral (± pulmonary embolism)	17 (53.1)	n/a	–
- Contralateral (± pulmonary embolism)	9 (28.1)	n/a	–
- Pulmonary embolism	6 (18.8)	n/a	–
History of pulmonary embolism	8 (25.0)[a]	4 (16.7)[b]	0.525
Family history of DVT	10 (31.3)	3 (12.5)	0.122
Antithrombotic therapy	32 (100.0)	17 (70.8)	0.001
Antithrombotic therapy, type			0.071
- VKA	26 (81.3%)	16 (66.7)	0.212
- DOAC[c]	6 (18.8%)	0 (0.0)	0.035
Elastic compression stockings, use	19 (59.4)	3 (12.5)	< 0.001

Data are n (%) or median (IQR)

DOAC Direct oral anticoagulant, DVT Deep venous thrombosis, LMWH Low Molecular Weight Heparin, n/a Not applicable, VKA Vitamin K Antagonist, VTE Venous Thrombo-Embolism

[a] All pulmonary embolisms were recurrent VTE which developed after the primary thrombo-embolic event. In 6 patients it presented as a solitary pulmonary embolism and in 2 patients it presented concurrent with a recurrent deep-vein thrombosis

[b] All pulmonary embolism were concurrent with the primary thrombo-embolic event

[c] The DOACs used were Rivaroxaban (n = 4), Apixaban (n = 1), and Dabigatran (n = 1)

[14]) was significantly higher in patients with reVTE (six (18.8%) versus none (0.0%); $p = 0.035$).

The current use of anticoagulant therapy and compression therapy was significantly higher in the reVTE-group: 100% (32 out of 32) versus 70.8% (17 out of 24), $p = 0.001$, and 59.4% (19 out of 32) versus 12.5% (three out of 24), $p < 0.001$, respectively. Most commonly used were the VKA: 26 out of 32 (81.3%) in patients with reVTE versus 16 (66.7%) out of 24 controls. A significant difference in the use of direct oral anticoagulants was seen, being restricted to patients with reVTE: six out of 32 (18.8%) versus none of the controls (0.0%), $p = 0.035$. Indication for indefinite treatment duration was more frequent in patients with reVTE: 30 out of 32 (93.8%) versus six out of 24 (25.0%), $p < 0.001$.

Study outcomes

There was no significant difference in the prevalence of VO between groups: six (18.8%) in patients who had experienced a recurrent event versus five (20.8%) in patients who did not; OR 0.88 (95%CI 0.23–3.30), $p = 1.000$ (Table 2). The presence of abnormalities on duplex findings such as extraluminal compression (four (12.5%) versus three (12.5%), OR 1.00 (95%CI 0.20–4.96), $p = 1.000$), intraluminal post-thrombotic sequelae (28 (87.5%) versus 18 (75.0%), OR 2.33 (95%CI 0.58–9.43), $p = 0.298$), or venous insufficiency (19 (59.4%) versus 10 (41.7%), OR 2.05 (95%CI 0.70–6.00), $p = 0.189$) did not differ either (Table 3).

Compression was seen solely in the caval and iliac tract: the ICVir (one (3.1%) versus two (8.3%) respectively, $p = 1.000$), the CIV (four (12.5%) versus three (12.5%), $p = 1.000$), and EIV (one (3.1%) versus none

(0.0%), $p = 0.126$). Trabeculations were most commonly seen in the popliteal (27 (79.4%) versus 16 (66.7%), $p = 0.200$) and femoral vein (18 (56.3%) versus 9 (37.5%), $p = 0.165$). In only two (6.3%) versus five (20.8%) patients all vein segments were free of anomalies ($p = 0.642$). There was no difference for any of the results whether the right or left leg was affected.

The mean Villalta score was 5.55 ± 3.02 in patients with reVTE compared to 5.26 ± 2.63 in patients without reVTE ($p = 0.909$), composed of objective (4.03 ± 3.07 versus 3.08 ± 1.74, $p = 0.519$) and subjective (1.63 ± 1.43 versus 2.22 ± 2.30, $p = 0.512$) components. No significant trends were seen in the mean total ($p = 0.909$), objective ($p = 0.519$), or subjective ($p = 0.512$) Villalta-score. PTS and PTS severity was similar between groups. There were no differences in the reported QoL according to the SF36v2, overall score ($p = 0.493$) as well as the scores per individual category (all $P > 0.156$), and the VEINES-QOL/Sym ($p = 0.518$ for the total score and $p = 0.966$ for the intrinsic score) (Table 4).

Furthermore, analyses regarding outcomes of the DUS assessment and the clinical assessments for the Villalta-score, PTS, PTS severity, and QoL were also performed for two subgroups: patients with or without an unprovoked cause for the primary DVT and patients with and without VO.

These analyses showed that patients with an unprovoked cause of the primary DVT ($n = 33$, 58.9%) did not differ from patients with a provoked primary event nor were there differences in outcomes.

VO was found in 11 (19.6%) of the 56 patients of which seven (12.5%) included extraluminal caval or iliac compression. Patients with VO were significantly younger than patients without VO (61.0 (IQR 32.0–69.0) versus 68.0 (IQR 59.5–72.0), $p = 0.046$). Apart from age there were no other

Table 2 Details in patients with central venous obstructions and anatomic anomalies

Recurrent VTE N = 32		No recurrent VTE N = 24		Total N = 56
6 (18.8)		5 (20.8)		11 (19.6)
Anatomic anomalies				
#1	Duplication of the VP, fibrosis of the VF	#1	Aneurysm VP	
#2	Duplication of the VF	#2	Duplication and fibrosis of the VF	
Central venous obstructions				
#3	Extraluminal compression: CIV and EIV	#3	Extraluminal compression: ICVir and CIV	
#4	Extraluminal compression: CIV[a]	#4	Extraluminal compression: ICVir and CIV	
#5	Extraluminal compression: ICVir and CIV[b]	#5	Extraluminal compression: CIV[c]	
#6	Extraluminal compression: CIV[c]			

Data are n (%)

ICVir Inferior caval vein, infra renal, *CIV* Common iliac vein, *EIV* External iliac vein, *FV* Femoral vein, *PV* Popliteal vein, *VTE* Venous thrombo-embolism

None of the variables mentioned in this table showed statistical significant difference between groups

Venous obstruction is defined as either extraluminal compression (e.g. due to May-Thurner Syndrome, adjacent anatomical structures, pelvic tumour) or the presence of anatomical anomalies (e.g. agenesis, hypoplasia, aneurysms, anatomical variances, and duplications) that might negatively influence the central venous flow

[a] Extraluminal compression caused by spondylosis

[b] Extraluminal compression caused by the left iliac artery

[c] Extraluminal compression caused by May Thurner Syndrome (compression by the right iliac artery)

Table 3 Results duplex assessment[a]

	Recurrent VTE N = 32	No recurrent VTE N = 24	Total N = 56	Odds ratio (95%CI)
Extraluminal compression	4 (12.5)	3 (12.5)	7 (12.5)	1.00 (0.20–4.96)
Extraluminal compression, per vein segment				
ICVir	1 (3.1)	2 (8.3)	3 (5.6)	0.36 (0.03–1.16)
CIV	4 (12.5)	3 (12.5)	7 (12.5)	1.00 (0.20–4.96)
EIV	1 (3.1)	0 (0.0)	1 (1.8)	2.33 (0.09–59.8)
Post-thrombotic sequalae[b]	28 (87.5)	18 (75.0)	46 (82.1)	2.33 (0.58–9.43)
Trabeculations, per vein segment				
ICVsr	1 (3.1)	0 (0.0)	1 (1.8)	2.33 (0.09–59.8)
ICVir	1 (3.1)	1 (4.2)	2 (3.6)	0.74 (0.04–12.5)
CIV	2 (6.3)	3 (12.5)	5 (8.9)	0.47 (0.07–3.04)
EIV	3 (9.4)	3 (12.5)	6 (10.7)	0.72 (0.13–3.95)
CFV	3 (9.4)	4 (16.7)	7 (12.5)	0.52 (0.10–2.57)
FV	18 (56.3)	9 (37.5)	27 (48.2)	2.14 (0.73–6.32)
DFV	1 (3.1)	1 (4.2)	2 (3.6)	0.74 (0.04–12.5)
PV	27 (79.4)	16 (66.7)	43 (76.8)	2.70 (0.75–9.68)
Venous insufficiency[c]	19 (59.4)	10 (41.7)	29 (51.8)	2.05 (0.70–6.00)
Venous insufficiency, per vein segment				
CFV	3 (9.4)	0 (0.0)	3 (5.6)	5.81 (0.29–118.1)
PV	19 (59.4)	10 (41.7)	29 (51.8)	2.05 (0.70–6.00)

Data are n (%)

None of the variables mentioned in this table showed statistical significant difference between groups

ICVsr Inferior caval vein, supra renal, *ICVir* Inferior caval vein, infra renal, *CIV* Common iliac vein, *EIV* External iliac vein, *CFV* Common femoral vein, *FV* Femoral vein, *DFV* Deep femoral vein, *PV* Popliteal vein, *VTE* Venous thrombo-embolism

[a] During the standardized duplex ultrasound study assessment the presence of extraluminal compression and/or trabeculations was assessed per individual vein segment of the affected leg(s) being the ICVsr, ICVir, CIV, EIV, CFV, FV, DFV, and PV. Venous insufficiency was assessed in the CFV and PV

[b]Post-thrombotic sequelae are defined as the presence of intraluminal trabeculations or synechiae

[c]Venous insufficiency was defined as a retrograde flow longer than 1 s [16]

differences between these groups. Based on the definition used, compression was seen only in the patients with VO: seven (63.6%) versus none (0.0%), OR 0.01 (95%CI 0.00–0.14), $p < 0.001$. No differences were seen regarding intra-luminal post-thrombotic trabeculations (nine (81.8%) versus 37 (82.2%), OR 1.03 (95%CI 0.19–5.70), $p = 1.000$) or venous insufficiency (six (54.5%) versus 23 (51.1%), OR 0.87 (95%CI 0.23–3.27), $p = 1.000$). The Villalta scores did not differ between groups (Total Villalta: 5.11 ± 2.80 versus 5.49 ± 2.87, $p = 0.639$; objective Villalta: 4.00 ± 3.02 versus 3.53 ± 2.53, $p = 0.748$; and subjective Villalta score: 1.50 ± 1.51 versus 1.96 ± 1.92, $p = 0.546$. Results regarding PTS, PTS severity, and QoL were also comparable between patients with and without VO.

Discussion

In this exploratory case-control study we did not find a difference in prevalence of VO between patients that did and patients that did not develop a recurrent thrombotic event. Moreover, no impact of the absence of either reVTE or VO was seen regarding the development of PTS or on the experienced QoL.

Also, the sub analysis comparing patients with VO to patients without VO showed no differences in post-thrombotic trabeculations or venous insufficiency on DUS assessment. This may indicate that there is no association between the presence of VO and long-term post-thrombotic intraluminal sequelae. No differences were seen for the prevalence of PTS, the severity of PTS, and QoL. However, we did find that patients with VO were younger than patients without VO, suggesting that these patients might be at risk for VTE development at an earlier age. This would be in line with the expected initial increased risk of thrombus formation under conditions of disturbed or turbulent blood flow.

However, our results do not indicate that VO increases the risk of developing reVTE. Furthermore, the presence of VO does not result in a worse clinical outcome regarding PTS and QoL in patients with recurrence. Therefore, one needs to critically consider whether DVT patients with objectified VO or patients with asymptomatic VO will benefit from prolonged anticoagulant therapy or more invasive treatments such as venous stenting.

Table 4 Long-term treatment outcomes

	Recurrent VTE $N = 32$	No recurrent VTE $N = 24$	Total $N = 56$	Odds ratio (95% CI)
Villalta score [15]	5.55 ± 3.02	5.26 ± 2.63	5.43 ± 2.84	–
- Subjective score	1.63 ± 1.43	2.22 ± 2.30	1.87 ± 1.85	–
- Objective score	4.03 ± 3.07	3.08 ± 1.74	3.62 ± 2.60	–
Post-Thrombotic syndrome[a] [15, 17]	20 (62.5)	14 (58.3)	34 (60.7)	1.19 (0.40–3.51)
- None (0–4)	11 (34.4)	9 (37.5)	20 (35.7)	0.87 (0.29–2.63)
- Mild (5–9)	17 (53.1)	11 (45.8)	28 (50.0)	1.34 (0.46–3.87)
- Moderate (10–14)	3 (9.4)	3 (12.5)	6 (10.7)	0.72 (0.13–3.95)
- Severe (≥15 or venous ulceration)	0 (0.0)	0 (0.0)	0 (0.0)	0.75 (0.01–39.3)
- Missing	1 (3.1)	1 (4.2)	2 (3.6)	0.74 (0.04–12.5)
SF-36[b] – Reported health transition	51.7 ± 18.5	52.1 ± 14.6	51.9 ± 16.7	–
VEINES QOL/Sym[c]	49.5 ± 11.1	51.5 ± 8.2	50.4 ± 9.9	–
VEINES QOL/Sym, intrinsic score[d]	71.3 ± 14.8	72.4 ± 12.2	71.8 ± 13.6	–

Data are n (%) or mean ± SD
None of the variables mentioned in this table showed statistical significant difference between groups
VTE Venous thrombo-embolism
[a] Post-thrombotic syndrome was defined according to the definition stated by the International Society of Thrombosis and Haemostasis. This definition requires a single Villalta-score ≥ 5 assessed at 6 months or more after the acute venous thrombo-embolic event [17]
[b]The SF-36 is a questionnaire aimed at the generic health-related quality of life as reported by the patients. It comprises 36 questions covering 8 different health-related dimensions: Physical functioning, Role limitations due to physical health, Role limitations due to emotional health, Energy/Fatigue, Emotional well-being, Social functioning, Bodily pain, and General health perceptions [18]
[c]The VEINES QOL/SYM is a questionnaire addressing the disease-specific self-reported quality of life in DVT patients. It entails 25 questions regarding the limitations, symptoms, and changes encountered as a result of the acute thromboembolic event. The final summarizing score is adapted to the study population [19, 20]
[d]By using the method by Bland et al. [21] the VEINES QOL/SYM summarizing score can be transformed into an intrinsic score which allows comparison to other quality of life scores

This study has several limitations. First of all, the number of included patients was low, this may especially affect the results of the sub analyses between patients with an unprovoked versus provoked VTE and between patients with and without VO. However, although it is an exploratory study and as such unable to be conclusive, its results can be used in the discussion regarding the need for long-term anticoagulation or indications for venous stenting. We found that VO is equally prevalent in patients with or without reVTE and as such VO is not a likely game changer for recurrent risk.

Second, the characteristics of the patients included in this study may differ from those in other post-thrombotic populations and therefore our findings might not be generalisable. Remarkable, yet without difference between the groups studied, was the high percentage of male patients (82.1%) and thrombosis with a right-sided (57.1%) thrombus localisation [5, 26, 27]. Also the incidence of PTS was high (60.7%) compared to the general post-thrombotic population [6–8] and was mainly based on high objective scores.

In addition, patients with reVTE differed from their age and sex matched controls regarding several baseline characteristics known to have a role in the pathophysiology of DVT and its post-thrombotic morbidity [5, 7, 8, 28–42]. This might have influenced the clinical outcomes. For example, the higher use of compression stockings in patients with a reVTE may have limited the development of PTS

and post-thrombotic signs or symptoms [33, 34]. The reason for a difference in compliance to compression therapy could not be determined based on the available data. Since all patients were treated according to international guidelines for post-thrombotic care, by definition the anticoagulant management following a reVTE differed from management following a single episode.

Nevertheless, since the influence of VO on the occurrence of reVTE had not been studied before, our study provides, to our knowledge, the first insight in the characteristics of patients with VO. Clearly defined inclusion criteria and selection from an existing cohort of patients that received standardized post-thrombotic care are some of the strengths of this study. Furthermore, all consultations and duplex assessments were performed by the same physician (RS) and a highly experienced registered vascular technologist (IT), respectively, who both had no involvement in the primary care process of these patients.

Conclusions

In conclusion, this exploratory study suggests that the presence of VO is not related to recurrent thrombotic events, nor to the clinical outcome following reVTE. Therefore, (asymptomatic) VO does not seem to provide a basis for specific treatment such as prolonged anticoagulant treatment or stenting, as means of reducing the risk of recurrent thrombosis.

Abbreviations

CFV: Common femoral vein; CIV: Common iliac vein; DFV: Deep femoral vein; DUS: Duplex ultrasonography; DVT: Deep-vein thrombosis; EIV: External iliac vein; FV: Femoral vein; ICV: Inferior caval vein; ICVir: Inferior caval vein, infra renal; ICVsr: Inferior caval vein, supra renal; IQR: Interquartile range; ISTH: International Society on Thrombosis and Haemostasis; OR: Odds ratio; PE: Pulmonary embolism; PTS: Post-thrombotic syndrome; PV: Popliteal vein; QoL: Quality of life; reDVT: Recurrent DVT; reVTE: Recurrent venous thromboembolism; VO: Venous obstruction; VTE: Venous thromboembolism; 95%CI: 95% confidence interval

Acknowledgements

Not applicable.

Authors' contributions

PN contributed to literature search, data collection, composition of the database, data analysis, data interpretation, composition of tables, and writing of the manuscript. RS and IT contributed to collection of the data and critical review of the manuscript. HtC contributed to study concept, study design, and critical review of the manuscript. AtCH conceived the study including protocol development, gaining ethical approval, and patient recruitment and contributed to data analysis, data interpretation, composition of tables, and writing of the manuscript. All authors read and approved the final manuscript.

Author details

[1]Department of Vascular Surgery, Maastricht University Medical Centre, P.O. Box 5800, Maastricht 6202 AZ, the Netherlands. [2]CARIM, Cardiovascular Research Institute Maastricht, School for Cardiovascular Diseases, Maastricht University Medical Centre, P.O. Box 616, Maastricht 6200 MD, the Netherlands. [3]Laboratory for Clinical Thrombosis and Hemostasis, Maastricht University, P.O. Box 616, Maastricht 6200 MD, The Netherlands. [4]Thrombosis Expertise Centre, Heart + Vascular Centre, Maastricht University Medical Centre, P.O. Box 5800, Maastricht 6202 AZ, the Netherlands. [5]Thrombosis Expertise Centre, Heart + Vascular Centre, Maastricht University Medical Centre, P. Debyelaan 25, Maastricht 6229 HX, the Netherlands.

References

1. Heit JA. Epidemiology of venous thromboembolism. Nat Rev Cardiol. 2015; 12(8):464–74.
2. Khan F, Rahman A, Carrier M, Kearon C, Weitz JI, Schulman S, et al. Long term risk of symptomatic recurrent venous thromboembolism after discontinuation of anticoagulant treatment for first unprovoked venous thromboembolism event: systematic review and meta-analysis. BMJ. 2019;366:I4363.
3. Prandoni P, Noventa F, Ghirarduzzi A, Pengo V, Bernardi E, Pesavento R, et al. The risk of recurrent venous thromboembolism after discontinuing anticoagulation in patients with acute proximal deep vein thrombosis or pulmonary embolism. A prospective cohort study in 1,626 patients. Haematologica. 2007;92(2):199–205.
4. Iorio A, Kearon C, Filippucci E, Marcucci M, Macura A, Pengo V, et al. Risk of recurrence after a first episode of symptomatic venous thromboembolism provoked by a transient risk factor: a systematic review. Arch Intern Med. 2010;170(19):1710–6.
5. Kahn SR, Comerota AJ, Cushman M, Evans NS, Ginsberg JS, Goldenberg NA, et al. The postthrombotic syndrome: evidence-based prevention, diagnosis, and treatment strategies: a scientific statement from the American Heart Association. Circulation. 2014;130(18):1636–61.
6. Prandoni P, Lensing AW, Prins MH, Pesavento R, Piccioli A, Sartori MT, et al. The impact of residual thrombosis on the long-term outcome of patients with deep venous thrombosis treated with conventional anticoagulation. Semin Thromb Hemost. 2015;41(2):133–40.
7. Kahn SR, Shrier I, Julian JA, Ducruet T, Arsenault L, Miron MJ, et al. Determinants and time course of the postthrombotic syndrome after acute deep venous thrombosis. Ann Intern Med. 2008;149(10):698–707.
8. Schulman S, Lindmarker P, Holmstrom M, Larfars G, Carlsson A, Nicol P, et al. Post-thrombotic syndrome, recurrence, and death 10 years after the first episode of venous thromboembolism treated with warfarin for 6 weeks or 6 months. J Thromb Haemost. 2006;4(4):734–42.
9. Kahn SR, Shbaklo H, Lamping DL, Holcroft CA, Shrier I, Miron MJ, et al. Determinants of health-related quality of life during the 2 years following deep vein thrombosis. J Thromb Haemost. 2008;6(7):1105–12.
10. Ten Cate-Hoek AJ, Toll DB, Buller HR, Hoes AW, Moons KG, Oudega R, et al. Cost-effectiveness of ruling out deep venous thrombosis in primary care versus care as usual. J Thromb Haemost. 2009;7(12):2042–9.
11. Meissner MH, Eklof B, Smith PC, Dalsing MC, DePalma RG, Gloviczki P, et al. Secondary chronic venous disorders. J Vasc Surg. 2007;46(Suppl S):68s–83s.
12. Neglen P, Thrasher TL, Raju S. Venous outflow obstruction: an underestimated contributor to chronic venous disease. J Vasc Surg. 2003;38(5):879–85.
13. Broholm R, Panduro Jensen L, Baekgaard N. Catheter-directed thrombolysis in the treatment of iliofemoral venous thrombosis. A review. Int Angiol. 2010;29(4):292–302.
14. Nagler M, Ten Cate H, Prins MH, Ten Cate-Hoek AJ. Risk factors for recurrence in deep vein thrombosis patients following a tailored anticoagulant treatment incorporating residual vein obstruction. Res Pract Thromb Haemost. 2018;2(2):299–309.
15. Villalta SB, Bagatella P, Piccioli A, Lensing A, Prins M, Prandoni P. Assessment of validity and reproducibility of a clinical scale for the post-thrombotic syndrome. Haemostasis. 1994;24(suppl 1):158a.
16. Wittens C, Davies AH, Baekgaard N, Broholm R, Cavezzi A, Chastanet S, et al. Editor's choice - management of chronic venous disease: clinical practice guidelines of the European Society for Vascular Surgery (ESVS). Eur J Vasc Endovasc Surg. 2015;49(6):678–737.
17. Kahn SR, Partsch H, Vedantham S, Prandoni P, Kearon C. Definition of post-thrombotic syndrome of the leg for use in clinical investigations: a recommendation for standardization. J Thromb Haemost. 2009;7(5):879–83.
18. Aaronson NK, Muller M, Cohen PD, Essink-Bot ML, Fekkes M, Sanderman R, et al. Translation, validation, and norming of the Dutch language version of the SF-36 Health Survey in community and chronic disease populations. J Clin Epidemiol. 1998;51(11):1055–68.
19. van der Velden SK, Biemans AA, Nijsten T, Sommer A. Translation and validation of the Dutch VEINES-QOL/Sym in varicose vein patients. Phlebology. 2014;29(4):227–35.
20. Lamping DL, Schroter S, Kurz X, Kahn SR, Abenhaim L. Evaluation of outcomes in chronic venous disorders of the leg: development of a scientifically rigorous, patient-reported measure of symptoms and quality of life. J Vasc Surg. 2003;37(2):410–9.
21. Bland JM, Dumville JC, Ashby RL, Gabe R, Stubbs N, Adderley U, et al. Validation of the VEINES-QOL quality of life instrument in venous leg ulcers: repeatability and validity study embedded in a randomised clinical trial. BMC Cardiovasc Disord. 2015;15:85.
22. Vedantham S, Thorpe PE, Cardella JF, Grassi CJ, Patel NH, Ferral H, et al. Quality improvement guidelines for the treatment of lower extremity deep vein thrombosis with use of endovascular thrombus removal. J Vasc Interv Radiol. 2009;20(7 Suppl):S227–39.
23. Linkins LA, Pasquale P, Paterson S, Kearon C. Change in thrombus length on venous ultrasound and recurrent deep vein thrombosis. Arch Intern Med. 2004;164(16):1793–6.
24. Prandoni P, Lensing AW, Bernardi E, Villalta S, Bagatella P, Girolami A. The diagnostic value of compression ultrasonography in patients with suspected recurrent deep vein thrombosis. Thromb Haemost. 2002;88(3):402–6.
25. Prandoni P, Cogo A, Bernardi E, Villalta S, Polistena P, Simioni P, et al. A simple ultrasound approach for detection of recurrent proximal-vein thrombosis. Circulation. 1993;88(4 Pt 1):1730–5.

26. Nordstrom M, Lindblad B, Bergqvist D, Kjellstrom T. A prospective study of the incidence of deep-vein thrombosis within a defined urban population. J Intern Med. 1992;232(2):155–60.

27. Johansson M, Johansson L, Lind M. Incidence of venous thromboembolism in northern Sweden (VEINS): a population-based study. Thromb J. 2014;12(1):6.

28. Bauersachs R, Berkowitz SD, Brenner B, Buller HR, Decousus H, Gallus AS, et al. Oral rivaroxaban for symptomatic venous thromboembolism. N Engl J Med. 2010;363(26):2499–510.

29. Tick LW, Kramer MH, Rosendaal FR, Faber WR, Doggen CJ. Risk factors for post-thrombotic syndrome in patients with a first deep venous thrombosis. J Thromb Haemost. 2008;6(12):2075–81.

30. Tick LW, Doggen CJ, Rosendaal FR, Faber WR, Bousema MT, Mackaay AJ, et al. Predictors of the post-thrombotic syndrome with non-invasive venous examinations in patients 6 weeks after a first episode of deep vein thrombosis. J Thromb Haemost. 2010;8(12):2685–92.

31. Stain M, Schonauer V, Minar E, Bialonczyk C, Hirschl M, Weltermann A, et al. The post-thrombotic syndrome: risk factors and impact on the course of thrombotic disease. J Thromb Haemost. 2005;3(12):2671–6.

32. Douketis JD, Crowther MA, Foster GA, Ginsberg JS. Does the location of thrombosis determine the risk of disease recurrence in patients with proximal deep vein thrombosis? Am J Med. 2001;110(7):515–9.

33. Ten Cate-Hoek AJ, Amin EE, Bouman AC, Meijer K, Tick LW, Middeldorp S, et al. Individualised versus standard duration of elastic compression therapy for prevention of post-thrombotic syndrome (IDEAL DVT): a multicentre, randomised, single-blind, allocation-concealed, non-inferiority trial. Lancet Haematol. 2018;5(1):e25–33.

34. Brandjes DP, Buller HR, Heijboer H, Huisman MV, de Rijk M, Jagt H, et al. Randomised trial of effect of compression stockings in patients with symptomatic proximal-vein thrombosis. Lancet. 1997;349(9054):759–62.

35. Galanaud JP, Monreal M, Kahn SR. Epidemiology of the post-thrombotic syndrome. Thromb Res. 2018;164:100–9.

36. Labropoulos N, Jen J, Jen H, Gasparis AP, Tassiopoulos AK. Recurrent deep vein thrombosis: long-term incidence and natural history. Ann Surg. 2010;251(4):749–53.

37. Kearon C, Akl EA, Ornelas J, Blaivas A, Jimenez D, Bounameaux H, et al. Antithrombotic therapy for VTE disease: CHEST guideline and expert panel report. Chest. 2016;149(2):315–52.

38. Appelen D, van Loo E, Prins MH, Neumann MH, Kolbach DN. Compression therapy for prevention of post-thrombotic syndrome. Cochrane Database Syst Rev. 2017;9:Cd004174.

39. Ten Cate-Hoek AJ, Prins MH, Wittens CH, ten Cate H. Postintervention duration of anticoagulation in venous surgery. Phlebology. 2013;28(Suppl 1):105–11.

40. Hull RD, Liang J, Townshend G. Long-term low-molecular-weight heparin and the post-thrombotic syndrome: a systematic review. Am J Med. 2011;124(8):756–65.

41. Schulman S, Kearon C, Kakkar AK, Mismetti P, Schellong S, Eriksson H, et al. Dabigatran versus warfarin in the treatment of acute venous thromboembolism. N Engl J Med. 2009;361(24):2342–52.

42. van Dongen CJ, Prandoni P, Frulla M, Marchiori A, Prins MH, Hutten BA. Relation between quality of anticoagulant treatment and the development of the postthrombotic syndrome. J Thromb Haemost. 2005;3(5):939–42.

8

The predictive value of D-dimer test for venous thromboembolism during puerperium in women age 35 or older

Wen Hu[†], Dong Xu[†], Juan Li, Cheng Chen, Yuan Chen, Fangfang Xi, Feifei Zhou, Xiaohan Guo, Baihui Zhao[*] and Qiong Luo[*] (iD)

Abstract

Background: This study aimed to investigate the predictive value of the D-dimer level for venous thromboembolism (VTE) events during puerperium of women age at 35 years or older, as well as to identify other risk factors associated with the occurrence of VTE.

Methods: It was a prospective observational cohort study, from January 2014 to December 2018, which involved 12,451 women age 35 or older who delivered at least 28 weeks of gestation at Women's Hospital of Zhejiang University, School of Medicine. The maternal and fetal demographic characteristics, pregnancy complications, imaging finding and results of laboratory test within postpartum 24 h including D-dimer level, platelet counts and fibrinogen level were collected for analyses.

Results: 30(2.4‰) women were identified as VTE, including 1 pulmonary embolism event and 29 deep venous thrombosis events. The receiver operating characteristic (ROC) curve analysis suggested the best cutoff point for D-dimer level within postpartum 24 h of women age 35 or older was 5.545 mg/L, with a specificity of 70.0% and a sensitivity of 75.4%. Besides, there was no statistical correlation between platelet counts and VTE, as well as between fibrinogen level and VTE. On multivariate analysis, D-dimer≥5.50 mg/L (OR = 5.874, 95%CI: 2.678–12.886) and emergency cesarean section (OR = 11.965, 95%CI: 2.732–52.401) were independently associated with VTE in puerperium of women age 35 or older.

Conclusions: We concluded that D-dimer≥5.50 mg/L was an independent predictor of VTE in puerperium with maternal age 35 or older and D-dimer testing was a necessary examination for perinatal women.

Keywords: D-dimer, Venous thromboembolism, Women age at 35 years or older, Puerperium

* Correspondence: zhaobh@zju.edu.cn; luoq@zju.edu.cn
[†]Wen Hu and Dong Xu contributed equally to this work.
Department of Obstetrics, Women's Hospital, Zhejiang University, School of Medicine, 1st Xueshi Road, Hangzhou 310006, Zhejiang, China

Background

Venous thromboembolism (VTE) remains one of the leading causes of maternal mortality [1], taking the place of postpartum hemorrhage, which has been highly prevented and treated. The incidence is 4 to 5 times higher among pregnant and postpartum women than that of non-pregnant women [2]. Pregnancy is an acquired and independent risk factor for the development of VTE. Many other risk factors have been linked to VTE, such as advanced maternal age, thrombophilia, cesarean section, obesity, and a personal or family history of VTE [3, 4]. In recent years, maternal age at childbirth continues to increase worldwide, particularly in China, as a consequence of the changes in attitudes towards fertility and the adjustment of the birth policy. Increasing maternal age is associated with the increasing incidence of pregnancy complications, which together lead to the increasing incidence of VTE.

Among the screening tools for VTE, D-dimer testing has been proved its reliability in non-pregnant individuals by several studies, with high sensitivity and moderate specificity [5]. For pregnant women, D-dimer concentration increased progressively during the pregnancy and peaked at the first postpartum day [6]. Some studies proved the predictive value of D-dimer test for pregnant related VTE by raising the cutoff value or finding a higher D-dimer reference range [6–8]. D-dimer level also has been shown to increase by patient age [9]. However, there is a lack of research on the predictive value of D-dimer level for VTE in the women age 35 or older.

Therefore, we designed a prospective observational study to identify the incidence and risk factors of VTE during the postpartum period in women age 35 or older.

Furthermore, we investigated the predictive value of coagulation markers including D-dimer level, platelet counts and fibrinogen level, and attempted to determine a suitable threshold for the assessment in postpartum period of older mothers.

Methods

Patients

Women's Hospital, School of Medicine, Zhejiang University (WHZJU) has 460 maternity beds and serves many provinces of East China region. Approximately 20,000 births occur annually. As a first-class specialized hospital of obstetrics and gynecology in China and a nationally-known referral center, many of the pregnant women are complicated and high-risk.

We initiated the study in January 1st 2014 and continued until December 31st 2018, and we prospectively collected the data of women age 35 or older who gave birth at least 28 weeks of gestation at WHZJU. Women used anticoagulant or anti-platelet drugs before delivery or with incomplete clinical data were excluded from this study (Fig. 1). The sample size required for the study was calculated according to the following formula:

$$n = \frac{\left(Z_\alpha \sqrt{2pq} + Z_\beta \sqrt{p_0 q_0 + p_1 q_1}\right)^2}{(p_1 - p_0)^2}.$$

In this formula, p_0 indicated the incidence of VTE in D-dimer< 5.545 mg /L group (0.96‰); p_1 indicated the incidence of VTE in D-dimer≥5.545 mg /L group (6.8‰); p stood for the average value of p_0 and p_1; q = 1-p. We set α = 0.05 and β = 0.10 (power = 0.90); z_α = 1.96

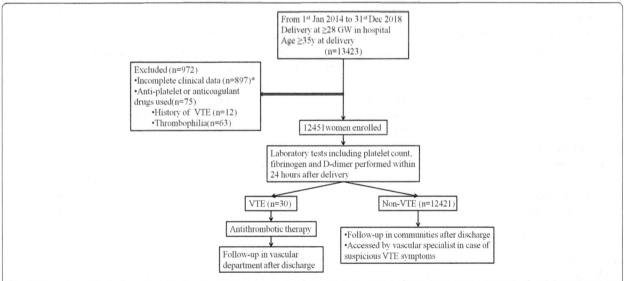

Fig. 1 Flow chart of indicating the patients included in and excluded from the study. * Lack of blood test data within 24 h after delivery because of delayed detection or patients' unwillingness to participate

and $z_\beta = 1.282$, which represented for the boundary value of normal distribution. The estimated sample size was 2380. The sample size of this study was larger than the estimated sample size. All clinical variables were recorded, including age, body mass index (BMI), pregnancy times, parity, gestational weeks of delivery, fetal position, mode of delivery, fetal birth weight, pregnancy complications, postpartum hemorrhage and predictive biomarkers within postpartum 24 h including D-dimer level, platelet counts and fibrinogen level. All biomarker values were obtained from the same laboratory affiliated to the hospital.

Clinical diagnosis of VTE

Imaging evidence was confirmed as the diagnostic criteria for VTE. Deep venous thrombosis (DVT) was diagnosed by upper and lower extremity venous color Doppler ultrasound and/or computed tomographic (CT) venography, and pulmonary embolism (PE) was diagnosed by CT pulmonary angiography.

Imaging examinations were required if the following conditions were present: (1) with suspicious symptoms of VTE, including pain or tenderness when move limbs, swelling of the limbs, measurement of inconsistencies in the circumference of the bilateral limbs, or unexplained dyspnea, chest pain or cough; or (2) with multiple high risk factors, and the clinician considered that the probability for VTE was great. Anticoagulation and antithrombotic therapy would be applied immediately when imaging examination indicated the diagnosis of VTE. All the VTE patients were told to follow up in the vascular department after discharge. Other women were followed up in the communities and would be accessed by vascular specialist in case of suspicious VTE symptoms (Fig. 1).

Laboratory assays

We performed laboratory tests including platelet counts, fibrinogen level and D-dimer level. The detection of platelet counts was measured by impedance (XN9000; Sysmex, Kobe, Japan). The detection of fibrinogen level was measured by the solidification (Stago-R, Paris, France). The detection of D-dimer level was measured by the latex-enhanced immunoturbidimetry (Stago-R, Paris, France) (normal reference range for non-pregnant adults is less than 0.5 mg/L).

Statistical analyses

Data inputting and statistical analysis were performed in SPSS 22.0 (IBM Corporation, New York, USA). Continuous variables were described as means ± standard deviation. The continuous variables were compared by Student's T test. The difference in the categorical variables was compared through Chi square test, Yate's correction of continuity or Fisher's exact test. Furthermore, to estimate the risk factors of VTE, the forward stepwise multiple logistic regression was performed. The associations between biomarkers and VTE were expressed as ROC curve analysis. Statistical significance was set at $p < 0.05$.

Results

Twelve thousand four hundred fifty-one women were enrolled in this study after screening (Fig. 1). In our cohort, 30 (2.4‰) women were identified as VTE, including 1 PE event and 29 DVT events. The DVT events included: 5 women with bilateral DVT of lower extremity, 11 women with DVT of right lower extremity and 13 with DVT of left lower extremity. VTE occurred at median of 3.5 days postpartum (range: 2–15 days).

All the D-dimer test results of VTE patients in this study exceeded the upper limit of the reference value (0.5 mg/L). The ROC curve analysis showed the best cutoff point for D-dimer level within postpartum 24 h of women age 35 or older was 5.545 mg/L, with a specificity of 70.0% and a sensitivity of 75.4%(Fig. 2). For convenience in clinical practice, the predefined cutoff value for dichotomized variables of D-dimer level was set at 5.50 mg/L. When the cutoff value was set at 6.475 mg/L, the specificity could increase to 80.0%, but the sensitivity would decrease to 53.3%; when the cutoff value was set at 9.875 mg/L, the specificity could increase to 90.0%, but the sensitivity would decrease to 36.7%.The AUCs of fibrinogen level and platelet counts were close to 0.5, indicating that there was no statistical correlation between them and VTE (Fig. 2).

Table 1 shows a comparison of maternal and fetal characteristics between VTE and non-VTE groups. Age, heights, gestational weeks of delivery, neonatal weight, fibrinogen level and platelet counts were not significantly associated with VTE. The average D-dimer level within postpartum 24 h with maternal age ≥ 35 in VTE group was significantly higher than that of non-VTE group (8.91 vs. 4.55 mg/L, $P < 0.001$).

The risk factors predisposing to VTE in puerperium of women age ≥ 35 were analyzed in Table 2. Mode of delivery, scared uterus, and D-dimer≥5.50 mg/L were significantly associated with VTE in puerperium of older mothers (Table 2).

A multivariate model using forward stepwise regression was constructed to identify the risk-factors associated with VTE in puerperium. D-dimer≥5.50 mg/L and emergency cesarean section were independently associated with VTE in puerperium (Table 3).

Discussion

VTE was reported 1.0–1.8/1000 in women during pregnancy and puerperium [10]. Our study showed that the rate of VTE during puerperium of women age ≥ 35

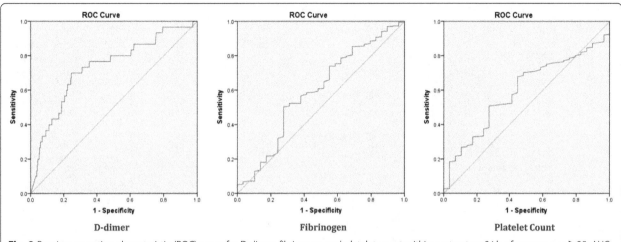

Fig. 2 Receiver operating characteristic (ROC) curve for D-dimer, fibrinogen, and platelet count within postpartum 24 h of women age ≥ 35. AUC (ROC of D-dimer): 0.732 (P < .001); AUC (ROC of fibrinogen): 0.592 (P = .086); AUC (ROC of platelet count): 0.594 (P = .081)

(2.4‰) was higher than that of younger mothers, which supported age was a risk factor for VTE, which had been proved by many other studies [3, 11–13]. It was noteworthy that even among the women age ≥ 35, age was almost significantly different between the VTE and non-VTE groups (p = 0.058). Considering the limitation of sample size, age difference between groups was likely to be statistically significant if the sample size was enlarged. It was considered that more cases of DVT events occured in the left lower extremity, which was related to the more serious venous stasis of the left lower extremity caused by the compression of the pregnant uterus [14]. But in our study, the proportion of DVT in the left lower extremity was only a little higher than that in the right. This may due to the limitation of the small sample size.

The diagnostic value of D dimer for pregnant related VTE is not clear up to now. For pregnant women, D-dimer concentration increased progressively during the pregnancy and peaked at the first postpartum day [6]. Most healthy pregnant women have higher D-dimer values during pregnancy and puerperium than the normal reference range [15]. A prospective study showed that in the first trimester, 84% women had normal D-dimer, in the second 33%, and by the third trimester only 1%, which suggests that D-dimer has no practical diagnostic use of VTE if the threshold for abnormal is used [7]. Guidelines from Royal College of Obstetricians and Gynaecologists recommended that D-dimer testing should not be performed in the investigation of acute VTE in pregnancy [16]. Guidelines from American College of Obstetricians and Gynecologists also recommended that the rise of D-dimer cannot predict VTE reliably [7, 17]. However, there still some studies supporting to perform D-dimer test and provide a higher threshold to increase the specificity of D-dimer without reducing the sensitivity [7, 8, 18–20]. Actually, D-dimer

Table 1 Comparison of general characteristics between VTE and non-VTE delivery women age ≥ 35(x ± SD)

	VTE (n = 30)	Non-VTE (n = 12,421)	t value	P value
Age (years)	38.10 ± 2.23	37.31 ± 2.29	1.893	.058
Height (cm)	161.13 ± 5.76	160.57 ± 4.71	0.650	.516
BMI before pregnancy	21.65 ± 2.96	21.05 ± 2.91	1.139	.255
BMI before delivery	26.70 ± 2.80	26.50 ± 2.99	0.363	.717
Gain weight during pregnancy (kg)	13.07 ± 3.19	14.04 ± 4.94	−1.067	.286
Gestational age at delivery (weeks)	37.83 ± 2.26	37.99 ± 1.95	−0.447	.655
Neonatal birth weight(g)	3114.67 ± 558.19	3203.16 ± 604.89	−0.800	.423
Laboratory test results within postpartum 24 h				
D-dimer (mg/L)	8.91 ± 6.16	4.55 ± 4.31	3.870	.001
Fibrinogen (g/L)	4.37 ± 0.85	4.63 ± 0.81	−1.706	.088
Platelet count (10^9/L)	172.00 ± 40.50	187.82 ± 53.53	−1.590	.112

Table 2 Risk factors predisposing to VTE in puerperium of women age ≥ 35

Risk factors	VTE(%) (n = 30)	Non-VTE(%) (n = 12,421)	χ^2 value	P value
Previous obstetric history				
0	11 (36.67)	2938 (23.65)	2.804	.094
≥ 1	19 (63.33)	9483 (76.35)		
Parity				
1	30 (100.00)	12,048 (97.00)		1.000[a]
≥ 2	0 (0.00)	373 (3.00)		
Fetal position of singleton cases				
Head	28 (93.33)	11,406 (94.67)		.385[a]
Breech	1 (3.33)	506 (4.20)		
Transverse	1 (3.33)	136 (1.13)		
Mode of delivery				
Vaginal delivery	2 (6.67)	4786 (38.53)	25.792	<.001
Emergency cesarean section	16 (53.33)	2399 (19.31)		
Elective caesarean section	12 (40.00)	5236 (42.15)		
In vitro fertilization (IVF)	0 (0.00)	678 (5.46)	0.834	.361
Scared uterus	20 (66.67)	5612 (45.18)	5.58	.018
Relative cephalopelvic disproportion	0 (0.00)	164 (1.32)		1.000[a]
Placenta previa	3 (10.00)	612 (4.93)	0.738	.390
Adherent placenta	4 (13.33)	610 (4.91)	2.910	.088
Fetal growth restriction	0 (0.00)	182 (1.47)		1.000[a]
Premature birth	5 (16.67)	1557 (12.54)	0.165	.684
Macrosomia (birthweight≥4000 g)	1 (3.33)	789 (6.35)	0.092	.762
Premature rupture of membranes	7 (23.33)	2184 (17.58)	0.682	.409
Fetal distress	5 (16.67)	1566 (12.61)	0.155	.694
Intrauterine infection	1 (3.33)	139 (1.12)		.288[a]
Postpartum hemorrhage	3 (10.00)	458 (3.69)	1.809	.179
Anemia	9 (30.00)	2654 (21.37)	1.327	.249
Intrahepatic cholestasis of pregnancy	3 (10.00)	398 (3.20)		.071[a]
Gestational diabetes mellitus	3 (10.00)	2951 (23.76)	3.130	.077
Hypertensive disorders of pregnancy	3 (10.00)	924 (7.44)	0.034	.853
Cardiac insufficiency	0 (0.00)	20 (0.16)		1.000[a]
Uterine rupture	0 (0.00)	84 (0.68)		1.000[a]
D-dimer≥5.545 mg /L	21 (70.00)	3057 (24.61)	33.130	<.001
D-dimer≥6.475 mg /L	16 (53.33)	2480 (19.97)	20.789	<.001
D-dimer≥9.88 mg /L	11 (36.67)	1242 (10.00)	20.661	<.001

[a] evaluated by Fisher's exact test

Table 3 Multivariate logistic regression of VTE risk factors during puerperium of women age ≥ 35

Risk factors	P value	OR	95% CI
Emergency cesarean section	.001	11.965	2.732–52.401
D-dimer≥5.545 mg /L	<.001	5.874	2.678–12.886

test is still being used by obstetricians. If the D-dimer level was abnormally high, the need for prophylactic use of low molecular weight heparin (LMWH) was decided by the doctors according to their own experiences.

However, up to now, there are few studies on the correlation between D-dimer level and VTE in delivery women age ≥ 35. The prevention of VTE in delivery women age ≥ 35 is particularly important because the risk of VTE increases with age. A variety of acquired prothrombotic risk factors (e.g., autoimmune disorders, diabetes and infection) also gradually develop with aging. Concurrently, aging is associated with a variety of coagulation and hemostasis changes in general population [21]. In our study, a large sample of older mothers was observed and we initially found the predictive value of D-dimer test for VTE during puerperium in women age ≥ 35. Although the specificity and sensitivity are not particularly high, the ROC curve analysis offered an even higher threshold of D-dimer in delivery women age ≥ 35. Multivariate analysis also indicated that D-dimer≥5.50 mg/L was independently associated with VTE in puerperium of older mothers. Therefore, we think it is necessary to perform the D-dimer test within postpartum 24 h of women age ≥ 35.

Elevated D-dimer level was not the only criterion for high risk of VTE. Our study revealed emergency cesarean section was another important independent risk factors of VTE in puerperium of women age ≥ 35, which was consistent with previous studies. A meta-analysis found that the risk of VTE was four fold greater following cesarean section than following vaginal delivery, and was greater following emergency cesarean section than following elective cesarean section [4]. Other studies also revealed several independent risk factors of VTE in puerperium such as higher BMI, thrombophilia, multiple pregnancy, gestational diabetes, premature birth, anemia, chorioamnionitis, in vitro fertilization with ovarian hyperstimulation, cardiac diseases and postpartum hemorrhage [11]. But we didn't find these risk factors because these factors may be age related and the objects of our study were older mothers while theirs were delivery women of all ages. Based on the results of this study, we recommend the use of LMWH to prevent VTE when the lever of D-dimer was higher than 5.50 mg/L of older mother, or the delivery mode of the older mother was emergency cesarean section.

The limitation of this study is that the sample size of VTE group is small, but this is consistent with the incidence of pregnancy-related VTE. Other limitations of this study include the effects of choice bias, for all the women in this study were at our hospital, and loss to follow-up bias, for we could hardly get the data of follow-up in communities and vascular department. Furthermore, this study did not discuss the predictive effect of D-dimer test for VTE during pregnancy and 24 h after postpartum, which need further study.

Conclusion

In summary, this study calculated that D-dimer≥5.50 mg/L was an independent factor associated with VTE in puerperium of women age ≥ 35, which confirmed the predictive value of D-dimer test for older delivery women. Another independent risk factor of VTE in puerperium of women age ≥ 35 was emergency cesarean section. We believe our study provides a new reliable evidence for clinicians to focus on the emphasis risk factors for VTE of older delivery women, which was expected to reduce the incidence of VTE.

Abbreviations
VTE: Venous thromboembolism; ROC: Receiver operating characteristic; BMI: Body mass index; CT: Computed tomographic; PE: Pulmonary embolism; DVT: Deep venous thrombosis; AUC: Area under the curve; LMWH: Low molecular weight heparin

Acknowledgements
Not applicable.

Authors' contributions
WH and DX wrote the manuscript. BZ and QL made critical revisions of the manuscript for important intellectual content and contributed to the study concept, design and implementation. JL, CC, YC and FX were responsible for data collection, input and correction. FZ and XG contributed to data statistics and analysis. All the authors discussed the first draft of the paper and put forward suggestions for revision. All authors read and approved the final manuscript.

References
1. Abe K, Kuklina EV, Hooper WC, Callaghan WM. Venous thromboembolism as a cause of severe maternal morbidity and mortality in the United States. Semin Perinatol. 2019;43:200–4.
2. Heit JA, Kobbervig CE, James AH, et al. Trends in the incidence of venous thromboembolism during pregnancy or postpartum: a 30-year population-based study. Ann Intern Med. 2005;143:697–706.
3. James AH, Jamison MG, Brancazio LR, Myers ER. Venous thromboembolism during pregnancy and the postpartum period: incidence, risk factors, and mortality. Am J Obstet Gynecol. 2006;194:1311–5.
4. Blondon M, Casini A, Hoppe KK, et al. Risks of venous thromboembolism after cesarean sections: a meta-analysis. Chest. 2016;150:572–96.
5. Johnson ED, Schell JC, Rodgers GM. The D-dimer assay. Am J Hematol. 2019;94:833–9.
6. Wang M, Lu S, Li S, Shen F. Reference intervals of D-dimer during the pregnancy and puerperium period on the STA-R evolution coagulation analyzer. Clin Chim Acta. 2013;425:176–80.
7. Kovac M, Mikovic Z, Rakicevic L, et al. The use of D-dimer with new cutoff can be useful in diagnosis of venous thromboembolism in pregnancy. Eur J Obstet Gynecol Reprod Biol. 2010;148:27–30.
8. Xu D, Cai SP, Xu JW, Liang C, He J. Study on the dynamic changes of D-dimer during pregnancy and early puerperium. Zhonghua Fu Chan Ke Za Zhi. 2016;51:666–71.
9. Haase C, Joergensen M, Ellervik C, Joergensen MK, Bathum L. Age- and sex-dependent reference intervals for D-dimer: evidence for a marked increase by age. Thromb Res. 2013;132:676–80.
10. Meng K, Hu X, Peng X, Zhang Z. Incidence of venous thromboembolism during pregnancy and the puerperium: a systematic review and meta-analysis. J Matern Fetal Neonatal Med. 2015;28:245–53.
11. Galambosi PJ, Gissler M, Kaaja RJ, Ulander VM. Incidence and risk factors of venous thromboembolism during postpartum period: a population-based cohort-study. Acta Obstet Gynecol Scand. 2017;96:852–61.
12. Sharma S, Monga D. Venous thromboembolism during pregnancy and the post-partum period: incidence and risk factors in a large Victorian health service. Aust N Z J Obstet Gynaecol. 2008;48:44–9.
13. Jensen TB, Gerds TA, Gron R, et al. Risk factors for venous thromboembolism during pregnancy. Pharmacoepidemiol Drug Saf. 2013; 22:1283–91.

14. James AH, Tapson VF, Goldhaber SZ. Thrombosis during pregnancy and the postpartum period. Am J Obstet Gynecol. 2005;193:216–9.

15. Reger B, Peterfalvi A, Litter I, et al. Challenges in the evaluation of D-dimer and fibrinogen levels in pregnant women. Thromb Res. 2013;131:e183–7.

16. Gynaecologists RCOO, editor. Thromboembolic disease in pregnancy and the puerperium: acute management. Green top guideline no.37b. London: Royal College of Obstetricians and Gynaecologists; 2015.

17. ACOG Practice Bulletin No. 196. Thromboembolism in pregnancy. Obstet Gynecol. 2018;132:e1–e17.

18. Parilla BV, Fournogerakis R, Archer A, et al. Diagnosing pulmonary embolism in pregnancy: are biomarkers and clinical predictive models useful? AJP Rep. 2016;6:e160–4.

19. Murphy N, Broadhurst DI, Khashan AS, et al. Gestation-specific D-dimer reference ranges: a cross-sectional study. BJOG. 2015;122:395–400.

20. Tang J, Lin Y, Mai H, et al. Meta-analysis of reference values of haemostatic markers during pregnancy and childbirth. Taiwan J Obstet Gynecol. 2019;58:29–35.

21. Favaloro EJ, Franchini M, Lippi G. Aging hemostasis: changes to laboratory markers of hemostasis as we age - a narrative review. Semin Thromb Hemost. 2014;40:621–33.

9

Association between cardiovascular risk-factors and venous thromboembolism in a large longitudinal study of French women

C. J. MacDonald[1,2], A. L. Madika[1,2,3], M. Lajous[4,5], M. Canonico[1,2], A. Fournier[1,2] and M. C. Boutron-Ruault[1,2*] ⓘ

Abstract

Background: Previous studies have shown conflicting results regarding the influence of cardiovascular risk-factors on venous thromboembolism. This study aimed to determine if these risk-factors, i.e. physical activity, smoking, hypertension, dyslipidaemia, and diabetes, were associated with the risk of venous thromboembolism, and to determine if these associations were confounded by BMI.

Methods: We used data from the E3N cohort study, a French prospective population-based study initiated in 1990, consisting of 98,995 women born between 1925 and 1950. From the women in the study we included those who did not have prevalent arterial disease or venous thromboembolism at baseline; thus 91,707 women were included in the study. Venous thromboembolism cases were self-reported during follow-up, and verified via specific mailings to medical practitioners or via drug reimbursements for anti-thrombotic medications. Hypertension, diabetes and dyslipidaemia were self-reported validated against drug reimbursements or specific questionnaires. Physical activity, and smoking were based on self-reports. Cox-models, adjusted for BMI and other potential risk-factors were used to determine hazard ratios for incident venous thromboembolism.

Results: During 1,897,960 person-years (PY), 1, 649 first incident episodes of thrombosis were identified at an incidence rate of 0.9 per 1000 PY. This included 505 cases of pulmonary embolism and 1144 cases of deep vein thrombosis with no evidence of pulmonary embolism. Hypertension, dyslipidaemia, diabetes, smoking and physical activity were not associated with the overall risk of thrombosis after adjustment for BMI.

Conclusions: Traditional cardiovascular risk factors were not associated with the risk of venous thromboembolism after adjustment for BMI. Hypertension, dyslipidaemia and diabetes may not be risk-factors for venous thromboembolism.

Keywords: Venous thromboembolism, Pulmonary embolism, Epidemiology, Prospective study

* Correspondence: marie-christine.boutron@gustaveroussy.fr
[1]INSERM (Institut National de la Santé et de la Recherche Médicale) U1018, Center for Research in Epidemiology and Population Health (CESP), Institut Gustave Roussy, Villejuif, France
[2]Université Paris-Saclay, Université Paris-Sud, Villejuif, France
Full list of author information is available at the end of the article

Introduction

Venous thromboembolism (VTE) is a multifactorial condition resulting from the formation of blood clots in the deep veins (deep vein thrombosis, DVT), or their migration to the lungs (pulmonary embolism, PE). Mortality rate estimates for the European Union give 500,000 VTE-related deaths per year [1]. VTE is considered a major global health burden, and a leading cause of lost disability-adjusted life years [2]. Established risk factors for VTE include long hospitalisations, surgery [3], and cancers [4]. Family history of VTE, non-O blood groups, and treatments such as menopausal hormone therapy (MHT) also increase the risk of VTE [5].

It is currently poorly understood how cardiovascular risk-factors contribute to VTE risk. Many common cardiovascular risk factors have been associated with VTE in meta-analyses including obesity, type 2 diabetes, smoking, non-O blood group, and high triglyceride concentrations [6, 7]. However, these associations are heterogeneous between studies [8, 9]. For example a recent cross-sectional study observed a positive association between hypertension and VTE [10]. However, a meta-analysis found that blood pressure was inversely associated with the risk of VTE [11], and a prospective study utilising time-varying covariates found no association [12]. Previous studies have failed to account for female specific risk-factors for VTE, such as parity, and the use of MHT [9]. As BMI is a major risk-factor for many of these conditions, it is possible that previous estimates not accounting for BMI are biased, and that common CVD risk-factors are not directly associated with the risk of VTE.

In this work, we aimed to explore the relationship between cardiovascular risk factors and VTE, in a large prospective study of middle-age, and older women controlling for specific female risk-factors for VTE. The hypothesis was that any associations between arterial risk-factors and VTE were confounded by BMI.

Methods
Study cohort

The E3N (Etude Epidémiologique auprès de femmes de la Mutuelle Générale de l'Education Nationale (MGEN)) cohort study was set up in 1990, and included 98,995 women born 1925–1950 and affiliated to the MGEN, a health insurance plan for workers in the education system and their spouses. The objective was to identify risk factors for cancer and chronic conditions in women. In 1990, participants signed an informed consent form in accordance to the French National Commission for Data Protection and Privacy. Part of this study is the French component of the European Prospective Investigation into Cancer (EPIC) [13].

Participants were asked every 2–3 years to complete self-administered questionnaires to provide and update medical events and lifestyle (1990, 1992, 1993, 1995, 1997, 2000, 2002, 2005, 2008, and 2011). The baseline for the current study was the date the participants answered the 1992 questionnaire. Participants were excluded from this study if they had stroke, coronary heart disease, cancer, death ($n = 6452$), or VTE ($n = 390$) before 1992. We excluded 721 participants with no reported baseline body mass index (BMI). The final study population included 91,707 women.

Assessment of venous thromboembolism cases

Non-fatal incident VTE cases were identified from self-reports in the follow-up questionnaires sent to the study participants after baseline. Before the 2008 questionnaire, participants were asked to report VTE events (without distinguishing between deep and superficial VTE) as yes/no, and the corresponding date, or pulmonary embolism (PE) and the corresponding date. From 2008 on, questionnaires were specific for DVT or PE, asking participants not to report superficial VTE. A flow-chart of case identification is presented in the supplementary material (sup. Fig. 1). All cases were considered validated, either by imaging procedures, or by reimbursement for anti-thrombotic medications following the event.

When participants reported VTE or PE events in the 2005 or preceding questionnaires, they were contacted via another letter, whereby they were asked to provide medical documents relating to the event. In addition, a questionnaire including information on potential predisposing factors (including surgeries, immobilisation over 8 days, cancers, long voyages on airplanes, or other factors) for thrombosis and characteristics of the event was sent to the medical doctors who followed these participants, permitting classification of the events as primary or secondary. To be validated, clinical events had to be diagnosed using an imaging procedure. PE was defined as the presence of either a positive pulmonary angiography or a positive helicoidal computed tomography or a high-probability ventilation/perfusion lung scan. DVT had to be diagnosed by use of compression ultrasonography or venography.

For DVT/PE identified from the 2008 and 2011 questionnaires, we confirmed that cases were associated with a relevant antithrombotic prescription (Heparin, Tinzaparin, Fragmin, Fraxiparin, Enoxaparin, Acénocoumarol, Fluindione, Warfarin, Dabigatran, Rivaroxaban, or Apixaban) at least twice in the year following the VTE using the MGEN database. Self-reported cases that were not validated with anti-thrombotic medications were not considered as valid cases. We cross-referenced self-reported VTE with self-reported hospital admissions, to determine if there was any associated cancer, immobilisation, hospitalisation, surgery (e.g. hip and knee surgeries), or trauma, which would indicate a secondary VTE. All other cases were considered a primary event with no obvious cause.

Fatal cases were identified from national death registers using International Classification of Diseases (ICD)-9 (codes 4151 and 4539) and ICD-10 (codes I26.0 and I26.9).

Amongst the 91,711 participants in the study, 1443 incident first cases of VTE were identified during follow-up (1992–2005) as previously described [14], and a further 1277 identified from in 2008 and 2011. Cases of superficial and upper extremity VT ($n = 848$) and cases for which the type could not be determined ($n = 223$) were not considered. As a result, 1649 incident cases of VTE consisting of 505 cases of PE and 1144 cases of DVT with no evidence of PE were considered.

Assessment of cardiovascular risk factors
All cardiovascular risk factors considered were updated at each questionnaire cycle for this study.

During the study period, women were asked if they had received a diagnosis of hypertension that required treatment in all questionnaires. In 2004, a drug reimbursement database became available for women in the study. Previously we have observed an 82% positive predictive value/agreement from self-reports when cross correlating with the drug reimbursement database for antihypertensive medications. (Anatomical Therapeutic Chemical Classification System codes C02, C03, C07, C08, and C09).

Type-2 diabetes cases were based on self-reports, which were then validated through a specific questionnaire mailed to women having reported type-2 diabetes, confirming either elevated glucose concentration at diagnosis (fasting ≥ 7.0 mmol/l or random glucose ≥ 11.1 mmol/l), treatment with diabetes drugs, and/or fasting glucose or HbA1c $\geq 7\%$,(53.0 mmol/mol), respectively [15]. Cases occurring after 2004 were identified using the MGEN reimbursement database. All women reimbursed for glucose lowering medications at least twice in a given year were classified as having type-2 diabetes.

Dyslipidaemia was self-reported at baseline, and at all follow up questionnaires. Participants in the study were asked if they had received a diagnosis of abnormal cholesterol from their doctor, or if they required treatment to control their cholesterol. Participants who did not provide information on dyslipidaemia were classified as unknown. The use of lipid-lowering medications was accounted for from 2004 onwards, using the MGEN database. Prior to 2004, statin use was considered unknown. As a secondary analysis, due to potential effects of statins on VTE risk, we considered the combination of self-reported dyslipidaemia, as well as statin reimbursement as 'treated dyslipidaemia'. Separate classes were also created for 'reported dyslipidaemia and no statin reimbursement' and 'no reported dyslipidaemia and statin reimbursement'.

We assessed usual physical activity from questionnaires that included questions on the time spent walking (to work, shopping, and leisure time), cycling (to work, shopping, and leisure time), housework, and sports activities. Metabolic equivalents (METs) per week were estimated by multiplying the hourly average METs for each item based on values from the Compendium of Physical Activities [16] by the reported activity duration. Physical activity was split into three tertiles depending on the population distribution. Blood ABO group and smoking were based on self-reports, and at each questionnaire participants were classified as smoker, ex-smoker, or never smoker.

Assessment of adjustment variables
Self-reported height and weight were used to calculate body mass index (BMI), defined as weight (kg) divided by squared height (m^2). In the cohort, self-reported anthropometry is considered reliable from a validation study [17].

Use of MHT was assessed using a booklet containing photos of all types of oestrogens and progestogens, as previously described [14]. Age at, and type of menopause was defined as either (in decreasing order of priority) age at last menstrual period, age at bilateral oophorectomy, self-reported age at menopause, age at start of MHT, or the age at the start of menopausal symptoms. If unavailable, the median age at menopause for the cohort (51 years for natural menopause, 47 years for artificial menopause) was imputed. Women were considered menopausal at baseline if any of these events occurred before the start of follow-up. Parity was based on self-reports. Family history of cardiovascular disease (stroke or coronary disease in either parent) was based on self-reports. Incident fractures, cancers, heart attacks, and strokes occurring during follow-up were based on cases validated by specific questionnaires to the women and their practitioners.

Statistical analysis
As risk-factor status can change over time, we updated values in modelling using information from follow-up questionnaires, similar to the method used by Wattanakit et at [12], i.e. the dataset contained multiple rows for each participant. If a participant reported hypertension, diabetes, or dyslipidaemia in one questionnaire, they were considered to have this condition for the remainder of follow-up.

Outcomes considered were the first VTE, then the first PE, or DVT; and then models considered the status of the event, i.e. primary VTE, and secondary VTE. In order to account for competing events when considering the specific types of VTE, the other types of VTE were censored from the analysis at the time of the competing event.

Potential confounders were selected with the help of directed acyclic graphs (supplementary Fig. 2). Risk-factors were assessed one by one, (i.e. we did not mutually adjust for hypertension, diabetes and dyslipidaemia), using Cox proportional hazard models with age as the time-scale in order to account for the effect of age. Models were initially assessed with age as the time scale (model 1), then on statin use (yes/no), for education level (high-school/no high-school/university), parity (0, 1, > 1), menopausal status (yes/no), ever use of MHT (yes/no), type of menopause (natural/artificial) (model 2), and finally BMI (model 3). Models were not mutually adjusted for the considered risk factors, in order to reduce the likelihood of introducing collider bias. Time at entry was the age at the beginning of follow-up (i.e., the age when the participants answered the questionnaire sent out in 1992); exit time was the age when participants were diagnosed with VTE, died (dates of death were obtained from the participants' medical insurance records), were lost to follow-up, or reached the end of the follow-up period (December 31, 2011), whichever occurred first.

As VTE can be provoked by bone fractures, other cardiovascular diseases, or cancer, we also considered a model controlled for incident fractures (time dependent, yes/no), cancers (time dependent, yes/no), and both heart attack and stroke (time dependent, yes/no), during follow-up as sensitivity analysis. The next sensitivity analysis excluded cases occurring after 2005 that were not part of the mailing conducted to validate the VTE cases. Another sensitivity analysis mutually adjusted for comorbid conditions at baseline, i.e. when considering hypertension, diabetes and dyslipidaemia were adjusted on at baseline. Finally, in the case of associations which were unexpected or suspected to be due to bias, we considered models using only baseline variables to determine if this was due to the inclusion of collider variables during follow-up.

When considering blood-groups 7834 participants were excluded from this analysis due to missing data on blood group. As a hypothesis generating exercise, we wished to determine if the associations between these risk factors were consistent over blood-groups, which are a major risk-factor for VTE. As blood-group is a determinant of blood lipid levels [18], hypertension [19], diabetes [20], and coagulation factors including von Willibrand factor [21], we considered effect modification

was plausible regarding dyslipidaemia, hypertension and diabetes.

Missing values (occurring in less than 5% of data) were imputed as the mean for continuous variables, and the median for categorical variables. During follow-up, if a value was missing, the previous value was imputed.

All statistical analyses were performed using R and R studio, with the 'Survival' package. A Bonferroni corrected p-value for statistical significance was 0.01. The proportional hazards assumption was assessed using the cox.zph function in R. A p-value is generated for the Person product-moment correlation between the scaled Schoenfeld residual, and the time transformation for each variable [22].

Results

During 1,897,960 person-years (PY) (mean follow-up of 20.7 years), 1649 first incident episodes of VTE were identified at an incidence rate of 0.9 per 1000 PY.

Table 1 displays data at baseline, and after 10 years of follow-up. The cardiovascular risk profile of the study participants worsened during follow-up, although total physical activity increased. BMI increased during follow-up from a mean of 22.9 kg / m^2 to 23.8 kg / m^2. Hypertension prevalence increased from 35.2 to 44.4%, diabetes from 1.0 to 2.2%, and self-reported dyslipidaemia from 7.8 to 25.4%. Smoking prevalence decreased during follow-up from 14.5 to 11.0%. At 2004, approximately 25% of study participants had been reimbursed for statins.

In unadjusted models, hypertension was associated with an increased risk of VTE (HR $_{HTA}$ = 1.21 (1.10: 1.34)), but this was not consistent after adjustment for BMI (HR $_{HTA}$ = 1.05 (0.95: 1.16)). Current smokers were associated with a lower risk of VTE in unadjusted models, but this was not observed after adjustment for BMI (HR $_{smokers}$ = 0.87 (0.73: 1.03)). Mean BMI among smokers at baseline was 22.5 (3.3) kg / m^2 compared to 22.9 (3.3) kg / m^2 among never smokers. Diabetes, dyslipidaemia, and physical activity were not associated with the risk of VTE in unadjusted or adjusted models (Table 2). Neither treated hypertension, nor treated dyslipidaemia were associated with the risk of VTE (not tabulated).

When considering VTE subtypes (Table 2), including PE, DVT, primary, and secondary VTE, hypertension showed a borderline positive association with PE (HR$_{hta}$ = 1.20 (0.99: 1.45)) after adjustment for BMI, and was consistent when considering treated hypertension, but not untreated hypertension (HR$_{hta\ trt}$ = 1.24 (0.99: 1.56), HR$_{hta\ untrt}$ = 1.16 (0.93: 1.45)). An inverse association with the highest tertile of physical activity was observed for primary VTE (HR$_{T3}$ = 0.71 (0.56: 0.90)) after adjustment for BMI. Dyslipidaemia was associated with

Table 1 Participant demographics at the beginning of followup, and mid-way through the study period

	Status at 1992 ($n = 91,711$)	Status at 2002 ($n = 88,302$)
Dynamic variables		
Age (years)	51.1 (6.6)	61.4 (6.6)
Declared hypertension (%)	35.2	44.4
Treated hypertension (%)*	Unknown	26.7
Diabetes (%)	1.0	2.2
Declared dyslipidaemia (%)	7.8	25.4
Statin user (%)*	Unknown	25.1
Treated dyslipidaemia (%)*	Unknown	12.9
BMI (kg / m^2)	22.9 (3.3)	23.8 (3.8)
BMI < 18.5 (%)	4.0	3.9
18.5–24.9 (%)	75.8	68.7
25.0–30.0 (%)	16.4	21.6
> 30.0 (%)	3.8	5.8
Physical activity (METs)	51.4 (30.2)	60.5 (37.6)
Physical activity < 34.3 METs (%)	33.1	33.5
Physical activity 34.3–57.8 METs (%)	33.0	32.1
Physical activity > 57.8 METs (%)	33.9	34.9
Current smoker (%)	14.5	11.8
Ex-smoker (%)	31.4	34.9
Never smoker (%)	54.1	53.3
Ever MHT use (%)	43.2	55.5
Static variables		
Education level (High-school / University (> = BAC + 4))	65.1 / 34.9	
Parity (number of pregnancies)	2.1	
Natural menopause (%)	88.0	
Family history CVD (%)	30.6	
Non-O blood group (%)	56.6	

*assessed in 2004
2488 participants died between 1992 and 2002

a reduced risk of primary VTE ($HR_{dys} = 0.68$ (0.52: 0.89)), and DVT ($HR_{dys} = 0.83$ (0.71: 0.97)), after adjustment for BMI. When the dyslipidaemia and statin treatment variables were combined, 'treated dyslipidaemia' was not significantly associated with a reduced risk of primary VTE ($HR_{treated\ dys} = 0.98$ (0.84: 1.16), not tabulated), compared to participants reporting no dyslipidaemia or statin reimbursement. This was also observed for DVT ($HR_{treated\ dys} = 0.85$ (0.68: 1.05), not tabulated). Diabetes was associated with a reduced risk of secondary VTE ($HR_{diab} = 0.66$ (0.44: 0.98)), but only 25 cases occurred among participants with diabetes, and was not significant after Bonferroni correction.

Results were similar when controlling for incident coronary disease, stroke, and cancer (supplementary Table 1). Association between hypertension and PE were consistent,

($HR_{hta} = 1.20$ (1.00: 1.45)), and similarly for dyslipidaemia and DVT ($HR_{dys} = 0.83$ (0.71: 0.97)) and primary VTE ($HR_{dys} = 0.68$ (0.52: 0.89)). Similarly, results were comparable when considering only cases that were validated by imaging procedures (Table 3), although the effect estimate confidence intervals were wider due to the reduced number of cases. Association between hypertension and PE were borderline, but of the same magnitude ($HR_{hta} = 1.22$ (0.95: 1.56)), and similarly for dyslipidaemia and DVT ($HR_{dys} = 0.86$ (0.71: 1.04)). Associations between dyslipidaemia and primary VTE were consistent ($HR_{dys} = 0.74$ (0.56: 0.99)), as were associations between physical activity and primary VTE ($HR_{T3} = 0.70$ (0.54: 0.90)). When mutually adjusting for comorbid conditions at baseline, results were similar to those presented in the main analysis (data not tabulated).

Table 2 Hazard ratio and 95 % confidence intervals for cardiovascular risk-factors and the risk of VTE, and VTE subtypes

	All VTE				Pulmonary embolism				Deep vein thrombosis			
	Cases	unadjusted	adjusted*	adjusted + BMI	Cases	unadjusted	adjusted*	adjusted + BMI	Cases	unadjusted	adjusted*	adjusted + BMI
physical activity T1	545	ref	ref	ref	166	ref	ref	ref	376	ref	ref	ref
physical activity T2	545	1.03 (0.91: 1.16)	1.00 (0.89: 1.12)	1.03 (0.92: 1.16)	160	1.02 (0.82: 1.26)	0.99 (0.80: 1.23)	1.04 (0.84: 1.29)	387	1.04 (0.90: 1.20)	1.01 (0.88: 1.16)	1.04 (0.90: 1.20)
physical activity T3	559	1.02 (0.90: 1.14)	0.98 (0.87: 1.10)	1.02 (0.90: 1.15)	179	0.98 (0.80: 1.21)	0.95 (0.77: 1.18)	1.01 (0.82: 1.25)	381	1.03 (0.90: 1.20)	0.99 (0.86: 1.14)	1.02 (0.89: 1.18)
Never smoker	946	ref	ref	ref	295	ref	ref	ref	652	ref	ref	ref
X smoker	557	0.97 (0.87: 1.08)	0.97 (0.87: 1.07)	0.94 (0.85: 1.05)	166	0.99 (0.82: 1.19)	0.98 (0.81: 1.18)	0.96 (0.70: 1.33)	392	0.96 (0.85: 1.09)	0.97 (0.85: 1.09)	0.95 (0.84: 1.07)
Smoker	146	0.80 (0.67: 0.95)	0.85 (0.71: 1.01)	0.87 (0.73: 1.03)	44	0.90 (0.66: 1.24)	0.93 (0.68: 1.28)	0.94 (0.78: 1.14)	100	0.76 (0.62: 0.94)	0.82 (0.67: 1.01)	0.94 (0.68: 1.03)
hypertension	827	1.21 (1.10: 1.34)	1.18 (1.07: 1.30)	1.05 (0.95: 1.16)	296	1.42 (1.18: 1.69)	1.41 (1.18: 1.69)	1.20 (0.99: 1.45)	532	1.13 (1.01: 1.27)	1.10 (0.98: 1.24)	0.99 (0.88: 1.12)
dyslipidaemia	354	0.92 (0.82: 1.03)	0.95 (0.84: 1.06)	0.90 (0.79: 1.01)	142	1.02 (0.83: 1.25)	1.05 (0.86: 1.29)	1.03 (0.84: 1.26)	212	0.84 (0.72: 0.98)	0.85 (0.73: 1.00)	0.83 (0.71: 0.97)
diabetes	36	0.98 (0.71: 1.37)	0.98 (0.71: 1.37)	0.73 (0.52: 1.02)	17	1.24 (0.76: 2.01)	1.26 (0.77: 2.04)	0.87 (0.53: 1.43)	19	0.83 (0.53: 1.31)	0.83 (0.52: 1.30)	0.63 (0.40: 1.00)

Table 2 Hazard ratio and 95 % confidence intervals for cardiovascular risk-factors and the risk of VTE, and VTE subtypes *(Continued)*

	Primary VTE				Secondary VTE			
	Cases	unadjusted	adjusted*	adjusted + BMI	Cases	unadjusted	adjusted*	adjusted + BMI
physical activity T1	163	ref	ref	ref	382	ref	ref	ref
physical activity T2	156	0.97 (0.78: 1.20)	0.95 (0.76: 1.18)	0.97 (0.78: 1.21)	389	1.06 (0.72: 1.21)	1.02 (0.89: 1.18)	1.06 (0.92: 1.22)
physical activity T3	113	0.70 (0.55: 0.89)	0.68 (0.54: 0.87)	0.71 (0.56: 0.90)	446	1.15 (1.00: 1.32)	1.10 (0.95: 1.26)	1.15 (0.99: 1.32)
Never smoker	253	ref	ref	ref	693	ref	ref	ref
X smoker	131	0.85 (0.69: 1.04)	0.86 (0.70: 1.06)	0.84 (0.68: 1.04)	426	1.02 (0.90: 1.14)	1.01 (0.89: 1.13)	0.98 (0.87: 1.11)
Smoker	48	0.91 (0.66: 1.24)	0.97 (0.71: 1.33)	0.99 (0.73: 1.36)	98	0.75 (0.61: 0.93)	0.79 (0.64: 0.98)	0.82 (0.66: 1.01)
hypertension	204	1.17 (0.97: 1.42)	1.13 (0.93: 1.38)	1.02 (0.84: 1.25)	623	1.23 (1.10: 1.38)	1.21 (1.08: 1.35)	1.06 (0.94: 1.20)
dyslipidaemia	69	0.67 (0.51: 0.88)	0.69 (0.53: 0.90)	0.68 (0.52: 0.89)	285	0.99 (0.86: 1.13)	1.00 (0.87: 1.15)	0.98 (0.85: 1.12)
diabetes	11	1.28 (0.70: 2.33)	1.24 (0.68: 2.27)	0.96 (0.52: 1.76)	25	0.89 (0.60: 1.33)	0.90 (0.61: 1.34)	0.66 (0.44: 0.98)

Table 3 Sensitivity analysis including cases occurring until 2005 which were strictly validated via mailing

	All VTE		Pulmonary embolism		DVT		Primary		Secondary	
	Cases	adjusted HR*	Cases	adjusted HR*	Cases	adjusted HR*	Cases	adjusted HR*	Cases	adjusted HR*
physical act T1	413	ref	97	ref	316	ref	154	ref	259	ref
physical activity T2	422	1.04 (0.90: 1.19)	97	1.05 (0.79: 1.39)	325	1.03 (0.88: 1.21)	148	0.97 (0.77: 1.22)	274	1.08 (0.91: 1.28)
physical activity T3	394	0.98 (0.85: 1.12)	96	1.00 (0.75: 1.33)	298	0.97 (0.83: 1.14)	107	0.70 (0.54: 0.90)	287	1.14 (0.96: 1.34)
Never smoker	721	Ref	172	ref	549	ref	241	ref	480	ref
X smoker	383	0.92 (0.82: 1.05)	88	0.93 (0.72: 1.20)	295	0.92 (0.80: 1.07)	120	0.87 (0.71: 1.09)	263	0.95 (0.82: 1.10)
smoker	125	0.89 (0.74: 1.08)	30	0.99 (0.67: 1.47)	95	0.86 (0.69: 1.07)	48	1.05 (0.77: 1.44)	77	0.81 (0.64: 1.04)
hypertension	583	1.02 (0.91: 1.15)	162	1.22 (0.95: 1.56)	421	0.97 (0.84: 1.11)	191	0.96 (0.78: 1.18)	392	1.05 (0.91: 1.22)
dyslipidaemia	189	0.86 (0.73: 1.01)	52	0.87 (0.64: 1.19)	137	0.86 (0.71: 1.04)	58	0.74 (0.56: 0.99)	131	0.93 (0.76: 1.13)
diabetes	21	0.71 (0.46: 1.11)	6	0.68 (0.30: 1.54)	15	0.73 (0.44: 1.22)	10	1.01 (0.54: 1.92)	11	0.56 (0.31: 1.03)

*adjusted on education level, statin use, menopause, MHT use, parity, type of menopause, family history of CVD and BMI

Associations between hypertension, dyslipidaemia and VTE differed slightly depending on ABO blood group (Table 4). Hypertension was associated with a higher risk of primary VTE amongst O-group participants (HR_{HTA} = 1.56 (1.07: 2.27)), and a non-significant increased risk of PE (HR_{HTA} = 1.21 (0.88: 1.68)). Dyslipidaemia was associated with a reduced risk of VTE amongst O-group participants (HR_{DYS} = 0.78 (0.63: 0.98), Table 3), with similar associations for all types of VTE (Table 4), but these associations were not consistent when considering the 'treated dyslipidaemia' variable, and showed no significant deviation from HR = 1 (not tabulated).

Discussion

In this large cohort of women, hypertension, dyslipidaemia, and diabetes were not associated with the risk of all-VTE after adjustment for BMI. We observed negative associations between physical activity and the risk of primary VTE, and potential negative associations between dyslipidaemia and primary VTE.

In this study, no evidence for associations between cardiovascular risk-factors and all-VTE was observed, or disappeared after adjustment for BMI. BMI has been identified as a major risk-factor for VTE in multiple

previous studies [12, 23–26], and confounded associations assessed in this study. BMI possibly explains previous positive associations between cardiovascular risk-factors and VTE in studies that were not adjusted for BMI. Studies of genetic variations using Mendelian randomisation provide evidence of the causal link between increased weight and VTE [27, 28]. These results suggest that people with metabolic conditions such as hypertension, diabetes and dyslipidaemia may not be at increased risk of VTE, given that they have a BMI within the healthy range.

VTE commonly presents with comorbid conditions such as endothelial dysfunction [29], and signs of atherosclerosis [30]. Prospective studies into risk factors for VTE provided conflicting results. A 2017 meta-analysis of prospective studies identified an inverse association between systolic blood pressure and VTE risk [11]. This inverse association was strongest in the highest range of systolic pressure (140–200 mmHg), but considering participants who may be approaching hypertensive crises (> 180 mmHg) may not represent the general population, and could be affected by bias due to unmeasured confounding from hypertension medications, lifestyle changes to reverse hypertension, diagnosis biases, or specific surveillance

Table 4 Hazard ratio and 95% confidence intervals for cardiovascular risk factors and specific VTE type in strata of blood ABO group for metabolic conditions

	p-interaction*	All VTE	Pulmonary Embolism	Deep vein thrombosis	Primary	Secondary
Group O						
hypertension	0.01	1.14 (0.95: 1.38)	1.21 (0.88: 1.68)	1.10 (0.88: 1.39)	1.56 (1.07: 2.27)	1.03 (0.83: 1.28)
dyslipidaemia	0.78	0.70 (0.58: 0.85)	1.10 (0.78: 1.53)	0.60 (0.44: 0.83)	0.67 (0.42: 1.09)	0.82 (0.64: 1.06)
diabetes	0.82	0.68 (0.36: 1.29)	0.55 (0.20: 1.50)	0.79 (0.35: 1.80)	1.31 (0.47: 3.66)	0.51 (0.23: 1.17)
Group non-O						
hypertension	–	0.97 (0.85: 1.11)	1.05 (0.82: 1.36)	0.95 (0.81: 1.10)	0.78 (0.60: 1.01)	1.05 (0.90: 1.23)
dyslipidaemia	–	0.78 (0.69: 0.88)	0.78 (0.63: 0.97)	0.78 (0.67: 0.90)	0.63 (0.48: 0.83)	0.83 (0.72: 0.95)
diabetes	–	0.78 (0.51: 1.18)	1.19 (0.66: 2.15)	0.56 (0.31: 1.01)	1.02 (0.47: 2.19)	0.71 (0.43: 1.16)

* interaction with all-VTE
* adjusted on education level, statin use, menopause, MHT use, parity, type of menopause, family history of CVD and BMI

for cardiovascular conditions. Another meta-analysis in 2016 of prospective and case-control studies has indicated that hypertension is associated with an increased risk for VTE compared to non-hypertensive subjects [31]. In the Nurses' Health Study [32], hypertension was identified as a risk factor for VTE, with a relative risk of 1.9; however, hypertension was not identified as risk factor in the Framingham Heart Study [33]. Our study of French women observed no associations between hypertension and all-VTE, but a weak association between hypertension and PE was identified. It is possible that these results could be explained by uncontrolled confounding from conditions such as pulmonary disease (or other respiratory conditions), which could be associated with both hypertension [34], and the risk of PE [35]. Similarly, isolated PE has been associated with a higher risk of arterial thrombotic events [36], which could possibly be explained by underlying hypertension among people with PE as reported in our results.

Previous studies have mostly shown that neither diabetes nor dyslipidaemia are associated with the risk of VTE [24, 26, 37]. The LITE study identified a slightly increased risk of VTE amongst participants with diabetes (HR = 1.5 (95% CI: 1.0–2.1)) [25]. One meta-analysis [38] of 19 prospective cohort and case control studies found a weak positive, but non-significant association between diabetes and VTE risk (HR = 1.10 (95% CI: 0.94–1.29)). The authors conclude that diabetes is unlikely to play a major role in VTE development, which our study supports. We were however limited by the number of cases which occurred amongst diabetic women, and the relatively low number of diabetic women in the cohort.

We observed a weak association between dyslipidaemia and the risk of primary VTE. Despite controlling for statins, it is possible that this relationship could be confounded by treatment for dyslipidaemia other than statins, or for behavioural changes provoked by a diagnosis of dyslipidaemia. These associations were not consistent when considering self-reported dyslipidaemia cross-referenced with statin reimbursement. Interestingly Wattanakit et al. [12] also observed a weak negative association between high concentrations of LDL-C, and all VTE (HR $_{LDL > 160}$ = 0.73 (0.54: 0.98)), and the UK biobank study observed inverse associations between apolipoprotein B, lipoprotein(a), and the risk of VTE [9]. Further research should be conducted to further understand these observations, which could possibly be resulting from bias after adjusting on an intermediate variable during follow-up, or due to time-varying confounding which may not be appropriately controlled for under the modelling strategy used [39]. It is unclear whether any independent protective effect from statins exists, despite Rovustatin having been shown to reduce the likelihood of VTE in a large RCT [40]. Statins are theorised to

reduce the risk of VTE through mechanisms independent to the lowering of LDL-C [41], such as increased anticoagulant activity. Elevated or oxidised low density lipoprotein (LDL) can promote thrombin formation [42], thus an imbalance in lipids may result in a hypercoagulative state.

In this study, we observed no association between smoking, and the risk of VTE. This is in opposition to previous studies [43, 44] including the large UK biobank study that observed convincing associations between smoking and the risk of VTE [9]. A previous meta-analysis [7] of 32 observational studies has shown that smoking is associated with an increased risk of VTE, with a risk ratio of 1.19 as well as linear responses from pack-years and cigarettes per day. We were unable to reproduce this observation perhaps due to the low number of smokers in this cohort, and that many participants quit smoking during follow-up. It is also possible that the effect of smoking could be mediated, or masked, by a lower BMI among smokers.

Total physical activity as estimated by METS was not associated with the overall risk of VTE, although the highest levels of physical activity were associated with a reduced risk of primary VTE. Previous prospective studies have shown similar results regarding all VTE, and data from the Nurses' Health Study [45] have shown that time spent inactive (but not total physical activity) is associated with an increased risk of pulmonary embolism. Physical activity could reduce the risk of VTE by improving circulation and the quality of blood-vessels, and lowering the likelihood of blood stagnation in the lower extremities which can lead to deep vein thrombosis. It is possible that time spent stationary could be a more important predictor of VTE than total physical activity.

Regarding ABO group, associations between hypertension and primary VTE were higher within the O group. The AB blood group is associated with an increased risk for VTE, through increased von Willebrand factor (VWF) [46]. Hypertension is also associated with increased VWF concentrations [47], and the O-group is associated with higher rates of hypertension [19]. It is possible that patients with O blood group and hypertension have similar VWF levels as patients with AB blood group and no hypertension, and that further increases in VWF in AB/hypertensive cases are limited. It is less clear why dyslipidaemia appeared associated with a reduced risk only amongst O-group participants, and these observations may have occurred by chance as the p-values were non-significant.

Strengths and limitations
This study has a number of strengths, notably a long follow-up, large number of participants and cases, control for a large set of potential confounders, detailed

reporting on the type of VTE, and a validation procedure used for all cases. Exposures of metabolic conditions were verified against specific treatment reimbursements. Regarding hypertension and diabetes, self-reported hypertension showed strong correlation with reimbursements for blood-pressure lowering medications, and diabetes cases were validated via a specific questionnaire. Measured blood pressure values, and cholesterol values were not available for the majority of study participants, thus it was not possible to determine if there is some non-linear relationship between blood-pressure levels/serum cholesterol and the risk of VTE. The dichotomisation of these variables should be considered a major limitation of the current approach.

As later VTE cases were based on self-reports verified by drug reimbursement, it is possible that a number of cases were misdiagnosed, or that cases were missed. Regarding DVT, it is possible that misclassification between superficial and deep thrombosis could occur. Baseline dyslipidaemia cases were based on self-reports, but later cases were verified by treatment reimbursements in secondary analysis. Smoking data was based on self-reports, and included a low number of current smokers, resulting in a lower statistical power to investigate associations among smokers. Similarly, physical activity data was based on self-report and may be subject to error. However, these data were assessed prior to the VTE event, and any error should be independent of the event.

A major strength is the consideration of risk-factors as time dependent variables, as a large number of participants developed hypertension and dyslipidaemia during follow up. However, this method can also introduce bias, through the inclusion of time-varying covariates or potential mediators in the model [39, 48]. Future studies should address this limitation using g-methods [49], which can take into account time-varying confounding without potentially introducing bias from time-varying covariates. Due to this possibility, models considering only baseline data were considered in sensitivity analysis, and showed no major differences. Limitations include the lack of data on medications at study baseline, and the fact that later cases of VTE were validated only via drug reimbursements, and not on information from imaging procedures. Reassuringly, we did observe similar results when only considering cases strictly validated via specific mailings to medical practitioners. The E3N cohort is rather homogenous, and the majority of participants are at a low-risk of non-communicable diseases such as VTE, and cardiovascular disease, thus it is unclear how these observations may translate to higher-risk populations.

As treatments for hypertension, diabetes, and dyslipidaemia are commonly long-term [50], we are confident that these exposures are true representations of these metabolic conditions. Although these conditions are potentially reversible with weight loss and changes in the diet, this would be hard to verify. It is possible that some residual confounding from other lifestyle factors could drive some of the associations observed, especially for the negative associations between dyslipidaemia and primary VTE. The modelling approach chosen, i.e. not mutually adjusting for all considered risk-factors reduces the likelihood of including mediators as in the model, which could introduce collider bias (for example baseline physical activity may influence the future risk of hypertension). Unmeasured confounding is another major concern. For example, certain auto-immune conditions such as rheumatoid arteritis are associated with hypertension [51], and with the risk of VTE [52]. Assuming that these types of conditions can cause hypertension, then associations between hypertension and VTE may be positively biased, which could potentially explain the observations between hypertension and PA. However as these conditions are relatively rare in the general population, we believe that this is a low risk of bias. Similarly, medications that can provoke VTE were unadjusted for, but unless they are causally related to the considered exposures and the thrombotic events, then they should not majorly bias the results. The lack of control for factors such as these is a common limitation in many previous cohort studies of VTE [12, 25].

Conclusion

Altogether these results suggest that the common risk-factors for CVD are not risk factors for VTE. Regular physical activity may reduce the risk of primary VTE. We confirm previous observations linking dyslipidaemia to a reduced risk of VTE, which should be investigated in future studies. People with metabolic conditions, but with a healthy BMI may not be at higher risk of VTE.

Abbreviations
CVD: Cardiovascular disease; VTE: venous thromboembolism; PE: pulmonary embolism; DVT: deep vein thrombosis; E3N: Etude Epidémiologique auprès de femmes de la Mutuelle Générale de l'Education Nationale; MGEN: Mutuelle Générale de l'Education Nationale; MHT: menopausal hormone therapy; BMI: body mass index

Acknowledgements
We gratefully acknowledge the contribution of all the participants in the E3N study for their diligence and their answers. The authors have no conflicts of interest to declare.

Authors' contributions

C J MacDonald – study design, conducting research, writing. AL Madika – conducting research, writing, approval of final draft. M Lajous - study design, conducting research, writing, approval of final draft. M Canonico – study design, approval of final draft. A Fournier – study design, approval of final draft. MC Boutron-Ruault – supervision, approval of final draft.

Author details

[1]INSERM (Institut National de la Santé et de la Recherche Médicale) U1018, Center for Research in Epidemiology and Population Health (CESP), Institut Gustave Roussy, Villejuif, France. [2]Université Paris-Saclay, Université Paris-Sud, Villejuif, France. [3]Université de Lille, CHU Lille, EA 2694 - Santé publique : épidémiologie et qualité des soins, F-59000 Lille, France. [4]Center for Research on Population Health, INSP (Instituto Nacional de Salud Pública), Cuernavaca, Mexico. [5]Department of Global Health and Population, Harvard T.H. Chan School of Public Health, Boston, MA, USA.

References

1. Cohen AT, Agnelli G, Anderson FA, Arcelus JI, Bergqvist D, Brecht JG, Greer IA, Heit JA, Hutchinson JL, Kakkar AK, Mottier D, Oger E, Samama M-M, Spannagl M, VTE Impact Assessment Group in Europe (VITAE). Venous thromboembolism (VTE) in Europe. The number of VTE events and associated morbidity and mortality. Thromb Haemost. 2007;98:756–764.

2. Raskob GE, Angchaisuksiri P, Blanco AN, Buller H, Gallus A, Hunt BJ, et al. Thrombosis: a major contributor to global disease burden. Arterioscler Thromb Vasc Biol. 2014;34(11):2363–71. https://doi.org/10.1161/ATVBAHA.114.304488.

3. Lijfering WM, Rosendaal FR, Cannegieter SC. Risk factors for venous thrombosis - current understanding from an epidemiological point of view: review. Br J Haematol. 2010;149(6):824–33. https://doi.org/10.1111/j.1365-2141.2010.08206.x.

4. Ay C, Pabinger I, Cohen AT. Cancer-associated venous thromboembolism: burden, mechanisms, and management. Thromb Haemost. 2017;117(2):219–30. https://doi.org/10.1160/TH16-08-0615.

5. Heit JA. Epidemiology of venous thromboembolism. Nat Rev Cardiol. 2015; 12(8):464–74. https://doi.org/10.1038/nrcardio.2015.83.

6. Ageno W, Becattini C, Brighton T, Selby R, Kamphuisen PW. Cardiovascular risk factors and venous thromboembolism: a Meta-analysis. Circulation. 2008;117(1):93–102. https://doi.org/10.1161/CIRCULATIONAHA.107.709204.

7. Cheng Y-J, Liu Z-H, Yao F-J, Zeng W-T, Zheng D-D, Dong YG, et al. Current and Former Smoking and Risk for Venous Thromboembolism: A Systematic Review and Meta-Analysis. PLoS Med. 2013;10:e1001515.

8. Holst AG, Jensen G, Prescott E. Risk factors for venous thromboembolism: results from the Copenhagen City heart study. Circulation. 2010;121(17): 1896–903. https://doi.org/10.1161/CIRCULATIONAHA.109.921460.

9. Gregson J, Kaptoge S, Bolton T, Pennells L, Willeit P, Burgess S, et al. Cardiovascular Risk Factors Associated With Venous Thromboembolism. JAMA Cardiol. 2019;4:163.

10. Zhang Y, Yang Y, Chen W, Liang L, Zhai Z, Guo L, et al. Hypertension associated with venous thromboembolism in patients with newly diagnosed lung cancer. Sci Rep. 2016;6:19603.

11. Mahmoodi BK, Cushman M, Anne Næss I, Allison MA, Bos WJ, Bråekkan SK, et al. Association of Traditional Cardiovascular Risk Factors With Venous Thromboembolism: An Individual Participant Data Meta-Analysis of Prospective Studies. Circulation. 2017;135:7–16.

12. Wattanakit K, Lutsey PL, Bell EJ, Gornik H, Cushman M, Heckbert SR, et al. Association between cardiovascular disease risk factors and occurrence of venous thromboembolism. A time-dependent analysis. Thromb Haemost. 2012;108(3):508–15. https://doi.org/10.1160/TH11-10-0726.

13. van Liere MJ, Giubout C, Niravong MY, Goulard H, Corre CL, Hoang LA, et al. E3N, a French cohort study on cancer risk factors. European Journal of Cancer Prevention. 1997;6:473–8.

14. Canonico M, Fournier A, Carcaillon L, Olié V, Plu-Bureau G, Oger E, et al. Postmenopausal hormone therapy and risk of idiopathic venous thromboembolism: results from the E3N cohort study. ATVB. 2010;30(2):340–5. https://doi.org/10.1161/ATVBAHA.109.196022.

15. Fagherazzi G, Vilier A, Bonnet F, Lajous M, Balkau B, Boutron-Ruault M-C, et al. Dietary acid load and risk of type 2 diabetes: the E3N-EPIC cohort study. Diabetologia. 2014;57(2):313–20. https://doi.org/10.1007/s00125-013-3100-0.

16. Ainsworth BE, Haskell WL, Whitt MC, Irwin ML, Swartz AM, Strath SJ, et al. Compendium of Physical Activities: an update of activity codes and MET intensities. Medicine & Science in Sports Exercise. 2000;32:S498–516.

17. Tehard B, Liere MJV, Nougué CC, Clavel-Chapelon F. Anthropometric measurements and body Silhouette of women. J Am Diet Assoc. 2002; 102(12):1779–84. https://doi.org/10.1016/S0002-8223(02)90381-0.

18. Langman MJS, Foote J, Elwood PC, Ryrie DR. Abo and LEWIS blood-groups and serum-cholesterol. Lancet. 1969;294(7621):607–9. https://doi.org/10.1016/S0140-6736(69)90323-7.

19. Groot HE, Villegas Sierra LE, Said MA, Lipsic E, Karper JC, van der Harst P. Genetically determined ABO blood group and its associations with health and disease. ATVB. 2020;40(3):830–8. https://doi.org/10.1161/ATVBAHA.119.313658.

20. Fagherazzi G, Gusto G, Clavel-Chapelon F, Balkau B, Bonnet F. ABO and Rhesus blood groups and risk of type 2 diabetes: evidence from the large E3N cohort study. Diabetologia. 2015;58(3):519–22. https://doi.org/10.1007/s00125-014-3472-9.

21. Larson NB, Bell EJ, Decker PA, Pike M, Wassel CL, Tsai MY, et al. ABO blood group associations with markers of endothelial dysfunction in the multi-ethnic study of atherosclerosis. Atherosclerosis. 2016;251:422–9. https://doi.org/10.1016/j.atherosclerosis.2016.05.049.

22. Grambsch PM, Therneau TM. Proportional hazards tests and diagnostics based on weighted residuals. Biometrika. 1994;81(3):515–26. https://doi.org/10.1093/biomet/81.3.515.

23. Kabrhel C, Varraso R, Goldhaber SZ, Rimm EB, Camargo CA. Prospective study of BMI and the risk of pulmonary embolism in women. Obesity. 2009; 17(11):2040–6. https://doi.org/10.1038/oby.2009.92.

24. Glynn RJ, Rosner B. Comparison of risk factors for the competing risks of coronary heart disease, stroke, and venous thromboembolism. Am J Epidemiol. 2005;162(10):975–82. https://doi.org/10.1093/aje/kwi309.

25. Tsai AW, Cushman M, Rosamond WD, Heckbert SR, Polak JF, Folsom AR. Cardiovascular risk factors and venous thromboembolism incidence: the longitudinal investigation of thromboembolism etiology. Arch Intern Med. 2002;162(10):1182–9. https://doi.org/10.1001/archinte.162.10.1182.

26. Bræekkan SK, Hald EM, Mathiesen EB, Njølstad I, Wilsgaard T, Rosendaal FR, et al. Competing risk of atherosclerotic risk factors for arterial and venous thrombosis in a general population: the Tromsø study. Arterioscler Thromb Vasc Biol. 2012;32(2):487–91. https://doi.org/10.1161/ATVBAHA.111.237545.

27. Klovaite J, Benn M, Nordestgaard BG. Obesity as a causal risk factor for deep venous thrombosis: a Mendelian randomization study. J Intern Med. 2015; 277(5):573–84. https://doi.org/10.1111/joim.12299.

28. Lindström S, Germain M, Crous-Bou M, Smith EN, Morange P-E, van Hylckama VA, et al. Assessing the causal relationship between obesity and venous thromboembolism through a Mendelian randomization study. Hum Genet. 2017;136(7):897–902. https://doi.org/10.1007/s00439-017-1811-x.

29. Poredos P, Jezovnik MK. Endothelial dysfunction and venous thrombosis. Angiology. 2018;69(7):564–7. https://doi.org/10.1177/0003319717732238.

30. Prandoni P, Bilora F, Marchiori A, Bernardi E, Petrobelli F, Lensing AWA, et al. An association between atherosclerosis and venous thrombosis. N Engl J Med. 2003;348(15):1435–41. https://doi.org/10.1056/NEJMoa022157.

31. Mi Y, Yan S, Lu Y, Liang Y, Li C. Venous thromboembolism has the same risk factors as atherosclerosis: a PRISMA-compliant systemic review and meta-analysis. Medicine. 2016;95(32):e4495. https://doi.org/10.1097/MD.0000000000004495.

32. Goldhaber SZ, Grodstein F, Stampfer MJ, Manson JE, Colditz GA, Speizer FE, et al. A prospective study of risk factors for pulmonary embolism in women. JAMA. 1997;277(8):642–5. https://doi.org/10.1001/jama.1997.03540320044033.

33. Puurunen MK, Gona PN, Larson MG, Murabito JM, Magnani JW, O'Donnell CJ. Epidemiology of venous thromboembolism in the Framingham heart study. Thromb Res. 2016;145:27–33. https://doi.org/10.1016/j.thromres.2016.06.033.

34. Kim S-H, Park J-H, Lee J-K, Heo EY, Kim DK, Chung HS. Chronic obstructive pulmonary disease is independently associated with hypertension in men: A survey design analysis using nationwide survey data. Medicine (Baltimore). 2017;96:e6826.

35. de Miguel Diez J, Albaladejo-Vicente R, Jiménez-García R, Hernandez-Barrera V, Villanueva-Orbaiz R, Carabantes-Alarcon D, et al. The effect of COPD on the incidence and mortality of hospitalized patients with pulmonary embolism: A nationwide population-based study (2016–2018). Eur J Intern Med. 2021;84:18–23.

36. ten Cate V, Eggebrecht L, Schulz A, Panova-Noeva M, Lenz M, Koeck T, et al. Isolated pulmonary embolism is associated with a high risk of arterial thrombotic disease. Chest. 2020;158(1):341–9. https://doi.org/10.1016/j.chest.2020.01.055.

37. Quist-Paulsen P, Naess IA, Cannegieter SC, Romundstad PR, Christiansen SC, Rosendaal FR, et al. Arterial cardiovascular risk factors and venous thrombosis: results from a population-based, prospective study (the HUNT 2). Haematologica. 2010;95(1):119–25. https://doi.org/10.3324/haematol.2009.011866.

38. Bell EJ, Folsom AR, Lutsey PL, Selvin E, Zakai NA, Cushman M, et al. Diabetes mellitus and venous thromboembolism: a systematic review and meta-analysis. Diabetes Res Clin Pract. 2016;111:10–8. https://doi.org/10.1016/j.diabres.2015.10.019.

39. Doosti-Irani A, Mansournia MA, Collins G. Use of G-methods for handling time-varying confounding in observational research. Lancet Glob Health. 2019;7(1):e35. https://doi.org/10.1016/S2214-109X(18)30471-6.

40. Glynn RJ, Danielson E, Fonseca FAH, Genest J, Gotto AM, Kastelein JJP, et al. A randomized trial of rosuvastatin in the prevention of venous thromboembolism. N Engl J Med. 2009;360(18):1851–61. https://doi.org/10.1056/NEJMoa0900241.

41. Zaccardi F, Kunutsor SK, Seidu S, Davies MJ, Khunti K. Is the lower risk of venous thromboembolism with statins related to low-density-lipoprotein reduction? A network meta-analysis and meta-regression of randomised controlled trials. Atherosclerosis. 2018;271:223–31. https://doi.org/10.1016/j.atherosclerosis.2018.02.035.

42. Griffin J, Fernández J, Deguchi H. Plasma Lipoproteins. Hemostasis and Thrombosis Thromb Haemost. 2001;86(1):386–94.

43. Lutsey PL, Virnig BA, Durham SB, Steffen LM, Hirsch AT, Jacobs DR, et al. Correlates and consequences of venous thromboembolism: the Iowa Women's health study. Am J Public Health. 2010;100(8):1506–13. https://doi.org/10.2105/AJPH.2008.157776.

44. Enga KF, Braekkan SK, Hansen-Krone IJ, le Cessie S, Rosendaal FR, Hansen J-B. Cigarette smoking and the risk of venous thromboembolism: the Tromsø study. J Thromb Haemost. 2012;10(10):2068–74. https://doi.org/10.1111/j.1538-7836.2012.04880.x.

45. Kabrhel C, Varraso R, Goldhaber SZ, Rimm E, Camargo CA. Physical inactivity and idiopathic pulmonary embolism in women: prospective study. BMJ. 2011;343(jul04 1):d3867. https://doi.org/10.1136/bmj.d3867.

46. Brill A, Fuchs TA, Chauhan AK, Yang JJ, De Meyer SF, Köllnberger M, et al. von Willebrand factor–mediated platelet adhesion is critical for deep vein thrombosis in mouse models. Blood. 2011;117(4):1400–7. https://doi.org/10.1182/blood-2010-05-287623.

47. van den Born B-JH, van der Hoeven NV, Groot E, Lenting PJ, Meijers JCM, Levi M, et al. Association between thrombotic microangiopathy and reduced ADAMTS13 activity in malignant hypertension. Hypertension. 2008;51(4):862–6. https://doi.org/10.1161/HYPERTENSIONAHA.107.103127.

48. Robins JM. Causal models for estimating the effects of weight gain on mortality. Int J Obes. 2008;32(Suppl 3):S15–41. https://doi.org/10.1038/ijo.2008.83.

49. Naimi AI, Cole SR, Kennedy EH. An introduction to g methods. Int J Epidemiol. 2017;46(2):756–62. https://doi.org/10.1093/ije/dyw323.

50. Cubeddu LX, Seamon MJ. Statin withdrawal: clinical implications and molecular mechanisms. Pharmacotherapy. 2006;26(9):1288–96. https://doi.org/10.1592/phco.26.9.1288.

51. Panoulas VF, Metsios GS, Pace AV, John H, Treharne GJ, Banks MJ, et al. Hypertension in rheumatoid arthritis. Rheumatology. 2008;47(9):1286–98. https://doi.org/10.1093/rheumatology/ken159.

52. Li L, Lu N, Avina-Galindo AM, Zheng Y, Lacaille D, Esdaile JM, et al. The risk and trend of pulmonary embolism and deep vein thrombosis in rheumatoid arthritis: a general population-based study. Rheumatology (Oxford). 2021;60:188–95.

10

Successful venous thromboprophylaxis in a patient with vaccine-induced immune thrombotic thrombocytopenia (VITT)

Archrob Khuhapinant, Tarinee Rungjirajittranon, Bundarika Suwanawiboon, Yingyong Chinthammitr and Theera Ruchutrakool* ⓘ

Abstract

Background: Vaccine-induced immune thrombotic thrombocytopenia (VITT) is a rare but fatal complication of the Coronavirus Disease 2019 vaccine. The many reports of VITT have mostly been in the Caucasian population. Here, we present the first reported case in an Asian population.

Case presentation: A 26-year-old female had severe headache and severe thrombocytopenia 8 days after administration of the ChAdOx1 nCoV-19 vaccine developed by AstraZeneca. Although no thrombosis was demonstrated by imaging studies, she had very highly elevated d-dimer levels during hospitalization. Serology for antibodies against platelet factor 4 was positive on several days with very high optical density readings. We found that the antibody could induce spontaneous platelet aggregation without the presence of heparin. We decided to treat her with intravenous immunoglobulin, high-dose dexamethasone, and a prophylactic dose of apixaban. She improved rapidly and was discharged from the hospital 6 days after admission. Neither thrombocytopenia nor thrombosis was subsequently detected at the three-week follow-up.

Conclusions: Despite the lower rate of thrombosis, VITT can occur in the Asian population. Early detection and prompt treatment of VITT can improve the patient's clinical outcome. Thromboprophylaxis with nonheparin anticoagulants also prevents clot formation.

Keywords: COVID-19 vaccine, Thrombocytopenia, Thrombosis, Vaccine-induced immune thrombotic thrombocytopenia

Background

The Coronavirus Disease 2019 (COVID-19) pandemic has affected health and economic systems globally. Shortly after the first case series was reported in China in December 2019 [1], the number of new cases increased exponentially. COVID-19 is a serious infectious disease with a high mortality rate of up to 2% among infected patients [2]. Although the disease can be controlled by social distancing and wearing masks and face shields, immunization with a vaccine against severe acute respiratory syndrome coronavirus 2 (SARS-CoV-2) should be the method of choice to combat the COVID-19 pandemic. Four different types of vaccines are currently available [3], and vaccination was started in March 2021, with most adverse event reports indicating minor side effects. However, several groups of people receiving

* Correspondence: truchutrakool@gmail.com
Division of Hematology, Department of Medicine, Faculty of Medicine Siriraj Hospital, Mahidol University, 2 Wanglang Road, Bangkok Noi, Bangkok 10700, Thailand

the ChAdOx1 nCoV-19 vaccine, an engineered nonreplicating viral vector vaccine using an adenovirus developed by AstraZeneca, developed a vaccine type-specific complication named vaccine-induced immune thrombotic thrombocytopenia (VITT). Patients usually develop thrombocytopenia and thrombosis [4–6] within 4–28 days after the first dose of vaccine [4–6]. Most of the cases were among young and previously healthy females [4–6]. Up to 38–80% of reported cases had severe thrombosis in the venous sinus system of the brain [4–6]. The mortality rate of VITT was high and reached 18% (71 of 390) in the United Kingdom, the country with the highest number of reported cases in the world [7]. Although the association between adenovirus viral vector vaccines and thrombocytopenia along with thrombosis is uncertain, it is believed that certain components of the vaccine could induce platelet aggregation and cause thrombocytopenia, eventually leading to thrombosis [6]. Moreover, it has been assumed that the mechanisms of VITT and autoimmune/spontaneous heparin-induced thrombocytopenia/thrombosis (HIT/T) are similar [6]. Although VITT has been mostly reported in the Caucasian population, there have been no reports in an Asian population receiving this type of vaccine. In Thailand, the vaccination program for COVID-19 was launched in May 2021, and mass vaccination with the ChAdOx1 nCoV-19 vaccine developed by AstraZeneca has been gradually rolled out to the Thai population since June 2021. Shortly after the start of this roll out, the first patient with VITT in Thailand presented to our institution.

Case presentation

A 26-year-old female presented with severe headache for 5 days. She had been previously healthy without comorbidities 8 days earlier when she had been scheduled for the first dose of ChAdOx1 nCoV-19 vaccine (AstraZeneca) vaccination. She had no adverse events following immunization until 3 days later, when she developed a severe headache. She did not report any fever, myalgia, blurred vision, nausea, or vomiting. Her headache was not improved by acetaminophen and mefenamic acid. One day prior to admission, she noticed multiple discrete reddish spots on both legs without bleeding gums or epistaxis. On examination, mildly pale conjunctiva and petechiae on both legs were noted, while other examinations were unremarkable. The initial complete blood count showed a hemoglobin of 9.7 g/dL, mean corpuscular volume of 71.5 fL, white blood cell count of 3.66×10^9/L (neutrophil 75%, lymphocyte 18%, monocyte 4.7%, eosinophil 2% basophil 0.3%), and platelet count of 22×10^9/L. The prothrombin time was 11.9 s (normal range, 9.8–12.9 s), the activated partial thromboplastin time was 25.8 s (normal range, 21.8–30.2 s), and the fibrinogen level was 173.8 mg/dL. D-dimer was 9452 ng/mL (normal d-dimer, < 500 ng/mL). NS-1 antigen, dengue IgM, and IgG serologic testing for the diagnosis of dengue hemorrhagic fever were negative. SARS-CoV2 RNA test was negative. Lupus anticoagulants, anticardiolipin IgM, IgG, and anti-β_2 glycoprotein I IgM and IgG were negative. Magnetic resonance imaging, angiography, and venography of the brain were normal without evidence of thrombosis. Computed tomography angiography of the pulmonary arteries showed no pulmonary embolism, and computed tomography of the abdomen was unremarkable.

Due to the high degree of suspicion of VITT, we performed a test for antibody against platelet factor 4 (PF4) by enzyme-linked immunosorbent assay-based assay (Zymutest HIA IgG, HYPHEN BioMed, Neuville-sur-Oise, France), and the result was positive with an optical density (OD) of 2.10 (normal OD, < 0.4) (Fig. 1). After we added heparin at a concentration of 100 units/mL, the OD was lower at 0.09 (Fig. 1). We then demonstrated a functional test of antibodies by a heparin-induced platelet aggregation (HIPA) test. Platelet-rich plasma from a healthy volunteer with blood Group O was incubated with the patient's serum for 1 h. Low doses (0.1 and 0.5 unit/mL) and a high dose (100 units/mL) of heparin and normal saline were added to the mixture. Platelet aggregation was assessed by light transmission (AggRAM Analyzer®, Helena Laboratories, Beaumont, Texas). After adding 0.1 and 0.5 units of heparin for final concentrations, 31.8 and 46% platelet aggregation was detected, respectively. After adding high-dose heparin (100 units of heparin for final concentration), platelet aggregation was 15.9%. Interestingly, spontaneous aggregation (30% aggregation) was found after saline was added instead of heparin (Table 1). After discussion with the patient, we promptly started treatment with 2 days (Day 1- Day 2 of hospital admission) of 1 g/kg intravenous immunoglobulin (IVIG) infusion and dexamethasone 40 mg per day for 4 days (Day 1- Day 4 of hospital admission). Apixaban was given to the patient beginning on Day 1 of hospital admission, and we planned to extend it for a total of 3 months. Despite a low platelet count, we were strongly against platelet transfusion, which may have worsened any thrombosis in the patient. We opted to monitor thrombus formation at the d-dimer level because we did not find evidence of thrombosis by imaging studies, and the d-dimer level gradually decreased during the hospital course after treatment (Fig. 2). After 6 days of IVIG and dexamethasone treatment, the platelet count slowly increased to 97×10^9/L (Fig. 2). The patient's symptoms improved, and she was discharged from the hospital on Day 6. At the three-week follow-up, her platelet count was 134×10^9/L (Fig. 2), and no clinical thrombosis was detected while she was taking 5 mg per day of apixaban.

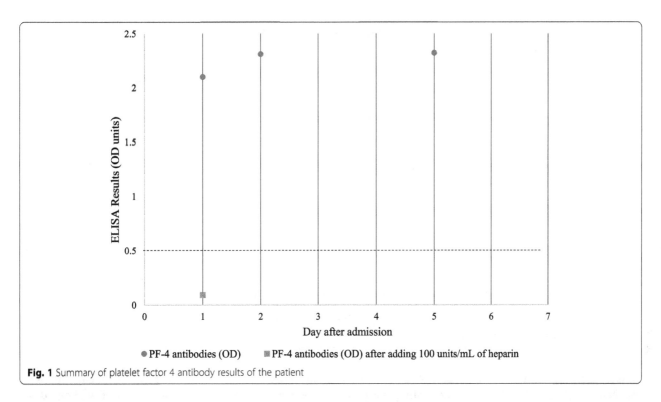

Fig. 1 Summary of platelet factor 4 antibody results of the patient

Because our patient had a serious adverse event and it was a reaction to a COVID-19 vaccine, we reported our case to the National Immunization Center of the Thai Ministry of Public Health. Currently, there are three reporting systems in Thailand: the AEFI (Adverse Events Following Immunization) surveillance system, which is a passive surveillance system reported to by medical personnel; the Active Surveillance System for COVID-19 Vaccine, which is an active surveillance system reported to by vaccine receivers; and the Adverse Event of Special Interest (AESI), which is a passive surveillance system reported to by specialists in university hospitals. Reported adverse events from these three systems are sent to the National Immunization Center of the Thai Ministry of Public Health.

Discussion

Since the first three independent reports of case series were published in April 2021, the number of patients

Table 1 Heparin-induce platelet aggregation results of the patient

Heparin for final concentration, units/mL	Platelet aggregation, %		
	D0	D1	D4
0.1	31.8	18.7	16.8
0.5	46.0	20.4	15.3
100	15.9	19.2	18.7
Saline	30.0	16.0	6.9

Abbreviations: *D#* Day after admission

diagnosed with VITT associated with the ChAdOx1 nCoV-19 vaccine developed by AstraZeneca has grown and continues to grow [4–6]. The Ad26.COV2.S vaccine, developed by Johnson and Johnson with similar adenovirus viral vector technology, was also reported to induce thrombocytopenia and thrombosis in the United States [8]. The ChAdOx1 nCoV-19 vaccine is a WHO-approved vaccine against SAR-CoV-2 and is widely used in Thailand. After the mass vaccination campaign was launched in May 2021, approximately two million doses of the ChAdOx1 nCoV-19 vaccine were administered. Thus, the incidence rate of VITT in the Thai population is approximately one in two million vaccinations, which is much lower than that reported in Caucasian populations [9]. There are several possible explanations for the lower incidence of VITT in the Thai population. First, Asian ethnicity is widely recognized to be associated with fewer thrombotic events than Caucasian ethnicity [10]. This could be due to a lower rate of inherited thrombophilia, such as prothrombin G20210A mutation or Factor V Leiden in Asian ethnicity [11], and Asian people requiring lower doses of warfarin treatment might imply an antithrombotic tendency [12]. Second, many reported cases of VITT had concomitant risks for thrombosis, such as antiphospholipid syndrome or oral contraceptive pill usage, which was not found in our patient.

Most patients with VITT present with an unusual site of thrombosis, such as the cerebral venous sinus or the splanchnic vein, with concomitant severe thrombocytopenia

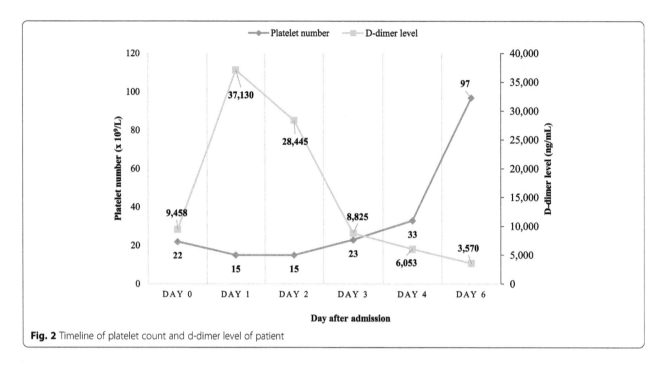

Fig. 2 Timeline of platelet count and d-dimer level of patient

[4–6, 8]. The onset of VITT is usually 4–28 days after vaccination [4–6, 8]. Although the pathogenesis of VITT is uncertain, there have been many laboratory findings supporting the hypothesis that the mechanism of thrombocytopenia and thrombosis is similar to that of autoimmune HIT/T in that the anti-PF4 antibody may be induced by polyanions, including lipid A, in bacterial surface nucleic acids instead of heparin [13]. For VITT, some components of the vaccine, for example, the adenovirus DNA, spike protein, and/or neoantigen induced by the vaccine, have been proposed to be key components that could induce PF4 release and anti-PF4 antibody production [14].

To the best of our knowledge, our patient is the first reported case of VITT in an Asian population, and she had severe thrombocytopenia 8 days after ChAdOx1 nCoV-19 vaccine administration. Pathologic anti-PF4 antibody was demonstrated by high OD and subsequently confirmed by functional HIPA test. Although most VITT cases developed thrombosis, as demonstrated by either clinical features or imaging studies, our patient did not have thrombosis after extensive investigations for occult clots. This might have been due to the high degree of suspicion and the early detection of VITT because some patients with VITT who come to the hospital early may not have clinical thrombosis despite having a high level of d-dimer detected [15]. Although a rare side effect of immunoglobulin is thrombosis, IVIG is still an essential treatment to slow the progression of this disease [16]. Immediate treatment with IVIG can decelerate the progression of the immune reaction and accelerate the recovery of the platelet count [17]. Many

guidelines also recommend starting treatment with IVIG in every case that is suspected of VITT without delay [18–20]. With lessons learned from our patient, we strongly support the use of anticoagulants other than heparin to prevent clot formation. Furthermore, the d-dimer level can be used to monitor thrombosis progression. Prophylactic anticoagulant for a duration of 3 months is recommended in patients with VITT [20].

Conclusions

Our case report highlights that VITT can occur in Asian populations. Prompt treatment with IVIG, dexamethasone, and prophylactic anticoagulants can improve the patient's outcome. More research data, especially about the risk factors and pathogenesis of the syndrome, are needed to encourage patients to be vaccinated confidently.

Abbreviations
COVID-19: Coronavirus Disease 2019; HIPA: Heparin-induced platelet aggregation; HIT/T: Heparin-induced thrombocytopenia/thrombosis; IVIG: Intravenous immunoglobulin; OD: Optical density; PF4: Platelet Factor 4; VITT: Vaccine-induced immune thrombotic thrombocytopenia; SARS-CoV-2: Severe Acute Respiratory Syndrome Coronavirus 2

Acknowledgments
The authors are grateful to Ms. Suthirak Sitaposa, Ms. Tussnem Binhama, and Mrs. Yupa Nakkinkun for their laboratory technical support. We would like to thank Mr. Anthony Tan for editing the manuscript for English language.

Authors' contributions
AK collected and provided all patient data and imaging. TR1 and TR2 drafted the manuscript. TR2 made critical revisions to the manuscript. All authors read and approved the final manuscript.

References

1. Huang C, Wang Y, Li X, Ren L, Zhao J, Hu Y, et al. Clinical features of patients infected with 2019 novel coronavirus in Wuhan. China Lancet. 2020;395(10223):497–506. https://doi.org/10.1016/S0140-6736(20)30183-5.

2. Coronavirus (COVID-19) Mortality Rate. https://www.worldometers.info/coronavirus/coronavirus-death-rate/. Accessed 20 June 2021.

3. Forni G, Mantovani A, Forni G, Mantovani A, Moretta L, Rappuoli R, et al. COVID-19 vaccines: where we stand and challenges ahead. Cell Death Differ. 2021;28(2):626–39. https://doi.org/10.1038/s41418-020-00720-9.

4. Scully M, Singh D, Lown R, Poles A, Solomon T, Levi M, et al. Pathologic antibodies to platelet factor 4 after ChAdOx1 nCoV-19 vaccination. N Engl J Med. 2021;384(23):2202–11. https://doi.org/10.1056/NEJMoa2105385.

5. Schultz NH, Sørvoll IH, Michelsen AE, Munthe LA, Lund-Johansen F, Ahlen MT, et al. Thrombosis and thrombocytopenia after ChAdOx1 nCoV-19 vaccination. N Engl J Med. 2021;384(22):2124–30. https://doi.org/10.1056/NEJMoa2104882.

6. Greinacher A, Thiele T, Warkentin TE, Weisser K, Kyrle PA, Eichinger S. Thrombotic thrombocytopenia after ChAdOx1 nCov-19 vaccination. N Engl J Med. 2021;384(22):2092–101. https://doi.org/10.1056/NEJMoa2104840.

7. Coronavirus Vaccine-Weekly Summary of Yellow Card Reporting. https://www.gov.uk/government/publications/coronavirus-covid-19-vaccine-adverse-reactions/coronavirus-vaccine-summary-of-yellow-card-reporting#yellow-card-reports. Accessed 20 June 2021.

8. See I, Su JR, Lale A, Woo EJ, Guh AY, Shimabukuro TT, et al. US Case Reports of Cerebral Venous Sinus Thrombosis With Thrombocytopenia After Ad26.COV2.S Vaccination, March 2 to April 21, 2021. JAMA. 2021;325(24):2448-56.

9. Chan BT, Bobos P, Oduyato A, et al. Meta-analysis of risk of vaccine-induced immune.thrombotic thrombocytopenia following ChAdOx1-S recombinant vaccine. Preprint. version. doi: https://doi.org/10.1101/2021.05.04.21256613.

10. White RH, Keenan CR. Effects of race and ethnicity on the incidence of venous thromboembolism. Thromb Res. 2009;123(Suppl 4):S11–7. https://doi.org/10.1016/S0049-3848(09)70136-7.

11. Klatsky AL, Baer D. What protects Asians from venous thromboembolism? Am J Med. 2004;116(7):493–5. https://doi.org/10.1016/j.amjmed.2004.01.005.

12. Klatsky AL, Armstrong MA, Poggi J. Risk of pulmonary embolism and/or deep venous thrombosis in Asian-Americans. Am J Cardiol. 2000;85(11):1334–7. https://doi.org/10.1016/S0002-9149(00)00766-9.

13. Warkentin TE, Greinacher A. Spontaneous HIT syndrome: knee replacement, infection, and parallels with vaccine-induced immune thrombotic thrombocytopenia. Thromb Res. 2021;204:40–51. https://doi.org/10.1016/j.thromres.2021.05.018.

14. Arepally GM, Ortel TL. Vaccine-Induced Immune Thrombotic Thrombocytopenia (VITT): What We Know and Don't Know. Blood. 2021. Epub ahead of print. https://doi.org/10.1182/blood.2021012152.

15. Thaler J, Ay C, Gleixner KV, Hauswirth AW, Cacioppo F, Grafeneder J, et al. Successful treatment of vaccine-induced prothrombotic immune thrombocytopenia (VIPIT). J Thromb Haemost. 2021. Epub ahead of print; 19(7):1819–22. https://doi.org/10.1111/jth.15346.

16. Rungjirajittranon T, Owattanapanich W. A serious thrombotic event in a patient with immune thrombocytopenia requiring intravenous immunoglobulin: a case report. J Med Case Rep. 2019;13(1):25. https://doi.org/10.1186/s13256-018-1955-x.

17. Bourguignon A, Arnold DM, Warkentin TE, Smith JW, Pannu T, Shrum JM, et al. Adjunct Immune Globulin for Vaccine-Induced Thrombotic Thrombocytopenia. N Engl J Med. 2021. Epub ahead of print. https://doi.org/10.1056/NEJMoa2107051.

18. Oldenburg J, Klamroth R, Langer F, Albisetti M, von Auer C, Ay C, et al. Diagnosis and Management of Vaccine-Related Thrombosis following AstraZeneca COVID-19 vaccination: guidance statement from the GTH. Hamostaseologie. 2021. Epub ahead of print;41(03):184–9. https://doi.org/10.1055/a-1469-7481.

19. American Society of Hematology. Vaccine-induced Immune Thrombotic Thrombocytopenia: Frequently Asked Questions. https://www.hematology.org/covid-19/vaccine-induced-immune-thrombotic-thrombocytopenia. Accessed 20 June 2021.

20. Guidance from the Expert Haematology Panel (EHP) on Covid-19 Vaccine-induced Immune Thrombocytopenia and Thrombosis (VITT) version 1.7. https://b-s-h.org.uk/media/19590/guidance-version-17-on-mngmt-of-vitt-20210420.pdf. Accessed 20 June 2021.

11

An independent, gender-dependent risk factor for venous thromboembolism

Vahideh Takhviji[1], Kazem Zibara[2], Asma Maleki[3], Ebrahim Azizi[4], Sanaz Hommayoun[1], Mohammadreza Tabatabaei[1], Seyed Esmaeil Ahmadi[5], Maral Soleymani[4], Omid Kiani Ghalesardi[5], Mina Farokhian[6], Afshin Davari[7], Pouria Paridar[8], Anahita Kalantari[9] and Abbas Khosravi[1][*] (iD)

Abstract

Background: Activated protein C resistance (APCR) due to factor V Leiden (FVL) mutation (R506Q) is a major risk factor in patients with venous thromboembolism (VTE). The present study investigated the clinical manifestations and the risk of venous thromboembolism regarding multiple clinical, laboratory, and demographic properties in FVL patients.

Material and methods: A retrospective cross-sectional analysis was conducted on a total of 288 FVL patients with VTE according to APCR. In addition, 288 VET control samples, without FVL mutation, were also randomly selected. Demographic information, clinical manifestations, family and treatment history were recorded, and specific tests including t-test, chi-square and uni- and multi-variable regression tests applied.

Results: APCR was found to be 2.3 times significantly more likely in men (OR: 2.1, $p < 0.05$) than women. The risk of deep vein thrombosis (DVT) and pulmonary embolism (PE) in APCR patients was 4.5 and 3.2 times more than the control group, respectively ($p < 0.05$). However, APCR could not be an independent risk factor for arterial thrombosis (AT) and pregnancy complications. Moreover, patients were evaluated for thrombophilia panel tests and showed significantly lower protein C and S than the control group and patients without DVT ($p < 0.0001$).

Conclusion: FVL mutation and APCR abnormality are noticeable risk factors for VTE. Screening strategies for FVL mutation in patients undergoing surgery, oral contraceptive medication, and pregnancy cannot be recommended, but a phenotypic test for activated protein C resistance should be endorsed in patients with VTE.

Keywords: APCR, Factor V Leiden, Thrombophilia, Venous thromboembolism, DVT, PE, Arterial thrombosis

Introduction

Thrombophilia, the most common hematologic disorder, is characterized by blood coagulation abnormalities that increases the risk of thrombosis events [1]. Venous Thrombosis (VT) is the third cause of death due to cardiovascular diseases [2]. VT occurs in two general forms known as pulmonary embolism (PE) and deep vein thrombosis (DVT) [3, 4]. Common predisposing factors include aging, surgery, pregnancy, cancer, recent myocardial infarction, hormone therapy in females, prolonged inertia and genetic factors. The latter genetic causes comprise non-O-blood groups, genetic mutations such as G20210A in prothrombin (PTM) gene, deficiencies in protein C (PC), protein S (PS), and antithrombin III (AT-III), as well as activated protein C resistance (APCR) associated with factor V Leiden (FVL) [2, 5–7]. An estimated 64% of patients with venous thromboembolism

* Correspondence: a-khosravi@razi.tums.ac.ir
[1]Transfusion Research center, High Institute for Research and Education in Transfusion, Tehran, Iran
Full list of author information is available at the end of the article

(VTE) have APCR as the most common associated clotting abnormality [8].

APCR is a hemostatic disorder characterized by the lack of adequate anticoagulant response to activated protein C (APC). More than 95% of cases with APCR abnormality are due to FVL mutation. Dahlback et al. in 1993 reported the first case of APCR created by FVL and in 1994; Bertina and colleagues discovered a single point mutation in the FV gene [7, 9]. APC, along with protein S as a cofactor, degrades Factor Va and Factor VIIIa by cleaving three arginine sites (R306, R506, and R679). The substitution mutation at G1691A results in an amino acid alteration (R506Q), leading to increased thrombin generation and a hypercoagulable state [9, 10]. The risk of thrombosis increase by 5 to 10 fold in patients with heterozygous FVL mutations while homozygotes have an increase of nearly 80 fold [7].

APCR screening tests are based on the anticoagulant activity of APC, and these include modified activated partial thromboplastin time (aPTT), prothrombin time (PT) and snake Russell Viper Venom (RVV) time for patients on heparin and a lupus anticoagulant (LA) [11]. A minimal prolongation of plasma clotting times by exogenous APC in the presence of FVL characterizes the APC-resistant phenotype. In addition, the R506Q mutation genetic defect can be unraveled by DNA techniques [10, 12]. However, the R506Q (FV $_{Leiden}$) is not the only cause of APCR since other mutations such as R306T (FV $_{Cambridge}$), R306G (FV $_{Hong Kong}$), and W1920R (FV $_{Nera}$) can also initiate APCR [13]. Demographics, ethnic, and coagulation factors can influence diagnostic tests and patients' clinical phenotype. Previous literature suggested a possible correlation between levels of factors V, VIII and IX with APCR parameters [14]. Protein S, protein C and antithrombin III levels may also affect APCR [15, 16]; however, they have not been evaluated before. In these patients, anticoagulants such as heparin, warfarin, or direct oral anticoagulants (DOACs) are used as a treatment. Notably, despite the relatively similar efficiency of all anticoagulants in treating VT, DOACs have shown a lower 2-year risk of VT recurrence after anticoagulant discontinuation [17].

To date, the majority of studies on this disease have been focused on the genotype component. However, clinical manifestations and disease characteristics were not assessed sufficiently, whether independently or in correlation. Given the above background, and due to concerns regarding assay limitations that could adversely affect clinical diagnosis, we aimed to evaluate inherited FV Leiden patients with VTE according to APCR and VET control samples without FV Leiden mutation. The APCR diagnostic and clinical parameters that were studied include the levels of thrombophilia panel, the frequency of adverse thrombotic outcomes, the frequency of adverse pregnancy outcomes associated with FV Leiden, and the influence of gender and age.

Material and methods
Study design and patients' enrollment
This study was designed as a case-control study survey conducted at the Coagulation Center of the Iranian Blood Transfusion Organization (IBTO) in Tehran, Iran. This center is a regional referral center for specialized coagulation testing and rare bleeding disorders. From 2013 to 2018, a total of 288 patients with confirmed FV Leiden abnormality with VTE according to APCR were recruited. Patients with the following criteria were included: 1) thrombotic symptoms (VTE like vein thrombosis and pulmonary embolism), 2) with reduced activity of APC, confirmed by APCR tests, and 3) who have tested for the presence of FV Leiden mutation. Patients excluded from the study were those having other hemostatic bleeding and thrombotic disorders such as an inherited deficiency of protein C, protein S, AT-III or FVIII as well as those who received anticoagulants (warfarin, heparin, etc...), or antiplatelet (aspirin, clopidogrel, etc...) therapies at least 72 h prior to blood sampling. Patients then undertook a detailed history assessment including demographical and clinical characteristics, age at first symptom, patient's chief complaint, familial history of thrombotic disorders, and their blood groups. In addition, clinical characteristics and laboratory investigations were determined. The control group included a total of 288 VTE patients who were reported negative for FV Leiden after confirmatory tests. This study was approved by the Medical Ethical Committee and the Institute Review Board (IRB) at IBTO. A written consent form was obtained and signed by all study participants for the collection of blood samples.

Thrombophilia occurrence in the year preceding the inclusion in the study
Before sample collection and in the year preceding the inclusion in the study, the patient's detailed history was obtained from all participants. This included demographic data, familial history of bleeding and thrombotic disorders, anticoagulants and antiplatelet drugs used, clinical phenotype and thrombotic events (VTE like vein thrombosis and pulmonary embolism), pregnancy complications (such as abortion, eclampsia, preeclampsia, stillbirth, infertility, abortion trimester) and a detailed clinical history of 12 bleeding episodes based on ISTH scoring [18].

Laboratory work-up
Peripheral venous blood was collected in 3.2% (0.105 M) sodium citrated tubes and centrifuged twice at 2200 x g for 10 min at room temperature to obtain citrated

platelet-poor plasma which was then stored at − 80 °C. As a principal challenge, complete assessments were performed in order to classify the patients' possible disorders and to discriminate between healthy subjects from mild thrombophilic disorders. Among all subjects assessed, those with thrombophilic disorders have been tested for APCR. Standard routine diagnostic assays were performed such as PT, International Normalized Ratio (INR), and aPTT. The presence of LA was confirmed with LA profile and PTT-LA and an abnormal dilute Russell Viper Venom (dRVV) time that demonstrated modification after the addition of the phospholipid rich dRVVT (LA Test and LA Confirm; Gradipore, Australia). Protein C activity was measured by the chromogenic protein C method (Chromogenix, USA) with the normal range being 70 ± 140%. On the other hand, Protein S activity was performed using the Elisa method (protein S normal range is 55 ± 150%). Finally, APC resistance was measured using the APCR test according to the manufacturer's instructions (Pefakit APC-R FVL, Pentapharm, Basel, CH). To finalize the diagnosis, the levels of Factor VIII, AT-III and fibrinogen were also assessed. FVIII and AT-III were assayed using deficient plasma (Diagnostica Stago, Asnieres, France) whereas Von clauss method was used for Fibrinogen assessment.

Statistical analysis

Descriptive analyzes were carried out and reported as frequencies and proportions (N, %). Data were analyzed by Kolomogorov-Smirnov test for normality checking. On the other hand, t-test and chi-square tests were used to compare variables in the studied groups (FV Leiden and Control and age and sex subgroups). Then, uni and multivariable ordinal logistic regression were performed to assess the relationship between the risk of FV Leiden and the studied variables. A correlation test was performed to evaluate the relationship between age and the thrombophilia panel. All tests were two-sided with the type I error rate fixed at 0.05 and the significant level for univariable and multivariable analyses assigned 0.25 and 0.05, respectively. Computations were performed using SAS (version 9.4; SAS Institute Inc., Cary, NC, USA) and SPSS for Windows (Version 19) (SPSS Inc., Chicago, IL, USA).

Results

A total of 288 FVL patients were investigated in this study of whom 189 patients (65.6%) were females and the remaining (99 patients) were males (34.4%) (Table 1). The age of patients ranged from 1 to 80 years old with a mean of 37.87 ± 13.67 years while the control group's age ranged from 2 to 84 years old with a mean of 33.58 ± 11.8 years. Patients with familial history of thrombosis were ~ 37.7%

Table 1 Characteristics of studied patients

Variable[a]		
Sex	–	
Female		424 (73.6%)
Male		152 (26.4%)
Age	35.34 ± 12.88	–
Familial History	–	167 (31%)
Manifestations	–	
Bleeding		5 (0.9%)
Thrombophilia		540 (93.8%)
Bleeding and Thrombophilia		16 (2.8%)
Laboratory Work-up	–	
PT	14.15 ± 3.7	
APTT	30.46 ± 3.3	
Protein C	117.76 ± 36.6	
Protein S	77.15 ± 22.9	
Anti-Thrombin	100.42 ± 14.3	
APCR	2.57 ± 1.3	
Clinical Manifestation	–	
Arterial Thrombosis		37 (6.4%)
DVT		149 (25.9%)
PE		39 (6.3%)
Abortion		199 (33.3%)
TUS		39 (6.8%)
Abortion Time	–	
First-trim		163 (28.3%)
Second-trim		24 (4.2%)
Third-trim		5 (0.9%)

PT prothrombin time, *APTT* activated partial thromboplastin time, *APCR* activated protein C resistance, *AT-III* antithrombin III, *DVT* deep vein thrombosis, *PE* pulmonary embolism, *TUS* thrombosis in unusual sites.
[a]Numerical data are expressed as mean/median and categorical with the percentage

whereas 66.3% of the patients were new cases with no family history. Demographic data are presented in Table 1.

Demographic characteristics of patients with FV Leiden abnormality

Regarding the presence or absence of FVL, this study contained two groups: APCR and the normal population. There was a significant correlation between gender and APCR abnormality. In fact, despite the significantly higher frequency of women in both groups, the ratio of women in the normal group was particularly (***, $p < 0.0001$) higher than that in the APCR patients (Table 2). Moreover, using the uni- and multivariate logistic regression model, APCR was found to be ~ 2.3 fold significantly higher in men than women, where female sex was

Table 2 Demographic, laboratory, and clinical status of patients with APCR abnormality and normal confirmed final diagnosis. (* $p < 0.05$, ** $p < 0.01$, *** $p < 0.001$)

Variable	Study Population		P-value
	APCR	Normal	
Sex			
Female	189 (65.6%)	233 (80%)	
Male	99 (55.6%)	52 (18%)	0.000***
Age (mean ± SD and range)	37 (1–80)	33.5 (2–84)	0.001***
Familial History of Thrombosis	87 (52.1%)	80 (47.9%)	0.18
Type of Disease			
Bleeding	5 (1%)	0 (0.0%)	0.99
Thrombophilia	261 (92.3%)	279 (92.7%)	
Bleeding and Thrombophilia	7 (2.5%)	9 (3.1%)	
Laboratory Findings			
PT	15.32 ± 4.14	13.13 ± 0.74	0.008***
APTT	36.44 ± 9.34	34.63 ± 3.26	0.92
Protein C	94.84 ± 46.58	125.89 ± 28.08	0.000***
Protein S	64.43 ± 29.96	82 ± 20.10	0.000***
Anti-Thrombin	97.58 ± 18.36	98.52 ± 11.64	0.189
APCR	1.47 ± 0.19	3.91 ± 0.78	0.000***
Pregnancy Complications			0.000***
Abortion	65 (22.5%)	127 (44%)	–
Eclampsia	0	0	0.25
Preeclampsia	3 (1%)	2 (0.6%)	0.23
Stillbirth	8 (2.7%)	11 (3.8%)	0.06
Infertility	4 (1.3%)	11 (3.8%)	
Abortion Time			0.17
First Trim	51 (17.7%)	112 (38.8%)	
Second Trim	11 (3.8%)	13 (4.5%)	
Third Trim	3 (1%)	2 (0.6%)	
Thrombotic Complications			
DVT	113 (39.2%)	36 (12.5%)	0.000***
PE	27 (9.3%)	9 (3.1%)	0.001***
Arterial Thrombosis	16 (5%)	21 (7.2%)	0.24

PT prothrombin time, APTT activated partial thromboplastin time, APCR activated protein C resistance, AT-III antithrombin III, DVT deep vein thrombosis, PE pulmonary embolism

a protective variable that remained significant after adjusting for other variables (OR: 2.1, $p < 0.05$) (Table 3).

The age of patients ranged from 1 to 80 years (median 37); however, 58.6% of patients were in the age interval of 20 to 50 years, whereas 20% were between 50 to 60 years. Regarding the autosomal recessive inheritance of this disease, the familial history was evaluated in APCR patients and controls. Indeed, the APCR abnormality was 1.2 times more likely to occur in individuals with family history (Odds ratio of 1.27, and a 75% CI of 0.63 to 0.87) (Table 3). As shown in this table, sex, young age, and familial history of thrombosis were predictive factors for FV Leiden.

Laboratory assessments

Results showed significant differences in laboratory findings between patients and controls. Overall, most APCR patients showed normal PT and aPTT with; respectively, only 10.8% and 5.6% of patients harboring abnormal interpretations. Similarly, all normal controls also revealed normal PT and aPTT results; however, their mean values were significantly lower than those in the APCR group (Table 2). Therefore, we measured the association of PT and PTT results with APCR abnormality by uni- and multivariable regression model. Increased PT in the APCR group was 1.43 fold more likely than the control group, which remained significant after adjustment for other variables in a multivariate analysis (Table 3). In addition, the risk of APCR diagnosis was increased three-fold in prolonged PTT situations (Table 3). Patients were then evaluated for thrombophilia panel tests; protein C, protein S and anti-thrombin. Interestingly, results showed that FV Leiden patients had significantly lower PC and PS levels than the control group (***, $p < 0.0001$), however, without a significant difference in anti-thrombin levels (Table 2). Using the logistic regression model, the thrombophilia panel was also identified as a highly valuable test (***, $p < 0.0001$) in univariate analysis (Table 3). Moreover, APCR patients experiencing DVT episodes had significantly lower levels of PC ($p = 0.003$), PS ($p = 0.000$) and, anti-thrombin III ($p = 0.007$) than patients without DVT. On the other hand, all thrombophilia tests including PC, PS, and anti-thrombin had a strong negative correlation with PT and aPTT results in both groups that were statistically significant in APCR patients only (data not shown). FVL patients also exhibited significantly lower levels of APCRPenta, used as a confirming test.

Thrombophilia panel and screening tests according to age and gender

Since APCR abnormality revealed a varied pattern in the age of manifestations and sex subgroups, compared to the normal group, therefore, changes in laboratory tests and thrombophilia panel were evaluated at different ages and sex subtypes. Thrombophilia panel in APCR patients showed a negative correlation with age, however, this did not reach statistical significance. There was no significant correlation between screening tests and sex subgroups except PrC, for which females showed a significantly higher mean rank range than males ($P = 0.000$).

Table 3 Crude and adjusted differences in APCR diagnosis according to demographic, laboratory, and clinical parameters

Variable	Univariable		Multivariable	
	Adjusted OR (75% CI)	P-value	Adjusted OR (95% CI)	P-value
Sex				
Female	1	–	–	–
Male	2.34	0.000*	**2.13**	**0.05****
Age (mean ± SD and range)	1.02	0.001*	1	0.92
Familial History of Thrombosis	1.27	0.18*	1.63	0.24
Laboratory Findings				
PT	1.43	0.001*	0.98	0.94
APTT	3.03	0.08*	0.99	0.97
Protein C	0.97	0.000*	0.99	0.20
Protein S	0.95	0.000*	0.98	0.10
Anti-Thrombin	0.98	0.09*	1	0.70
APCR	0.00	0.95	–	–
Thrombotic Complications				
DVT	4.52	0.000*	**3.53**	**0.006****
PE	3.2	0.003*	3.25	0.19
AT-III	0.74	0.39	1.98	0.48
Abortion	0.37	0.000*	0.82	0.67
Abortion Time				
First Trim	–	0.185*		
Second Trim	1.85	0.162*		
Third Trim	3.29	0.199*		

PT prothrombin time, *APTT* activated partial thromboplastin time, *APCR* activated protein C resistance, *AT-III* antithrombin III, *DVT* deep vein thrombosis, *PE* pulmonary embolism

Thrombotic clinical manifestations

Patients were divided into 3 groups according to their type of symptoms: bleeding disorder, thrombophilia, and bleeding and thrombophilia. More than 94% of subjects were thrombophilic and about 3% were thrombophilic-hemorrhagic. In the APCR group, 5 patients had just bleeding symptoms such as menorrhagia, coetaneous bleeding, epistaxis, GI bleeding, bleedings after tooth extraction and surgery. In fact, one patient had a total score of 21, three patients with a score of 3, and one patient with a score of 2.

The frequency of each clinical symptom was assessed and compared between the two groups. The most common manifestations in patients with APCR abnormality were DVT (39.2%) followed by abortion (22.6%) and PE (9.4%) (Fig. 1). About 75% of DVT and PE were seen in APCR patients and the rest of them in normal controls. The frequency of DVT and PE in the APCR group was significantly higher than that in the control group. Moreover, using the uni- and multivariate logistic regression model, the risk of DVT and PE in APCR patients, was 4.5 and 3.2 times higher than the normal group, respectively. This risk remained significant after adjusting for other variables (Table 3).

Abortion, the second most common symptom in APCR patients, was the most common symptom in normal patients who showed ~ 66% of all abortions. Abortion in both groups occurred most frequently in the first trimester of pregnancy and the two groups did not show a significant difference in abortion trimester (Tables 2 and 3). Other pregnancy complications such as eclampsia, pre-eclampsia, stillbirth, and infertility were also assessed and there was no significant difference between the two groups (Table 2).

We then investigated separately all thrombotic symptoms in different demographic groups. Chi-Square test results revealed significant correlations between DVT and PE symptoms with sex subgroups. Despite the higher frequency of women, the incidence of DVT and PE symptoms was significantly higher in men ($p = 0.01$) (Fig. 2).

Finally, the incidence of symptoms at age intervals was assessed in both normal and APCR groups. All symptoms in APCR patients occurred at a young age. The inter-quartile range or the mean age dispersion of symptoms was low for FV Leiden patients and ranged between 30 to 50 years for all symptoms. Results showed that individuals with Arterial Thrombosis (AT) and

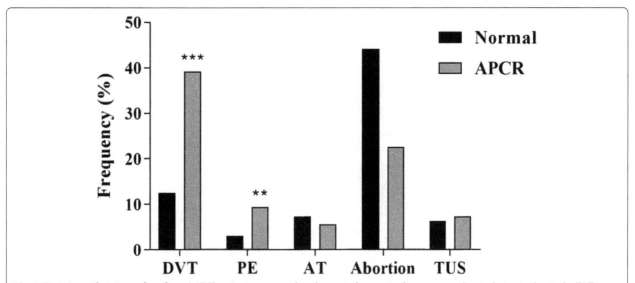

Fig. 1 Clinical manifestations of confirmed APCR patients compared to the control group in the year preceding inclusion in the study. (DVT: Deep Vein Thrombosis, PE: Pulmonary Embolism, AT: Arterial Thrombosis, TUS: Thrombosis in Unusual Sites) (* $p < 0.05$, ** $p < 0.01$, *** $p < 0.001$)

DVT in APCR patients had a mean age higher than normal controls (Fig. 3).

Discussion

APCR is the most common outcome in individuals with familial thrombophilia, as patients have a heightened risk of developing thrombosis [1]. The inheritance of this abnormality is autosomal recessive and its frequency varies between countries. The prevalence of FVL in some parts of the world, such as Japan and Africa, is null; however, it is 5–10% in Europe. In Tehran, a province with

different nations in Iran, the prevalence was reported to be ~ 5.5% [7, 12, 19, 20]. Consanguineous marriages in Iranian culture play an important role in the development of hereditary disorders [21]. Therefore, we focused in this study on the demographic, clinical and laboratory characteristics as well as on estimating the risk of venous thromboembolism in patients showing resistance to APC in the Iranian population.

APCR abnormality is associated not only with genetic mutations but also with a number of factors including sex, age, anticoagulant, and antiplatelet agents. Previous

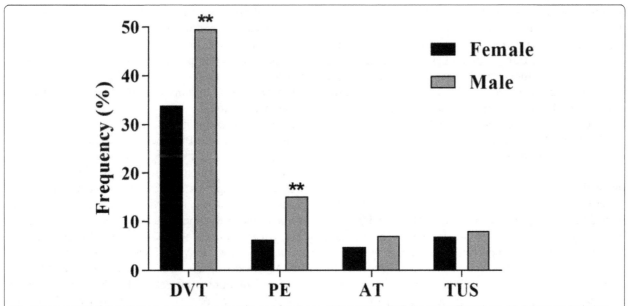

Fig. 2 Comparison of thrombotic symptoms among males and females in APCR patients. (DVT: Deep Vein Thrombosis, PE: Pulmonary Embolism, AT: Arterial Thrombosis, TUS: Thrombosis in Unusual Sites) (* $p < 0.05$, ** $p < 0.01$, *** $p < 0.001$)

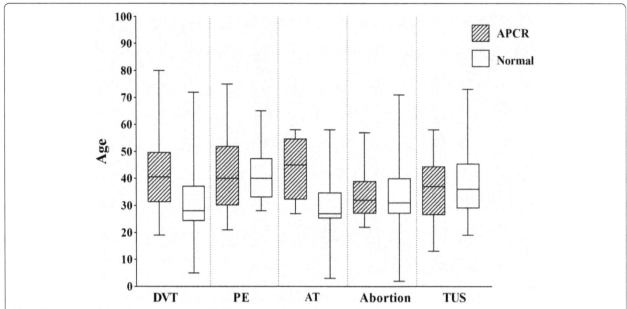

Fig. 3 The pattern of thrombotic symptoms in APCR patients and control groups of different ages. (DVT: Deep Vein Thrombosis, PE: Pulmonary Embolism, AT: Arterial Thrombosis, TUS: Thrombosis in Unusual Sites)

studies have shown that APCR along with the female gender, appeared to increase the risk of thrombosis and that the mean APC ratio is significantly lower in females than in males [22]. Interestingly, in the present study, despite the higher frequency of women in both APCR and control groups, more than 65% of men were resistant to APC which was found to be significantly more likely in men than women, in contradiction to other previous reports [23, 24]. Indeed, although twice as many females than males were included in the study; however, we found a gender-related difference for APCR which was more likely to develop in men. This could reflect the fact that women are generally more investigated than men for inherited thrombophilia [25]. We suggest that a comprehensive study should be performed on the gender-related differences of APCR abnormality. On the other hand, the onset of thrombosis in the APCR group occurred at a young age, with a narrower range of 20–50 years, than the control group. Our data is in accordance with previous studies which showed that APCR is a significant thrombosis cause in younger individuals [26, 27].

Here, we describe the association of resistance to APC with VTE. Participants bearing APCR abnormality had a clearly significant increased risk for VTE. The age and sex-adjusted incidence odds ratio for the first episode of VTE was 3.53, consistent with the data reported by Ridker and Francesco [28, 29]. The most common manifestations in patients with APCR abnormality were DVT followed by abortion and PE. Other reported symptoms were AT and TUS. Despite the higher frequency of

women, the second thrombotic symptom was miscarriage (22%) along with pregnancy complications (5%), accounting together for 27% of all symptoms. This percentage in the APCR group was significantly lower than that in normal women controls which harbored more than 66% of all abortions. Previous studies reported that APC-resistant women experience their first thrombotic event at fertility, associated with both oral contraceptive use and pregnancy [30–32]. This may in part explain that one of the relevant risk factors associated with the first event are oral contraceptive medication, pregnancy, and postpartum because women also had a lower average age than men [32]. However, given that abortions and pregnancy complications were higher in normal controls, FVL cannot be considered independently as the cause of these symptoms in APCR patients, but this is rather multifactorial.

In APC-resistant patients, only 11.8 and 9% of total events were AT and PE. The association of AT with resistance to APC is a controversial issue. In our study, the mean age of patients with AT was higher than those with other symptoms and also higher than the control group. In accordance, a previous study revealed that AT is associated with other risk factors at an advanced age [33]. All thrombotic symptoms were also compared in sex subgroups when gynecological symptoms were omitted. As mentioned above, despite the significantly higher frequency of women investigated, APCR was found significantly more likely in men. Moreover, thrombotic complications including DVT, PE, and AT were significantly higher in men than women. This could indicate a clinically relevant gender difference and reflect an increased DVT and PE risk in men, highlighting the low risk of VTE caused by oral contraceptive use in female carriers [34].

Conclusion

In conclusion, patients with phenotypic resistance to APC have an increased risk for VTE. This study suggests that women experience their first thrombotic event at a younger age; however, factor V Leiden cannot be independently the cause of abortion and pregnancy complications in APCR patients. Finally, thrombotic events are found to be significantly more likely in men. Screening strategies for factor V Leiden mutation in patients undergoing surgery, oral contraceptive medication, and pregnancy cannot be recommended, but a phenotypic test for activated protein C resistance should be endorsed in patients with VTE.

Limitations

The size of studied population and some incomplete questionnaires was the limitations of this study.

Abbreviations

VT: Venous Thrombosis; PE: Pulmonary embolism; DVT: Deep vein thrombosis; PTM: Prothrombin; PC: Protein C; PS: Protein S; AT-III: Antithrombin III; FVL: Factor V Leiden; APC: Activated protein C; aPTT: Activated Partial Thromboplastin Time; PT: Prothrombin time; RVV: Russell Viper Venom; LA: Lupus anticoagulant; IBTO: Iranian Blood Transfusion Organization; IRB: Medical Ethical Committee and the Institute Review Board; INR: International Normalized Ratio; dRVV: Dilute Russell Viper Venom

Acknowledgements

The authors would like to thank all colleagues at the Iranian Blood Transfusion Organization, Tehran, Iran.

Authors' contributions

Abbas Khosravi designed the study. Vahideh Takhviji, Asma Maleki, Sanaz Hommayoun, Mohammadreza Tabatabaei, Seyed Esmaeil Ahmadi and Omid Kiani Ghalesardi conceived and carried out the experiments. Afshin Davari, Ebrahim Azizi and Kazem Zibara analyzed the data. Mina Farokhian and Maral Soleimani validated the data. Vahideh Takhviji and Kazem Zibara finalized the figures and wrote the paper. Afshin Davari and Pouria Paridar revised the manuscript. All authors discussed the results and commented on the manuscript. The author(s) read and approved the final manuscript.

Author details

[1]Transfusion Research center, High Institute for Research and Education in Transfusion, Tehran, Iran. [2]PRASE and Biology Department, Faculty of Sciences, Lebanese University, Beirut, Lebanon. [3]Department of hematology, School of Allied Medical Sciences, Tehran University of Medical Sciences, Tehran, Iran. [4]Faculty of Medicine, Ahvaz Jundishapur University of Medical Sciences, Ahvaz, Iran. [5]Department of Hematology and Blood Banking, Faculty of Allied Medicine, Iran University of Medical Sciences, Tehran, Iran. [6]Hematology Department, Tarbiat Modares University, Tehran, Iran. [7]School of Public Health, Tehran University of Medical Sciences, Tehran, Iran. [8]Islamic Azad University, North-Tehran Branch, Tehran, Iran. [9]Department of Anesthesiology, Golestan Hospital, Ahvaz Jundishapur University of Medical Sciences, Ahvaz, Iran.

References

1. Buchholz T, et al. Polymorphisms in the ACE and PAI-1 genes are associated with recurrent spontaneous miscarriages. Hum Reprod. 2003;18(11):2473–7.
2. Byrnes JR, Wolberg AS. New findings on venous thrombogenesis. Hämostaseologie. 2017;37(01):25–35.
3. Members ATF, et al. 2014 ESC guidelines on the diagnosis and management of acute pulmonary embolism: the task force for the diagnosis and Management of Acute Pulmonary Embolism of the European Society of Cardiology (ESC) endorsed by the European Respiratory Society (ERS). Eur Heart J. 2014;35(43):3033–80.
4. Cushman M. Inherited risk factors for venous thrombosis. ASH Education Program Book. 2005;2005(1):452–7.
5. Walker I, Greaves M, Preston F. On behalf of the Haemostasis and thrombosis task force British Committee for Standards in Haematology. Investigation and management of heritable thrombophilia. Br J Haematol. 2001;114(3):512–28.
6. De Santis M, et al. Inherited and acquired thrombophilia: pregnancy outcome and treatment. Reprod Toxicol. 2006;22(2):227–33.
7. Singh D, et al. Genetics of hypercoagulable and Hypocoagulable states. Neurosurgery Clinics. 2018;29(4):493–501.
8. Sheppard DR. Activated protein C resistance: the most common risk factor for venous thromboembolism. J Am Board Fam Pract. 2000;13(2):111–5.
9. Dahlback B. Pro- and anticoagulant properties of factor V in pathogenesis of thrombosis and bleeding disorders. Int J Lab Hematol. 2016;38(Suppl 1):4–11.
10. Van Cott EM, Khor B, Zehnder JL. Factor VL eiden. Am J Hematol. 2016;91(1):46–9.
11. Campello E, Spiezia L, Simioni P. Diagnosis and management of factor V Leiden. Expert Rev Hematol. 2016;9(12):1139–49.
12. Amiral J, Vissac AM, Seghatchian J. Laboratory assessment of activated protein C resistance/factor V-Leiden and performance characteristics of a new quantitative assay. Transfus Apher Sci. 2017;56(6):906–13.
13. Nogami K, et al. Novel FV mutation (W1920R, FVNara) associated with serious deep vein thrombosis and more potent APC resistance relative to FVLeiden. Blood. 2014;123(15):2420–8.
14. Cumming A, et al. Development of resistance to activated protein C during pregnancy. Br J Haematol. 1995;90(3):725–7.
15. Freyburger G, et al. Proposal for objective evaluation of the performance of various functional APC-resistance tests in genotyped patients. Thromb Haemost. 1997;78(01):1360–5.
16. Ahmadi SE, et al. Congenital combined bleeding disorders, a comprehensive study of a large number of Iranian patients. Clin Appl Thromb Hemost. 2021;27:1076029621996813.
17. Campello E, et al. Direct Oral anticoagulants in patients with inherited thrombophilia and venous thromboembolism: a prospective cohort study. J Am Heart Assoc. 2020;9(23):e018917.
18. Moore GW, et al. Recommendations for clinical laboratory testing of activated protein C resistance; communication from the SSC of the ISTH. J Thromb Haemost. 2019;17(9):1555–61.
19. Laffan M. Activated protein C resistance and myocardial infarction. BMJ Publishing Group Ltd. 1998.
20. Rahimi Z, et al. Prevalence of factor V Leiden (G1691A) and prothrombin (G20210A) among Kurdish population from Western Iran. J Thromb Thrombolysis. 2008;25(3):280–3.

21. Hamamy H. Consanguineous marriages. J Community Genet. 2012;3(3): 185–92.
22. Svensson PJ, et al. Female gender and resistance to activated protein C (FV: Q506) as potential risk factors for thrombosis after elective hip arthroplasty. Thromb Haemost. 1997;78(3):993–6.
23. Favaloro EJ, et al. Activated protein C resistance: the influence of ABO-blood group, gender and age. Thromb Res. 2006;117(6):665–70.
24. Svensson P, et al. Female gender and resistance to activated protein C (FV: Q506) as potential risk factors for thrombosis after elective hip arthroplasty. Thromb Haemost. 1997;78(01):0993–6.
25. Hansen RS, Nybo M. The association between activated protein C ratio and factor V Leiden are gender-dependent. Clin Chem Lab Med (CCLM). 2019.
26. Kuhli C, et al. High prevalence of resistance to APC in young patients with retinal vein occlusion. Graefes Arch Clin Exp Ophthalmol. 2002;240(3):163–8.
27. Federici EH, Al-Mondhiry H. High risk of thrombosis recurrence in patients with homozygous and compound heterozygous factor V R506Q (factor V Leiden) and prothrombin G20210A. Thromb Res. 2019;182:75–8.
28. Rodeghiero F, Tosetto A. Activated protein C resistance and factor V Leiden mutation are independent risk factors for venous thromboembolism. Ann Intern Med. 1999;130(8):643–50.
29. Ridker PM, et al. Mutation in the gene coding for coagulation factor V and the risk of myocardial infarction, stroke, and venous thrombosis in apparently healthy men. N Engl J Med. 1995;332(14):912–7.
30. Thorogood M. Oral contraceptives and thrombosis. Curr Opin Hematol. 1998;5(5):350–4.
31. Gerhardt A, Scharf RE, Zotz RB. Effect of hemostatic risk factors on the individual probability of thrombosis during pregnancy and the puerperium. Thromb Haemost. 2003;90(07):77–85.
32. Faioni EM, et al. Resistance to activated protein C in unselected patients with arterial and venous thrombosis. Am J Hematol. 1997;55(2):59–64.
33. Yokus O, et al. Risk factors for thrombophilia in young adults presenting with thrombosis. Int J Hematol. 2009;90(5):583–90.
34. Favaloro EJ, et al. Laboratory identification of familial thrombophilia: do the pitfalls exceed the benefits? A reassessment of ABO-blood group, gender, age, and other laboratory parameters on the potential influence on a diagnosis of protein C, protein S, and antithrombin deficiency and the potential high risk of a false positive diagnosis. Lab Hematol. 2005;11(3): 174–84.

12

Optimal authoritative risk assessment score of Cancer-associated venous thromboembolism for hospitalized medical patients with lung Cancer

Wei Xiong[1*†] (ID), Yunfeng Zhao[2†], He Du[3†], Yanmin Wang[1], Mei Xu[4*] and Xuejun Guo[1*]

Abstract

Background: Cancer-associated venous thromboembolism (VTE) is common in patients with primary lung cancer. It has been understudied which authoritative risk assessment score of cancer-associated VTE is optimal for the assessment of VTE development in hospitalized medical patients with lung cancer.

Methods: Patients with lung cancer who had undergone computed tomography pulmonary angiography (CTPA), compression ultrasonography (CUS) of lower and upper extremities, and/or planar ventilation/perfusion (V/Q) scan to confirm the presence or absence of VTE during a medical hospitalization were retrospectively reviewed. Based on the actual prevalence of VTE among all patients, the possibility of VTE were reassessed with the Khorana score, the PROTECHT score, the CONKO score, the ONKOTEV score, the COMPASS-CAT score, and the CATS/MICA score, to compare their assessment accuracy for VTE development.

Results: A total of 1263 patients with lung cancer were incorporated into the final analysis. With respect to assessment efficiency for VTE occurrence, the scores with adjusted agreement from highest to lowest were the ONKOTEV score (78.6%), the PROTECHT score (73.4%), the CONKO score (72.1%), the COMPASS-CAT score (71.7%), the Khorana score (70.9%), and the CATS/MICA score (60.3%). The ONKOTEV score had the highest Youden index which was 0.68, followed by the PROTECHT score (0.58), the COMPASS-CAT score (0.56), the CONKO score (0.55), the Khorana score (0.53), and the CATS/MICA score (0.23).

Conclusions: Among the Khorana score, the PROTECHT score, the CONKO score, the ONKOTEV score, the COMPASS-CAT score, and the CATS/MICA score which are approved by authoritative guidelines, the ONKOTEV score is optimal for the assessment of VTE development in hospitalized medical patients with lung cancer.

Keywords: Lung cancer, Venous thromboembolism, Cancer-associated VTE, Risk assessment score, Hospitalized medical patients

* Correspondence: xiongwei@xinhuamed.com.cn; 15026472812@163.com; guoxuejun@xinhuamed.com.cn
Wei Xiong, Mei Xu and Xuejun Guo are co-corresponding authors.
†Wei Xiong, Yunfeng Zhao and He Du contributed equally to this work.
[1]Department of Pulmonary and Critical Care Medicine, Xinhua Hospital, Shanghai Jiaotong University School of Medicine,Shanghai, No. 1665, Kongjiang Road, Yangpu District, Shanghai 200092, China
[4]Department of General Medicine, North Bund Community Health Service Center, Hongkou District, Shanghai, China
Full list of author information is available at the end of the article

Introduction

Venous thromboembolism (VTE) is broadly defined as pulmonary embolism (PE), deep venous thrombosis (DVT), superficial vein thrombosis (SVT), and/or splanchnic vein thrombosis (SPVT), whereas narrowly defined as PE and/or DVT. Cancer-associated VTE is a common complication that threatens the life of adult patients with cancer. Patients with cancer are four to seven times more likely to develop cancer-associated VTE than patients without cancer. Established cancer-associated VTE is an important cause of morbidity and the second leading cause of mortality for patients with cancer [1–5]. Although its incidence and mortality have shown a declining trend, primary lung cancer still remains the second most common cancer type with the highest mortality rate globally [6, 7]. Rates of VTE prevalence ranged from 7 to 13% among patients with lung cancer [8]. The occurrence of VTE events was an indicator that was significantly associated with an increased risk of mortality in patients with lung cancer [9, 10]. Under such circumstances, missing a diagnosis of VTE or the need of thromboprophylaxis could be devastating, whereas frequent VTE diagnostic tests and/or thromboprophylaxis for all lung cancer patients would significantly increase unnecessary burden. Accordingly, the risk assessment of VTE is imperative prior to the diagnostic tests and/or thromboprophylaxis of cancer-associated VTE for patients with lung cancer.

A time-dependent association between VTE and cancer has been observed after cancer diagnosis [2]. Risk of VTE should be assessed initially and periodically thereafter for patients with cancer, particularly at the initiation of systemic anticancer therapy or during hospitalization [3]. The increased risk of VTE can be affected by a variety of risk factors such as cancer site, metastasis stage, surgery, hospitalization, central venous catheters, systemic anticancer therapy, history of previous VTE, obesity, immobility, platelet, leucocyte, and D-dimer [2]. However, single risk factor does not reliably identify patients with cancer at high risk of VTE development. In cancer patients treated with systemic therapy, the assessment of VTE development and thromboprophylaxis need are usually performed with validated risk assessment scores [2, 3].

The contemporary VTE risk assessment scores for ambulatory patients with cancer in the authoritative guidelines [2, 3] mainly comprise the Khorana score [11], the Vienna score [12], the PROTECHT score [13], the CONKO score [14], the ONKOTEV score, [15] the COMPASS-CAT score [16], the Tic-Onco score [17], and the CATS/MICA score [18]. The Vienna score, the PROTECHT score, the CONKO score, and the ONKOTEV score are modified Khorana risk score (KRS). A few studies compared the performance of different VTE risk assessment scores in patients with cancer. In a study

comparing the Khorana, Vienna, PROTECHT, and CONKO scores in a prospective cohort of 876 patients with advanced cancer, the results showed that the patients with high risk score had a significantly increased risk of VTE by using the Vienna or PROTECHT scores [19].

With respect to lung cancer, another study comparing the predictive efficiency among the Khorana, PROTECHT, CONKO and COMPASS-CAT scores in 118 lung cancer patients showed that only the COMPASS-CAT score identified 100% of patients who developed VTE, being the most accurate risk assessment model of VTE occurrence in patients with lung cancer [20]. Nevertheless, since routine VTE screening was not performed in the study, the asymptomatic VTE may have been missed, interfering with the confidence of the conclusion. Besides, the sample size($n = 118$) was too poor to draw a convincing conclusion.

Taken together, despite the aforementioned risk scores of VTE have been validated in ambulatory patients with cancer or lung cancer, their roles in hospitalized patients with cancer have been understudied. Besides, which of them is the most appropriate one to assess the VTE development for hospitalized patients with lung cancer remains unknown. Accordingly, the current study was performed to compare the assessment accuracy of VTE development by the risk assessment scores approved by the authoritative guidelines in hospitalized medical patients with lung cancer [2, 3].

Methods

Study design

A retrospective study was performed to explore which one of the currently authoritative risk assessment scores for VTE including PE and/or DVT had the optimal assessment accuracy for the development of VTE in hospitalized medical patients with primary lung cancer. We reviewed consecutive patients with lung cancer who had undergone VTE investigation including computed tomography pulmonary angiography (CTPA), compression ultrasonography (CUS) of lower and upper extremities, and/or planar ventilation/perfusion (V/Q) scan [21, 22] during a medical hospitalization which implied a higher probability of VTE than ambulatory outpatients. Medical hospitalization denotes the hospitalization in which chemotherapy, radiotherapy, targeted therapy, immunotherapy, and/or other medical treatment were administered to patients. Patients underwent all of the aforementioned three investigations unless there was a contraindication to CTPA. The patients were assigned into the lung cancer (LC) and lung cancer-VTE (LC-VTE) groups according to whether or not they had been diagnosed with VTE till the present study or death prior to the present study after the diagnosis of lung cancer. In the meantime of VTE diagnostic investigation, all patients received thromboprophylaxis through discharge unless there was a contraindication. The follow-up period commenced from the diagnosis of lung cancer to the present study or the death of patients, whereas the post hoc analysis period initiated from lung cancer diagnosis to the last time of VTE testing in hospitalization prior to the present study.

In the current study, the likelihood of VTE in patients were reassessed with the Khorana score, the PROTECHT score, the CONKO score, the ONKOTEV score, the COMPASS-CAT score, and the CATS/MICA score, thereby comparing their assessment accuracy for the development of VTE. The Khorana score comprises variables including primary site of cancer (very high risk [2 points] or high risk [1 point]), pre-chemotherapy platelet count of 350×10^9 /L or more (1 point), hemoglobin level less than 100 g/L and/or use of red cell growth factors (1 point), leukocyte count more than 11×10^9 /L (1 point), and body mass index (BMI) of 35 kg/m² or more (1 point). A total score of 3 or more was defined as high risk of VTE [11]. The PROTECHT score consists of Khorana score, gemcitabine chemotherapy (1point), and platinum-based chemotherapy (1point). A total score of 3 or more was defined as high risk of VTE [13]. The CONKO score is also a revised Khorana score in which BMI is replaced by the Eastern Cooperative Oncology Group (ECOG)/World Health Organization (WHO) performance status ≥2 (1 point). A total score of 3 or more was defined as high risk of VTE [14]. The ONKOTEV score is based on a Khorana score > 2(1 point), metastatic disease (1point), previous VTE (1point), and vascular/lymphatic macroscopic compression (1point). A total score of 2 or more was defined as high risk of VTE [15]. The COMPASS-CAT score includes anti-hormonal or anthracycline therapy (6 points), time since cancer diagnosis ≤6 months (4 points), central venous catheter (3 points), advanced stage of cancer (2 points), cardiovascular risk factors (5 points), recent hospitalization (5 points), personal history of VTE (1 point), and platelet count ≥350 × 10⁹ /L (2 points). A total score of 7 or more was defined as high risk of VTE [16]. The CATS/MICA score comprises one tumor-site category and D-dimer level. A 6-month cumulative risk of VTE ≥ 10%(or a total score ≥ 110) was defined as high risk of VTE [18].

The patients with high risk of VTE assessed by each score were defined as VTE likely, whereas those with non-high risk of VTE were defined as VTE unlikely. Then such dichotomy was contrasted with the actual presence and absence of VTE confirmed by CTPA, V/Q scan, and CUS, so as to compare the assessment accuracy for VTE development among these risk assessment scores. The parameter values at admission were adopted for the variables involved in these scores. For patients who had been diagnosed with VTE prior to the present study, the data of the hospitalization in which VTE was initially diagnosed was incorporated into the present study as one case, whereas for those who had not been diagnosed with VTE until the present study, the data in the hospitalization in which the last time of VTE

diagnostic testing was performed prior to the present study was adopted as one case. For each patient, all these VTE risk assessment scores were performed post hoc based on the data in the same hospitalization. One patient could not be counted as more than one case. All data were retrieved from the Electronic Medical Record (EMR) of three hospitals in Shanghai, including Shanghai Xinhua Hospital, Shanghai Pulmonary Hospital, and Shanghai Punan Hospital. The protocol was approved by the institutional review boards of these hospitals.

Study population
In terms of inclusion and exclusion criteria, we incorporated eligible patients into the current study. The inclusion criteria comprised: 1) all eligible patients were 18 years old or older; 2) all eligible patients had a definite histopathological diagnosis of primary lung cancer; 3) all eligible patients with lung cancer underwent CTPA, CUS and/or V/Q scan that could confirm the presence or absence of VTE during the hospitalizations of diagnoses or medical treatment of lung cancer, or an acute medical illness; 4) all eligible patients had complete information required for the study. The exclusion criteria comprised: 1) patients who had other known primary cancers apart from lung cancer were excluded; 2) patients who had a history of chronic VTE or thrombophilia were excluded; 3) patients who had undergone major surgery or trauma within previous month prior to the diagnoses of VTE were excluded.

Statistical analyses
Comparison of measurement data between groups was performed by using T-test. The comparison of rates was performed by Chi-square test. The number of true positive (TP), false positive (FP), false negative (FN), and true negative (TN) resulted from each risk score were compared between every two risk scores. The sensitivity, specificity, positive predictive value (PPV), negative predictive value (NPV), false positive rate (FPR), false negative rate (FNR), positive likelihood ratio (PLR), negative likelihood ratio (NLR), diagnostic odds ratio (DOR), crude agreement (CA), adjusted agreement (AA), and Youden index (YI) for the assessment of VTE development were compared among the Khorana score, the PROTECHT score, the CONKO score, the ONKOTEV score, the COMPASS-CAT score, and the CATS/MICA score. SPSS 26 was used for the statistical analysis. A P-value being less than 0.05 was defined as statistical significance.

Results
Demographics and characteristics of patients
A total of 1370 patients with lung cancer from Jan, 2013 through Dec, 2020 were incorporated into the current

study based on the inclusion criteria. According to the exclusion criteria, 29 patients who had other known primary cancers apart from lung cancer, 37 patients who had a history of chronic VTE or thrombophilia and 41 patients who had undergone major surgery or trauma within previous month prior to the diagnoses of VTE were excluded. Finally, 1263 patients were determined to be in the analysis of current study. The mean age of all patients was 70.4 years old. The number of female and male patients were 550 and 713, respectively. Among a total of 1263 patients with primary lung cancer who underwent VTE-confirming investigations, all patients underwent CUS and V/Q scan, and 1092 patients underwent CTPA whereas 171 patients did not due to contraindications.

Taken together, among 1263 patients with lung cancer, 173 patients (13.7%) had VTE, whereas 1090 ones had not. Among 173 patients with established VTE, 79 and 57 ones solely had PE and DVT, respectively, whereas 37 ones had both PE and DVT. For 173 patients with established PE, 155 patients were diagnosed with CTPA and/or V/Q scan, whereas 18 patients were diagnosed with sole V/Q scan due to the contraindications to CTPA. For 1090 patients whose VTE diagnoses were excluded, 937 patients had negative results of CTPA, V/Q scan and CUS, whereas 153 patients had negative results of V/Q scan and CUS due to the contraindications to CTPA. The median time from lung cancer diagnosis to the hospitalization in which the last time of VTE diagnostic testing was performed prior to the present study in LC and LC-VTE groups were 13.3(7.6–19.0) and 15.9(9.1–22.7) months, respectively.($p = 0.868$) The median time from lung cancer diagnosis to the hospitalization in which data were analyzed in LC and LC-VTE groups were 13.3(7.6–19.0) and 11.8(5.2–18.4) months, respectively ($p = 0.357$) The demographic and clinical characteristic of patients were summarized in Table 1.

True Positive, False Positive, False Negative, and True Negative of all Risk Scores.

The VTE possibility of all patients in the final analyses were reassessed with the Khorana score, the PROTECHT score, the CONKO score, the ONKOTEV score, the COMPASS-CAT score, and the CATS/MICA score, then were contrasted with the actual VTE establishment, to determine the number of TP, FP, FN, and TN resulted from each risk score. The number of TP, FP, FN, and TN of all risk scores are demonstrated in Table 2. In contrast with the actual VTE prevalence of 13.7%, the diagnostic VTE prevalence by the Khorana score, the PROTECHT score, the CONKO score, the ONKOTEV score, the COMPASS-CAT score, and the CATS/MICA score were 27.5, 26.5, 27.4, 22.6, 31.4, and 18.3%, respectively. The Pairwise difference of number of TP, FP, FN, TN between every two risk scores are demonstrated in Fig. 1.

Comparison of assessment accuracy for VTE development among all risk scores

Base on the number of TP, FP, FN, TN of each risk score, the assessment accuracy for VTE development among all risk scores were compared. The ratio of actual VTE prevalence in patients predicted as VTE-positive over that in those predicted as VTE-negative by the Khorana score, the PROTECHT score, the CONKO score, the ONKOTEV score, the COMPASS-CAT score, and the CATS/MICA score were 7.08(36.3% vs 5.13%), 9.21(39.7% vs 4.31%), 8.02(37.6% vs 4.69%), 15.1(49.5% vs 3.27%), 8.61(34.8% vs 4.04%), 2.75(28.6% vs 10.4%), respectively. The ratio of actual VTE exclusion in patients predicted as VTE-negative over that in those predicted as VTE-positive by the Khorana score, the PROTECHT score, the CONKO score, the ONKOTEV score, the COMPASS-CAT score, and the CATS/MICA score were 1.49(94.9% vs 63.7%), 1.59(95.7% vs 60.3%), 1.53(95.3% vs 62.4%), 1.91(96.7% vs 50.5%), 1.47(96.0% vs 65.2%), 1.25(89.6% vs 71.4%), respectively.

The sensitivity, specificity, PPV, NPV, FPR, FNR, PLR, NLR, DOR, CA, AA, and Youden index for VTE assessment by all VTE risk assessment scores involved in the present study are demonstrated in Table 3. The comparison of assessment efficiency for VTE occurrence showed that the adjusted agreement of the Khorana score, the PROTECHT score, the CONKO score, the ONKOTEV score, the COMPASS-CAT score, and the CATS/MICA score were 70.9, 73.4, 72.1, 78.6, 71.7, and 60.3%, respectively. The ONKOTEV score had the highest Youden index which was 0.68, followed by the PROTECHT score (0.58), the COMPASS-CAT score (0.56), the CONKO score (0.55), the Khorana score (0.53), and the CATS/MICA score (0.23).

Discussion

The results of current study revealed that the ONKOTEV score performed best in the assessment of VTE development in hospitalized medical patients with primary lung cancer, followed by the PROTECHT score, the COMPASS-CAT score, the CONKO score, the Khorana score, and the CATS/MICA score. Comparable studies similar to the current study are scarce except for the one of Rupa-Matysek et al., in which the COMPASS-CAT was most effective at predicting VTE in ambulatory outpatients with lung cancer, among the Khorana, PROTECHT, CONKO and COMPASS-CAT scores [20]. Nevertheless, the performance of COMPASS-CAT score for the assessment of VTE development was mediocre based on our findings. Since the study of Rupa-Matysek et al. did not include the ONKOTEV score, it is impossible to learn the results of comparison between the ONKOTEV score and the COMPASS-CAT score based on their study.

Table 1 Demographics and Characteristics of Patients

Variables	LC(n = 1090)	LC-VTE (n = 173)	P value
Age-years	68.5 (47.6–86.3)	72.2 (51.5–88.6)	0.723
Sex (female/male)-%	43.0/57.0	46.8/53.2	0.915
BMI-kg/m^2	21.9 (17.5–27.3)	29.6 (24.3–34.7)	0.013
Smoking (Y/N)-%	40.1/59.9	50.9/49.1	0.009
Smoking index-pack/year	33.6 (21.3–45.9)	47.3 (30.6–63.7)	0.001
Histopathology-no.(%)			
Adenocarcinoma	673 (61.7)	109 (63.0)	0.537
Squamous	269 (24.7)	40 (23.1)	0.941
SCLC	123 (11.3)	17 (9.80)	0.713
Others	25 (2.30)	7 (4.10)	0.025
Stage-no.(%)			
Stage I	199 (18.3)	3 (1.70)	< 0.001
Stage II	227 (20.8)	33 (19.1)	0.985
Stage III	257 (23.6)	44 (25.4)	0.836
Stage IV	407 (37.3)	93 (53.8)	0.001
High or intermediate			
C-PTP(Y/N)-%	45.2/54.8	74.6/25.4	< 0.001
D-dimer-mg/L	3713 (2336–5369)	1331 (854–1776)	< 0.001
Platelet-× 10^9/L	387 (226–543)	252 (157–357)	0.001
Hemoglobin-g/L	97 (83–114)	109 (91–127)	0.573
WBC-× 10^9/L	13.1 (7.62–18.6)	7.73 (4.38–11.1)	0.001
Chemotherapy(Y/N)-%	65.8/34.2	94.2/5.8	< 0.001
PS score-point	1.35 (0.66–2.25)	2.31 (1.23–3.47)	0.005
Metastasis(Y/N)-%	37.3/62.7	53.8/46.2	0.001
Previous VTE(Y/N)-%	9.9/90.1	17.9/82.1	0.001
Vascular/lymphatic compression(Y/N)-%	70.1/29.9	90.8/9.2	< 0.001
Anti-hormonal or anthracycline therapy(Y/N)-%	2.0/98.0	1.7/98.3	0.896
Time since cancer diagnosis≤6 months(Y/N)-%	49.8/50.2	52.6/47.4	0.916
CVC(Y/N)-%	3.9/96.1	9.8/90.2	< 0.001
Cardiovascular risk factors(Y/N)-%	15.0/85.0	29.5/70.5	< 0.001
Recent hospitalization (Y/N)-%	66.5/33.5	97.7/2.3	< 0.001

Note: LC: Lung Cancer, LC-VTE:Lung Cancer and Venous Thromboembolism, no.:number, BMI: Body Mass Index, kg/m^2: kilogram/meter^2, Y/N:Yes/No, SCLC: Small Cell Lung Cancer, C-PTP: Clinical Pretest Probability, mg/L:milligram/liter, L:liter, WBC: White Blood Cell, PS: Performance Status, VTE:Venous Thromboembolism, CVC: Central Venous Catheter

Table 2 True Positive, False Positive, False Negative, and True Negative of all Risk Scores

Variables	Khorana	PROTECHT	CONKO	ONKOTEV	COMPASS-CAT	CATS/MICA
True Positive-no.	126	133	130	141	138	66
False Positive,-no.	221	202	216	144	258	165
False Negative-no.	47	40	43	32	35	107
True Negative-no.	869	888	874	946	832	925
Diagnostic Prevalence-%	27.5	26.5	27.4	22.6	31.4	18.3
Actual Prevalence-%	13.7	13.7	13.7	13.7	13.7	13.7

Note: TP: True Positive, FP: False Positive, FN: False Negative, TN: True Negative, DP: Diagnostic Prevalence, AP: Actual Prevalence

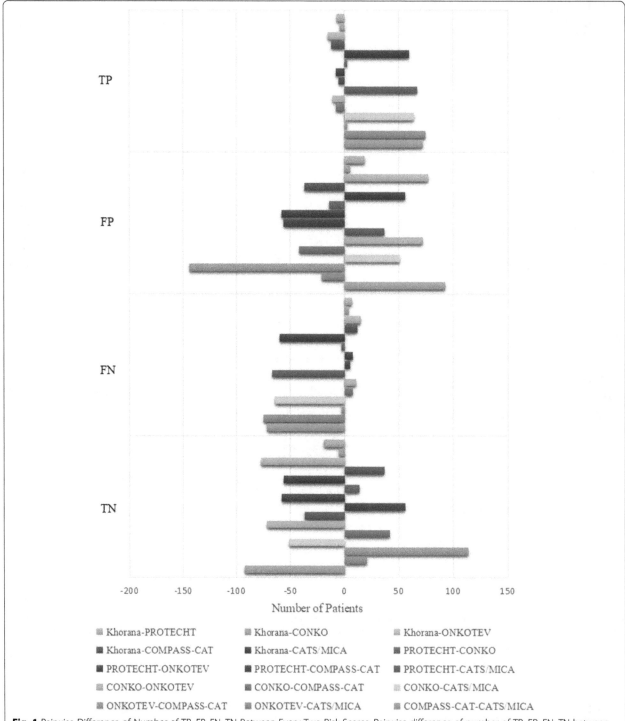

Fig. 1 Pairwise Difference of Number of TP, FP, FN, TN Between Every Two Risk Scores. Pairwise difference of number of TP, FP, FN, TN between every two risk scores are demonstrated in Fig. 1. For example, the gray bar at the top of the first row denotes the difference of number of TP between Khorana and PROTECHT, which is −7. The orange bar right below the gray one denotes the difference of number of TP between Khorana and CONKO, which is −4. The gray bar at the top of the second row denotes the difference of number of FP between Khorana and PROTECHT, which is 19. The rest bars can be interpreted in the same manner. Note: TP:True Positive, FP: False Positive, FN: False Negative, TN: True Negative.

The ONKOTEV score outperformed the other VTE risk assessment scores involved in the current study. In the ONKOTEV study, at a multivariate analysis, it was found that a Khorana score > 2, the presence of metastatic disease status, vascular/lymphatic compression, or previous history of VTE accurately predicted the

Table 3 Comparison of Assessment Accuracy for VTE Development Among all Scores

Variables	Khorana	PROTECHT	CONKO	ONKOTEV	COMPASS-CAT	CATS/MICA
Sensitivity -%	72.8	76.9	75.1	81.5	79.8	38.1
Specificity -%	79.7	81.5	80.2	86.8	76.3	84.9
PPV -%	36.3	39.7	37.6	49.5	53.5	28.6
NPV -%	94.9	95.7	85.9	96.7	96.0	89.6
FPR -%	20.3	18.5	19.8	13.2	23.7	15.1
FNR -%	27.2	23.1	24.9	18.5	20.2	61.8
PLR	3.59	4.16	3.79	6.17	3.37	2.52
NLR	0.34	0.28	0.31	0.21	0.27	0.73
DOR	10.5	14.7	12.2	29.0	12.7	3.5
CA -%	78.8	80.1	79.5	86.1	76.8	78.5
AA -%	70.9	73.4	72.1	78.6	71.7	60.3
YI	0.53	0.58	0.55	0.68	0.56	0.23

Note: PPV: Positive Predictive Value, NPV: Negative Predictive Value, FPR: False Positive Rate, FNR: False Negative Rate, PLR: Positive Likelihood Ratio, NLR: Negative Likelihood Ratio, DOR: Diagnostic Odds Ratio, CA: Crude Agreement, AA: Adjusted Agreement, YI: Youden Index

outcome of patients with cancer respectively, thereby establishing the ONKOTEV score with these four variables [15]. The Khorana score is the most classic, authoritative, and long-tested VTE risk assessment score, in which a total score > 2 represents a high risk of VTE [11]. Lung cancer patients with metastatic disease status are nearly 3 times likely to develop VTE, in contrast to those with non-metastatic status [23, 24]. In a study with respect to venous thrombosis in resected specimens for non-small cell lung cancer (NSCLC), 53.6% of cases with thrombosis were accompanied by tumor vascular infiltrating [25]. Another prospective study suggested monocyte tissue factor (TF) that was a source of TF-mediated thrombogenicity in NSCLC patients was significantly higher in patients with lymph node metastasis than those without lymph node metastasis [26]. In addition, for patients with advanced NSCLC, VTE development is associated with a previous history of VTE [27]. As a result, the combination of these three variables and a high Khorana score (> 2) could form an accurate risk assessment score for VTE development in patients with lung cancer.

Despite the authoritativeness of the Khorana score in the cancer-associated VTE risk assessment, a single Khorana score has poor performance in the assessment of VTE development for patients with lung cancer, especially for advanced lung cancer patients who may carried a high VTE risk [28–30]. Similarly, the Khorana score performed second worst in the current study. Due to a low VTE prevalence (2.2%) of the study of Khorana et al., in which the Khorana score was created, [11] the Khorana risk model appears to be a predictive tool for the identification of cancer patients at low risk of early VTE development, instead of one for patients at intermediate or high risk of VTE such as lung cancer patients.

Being basically consistent with the study of van Es N et al. [19], the PROTECHT score performed second best for the VTE assessment of patients with lung cancer in the current study. VTE is not uncommon in patients receiving chemotherapy especially platinum-based chemotherapy, of whom the majority of VTE events occur within 6 months after the initiation of chemotherapy [9, 31]. Nonetheless, since the variable "gemcitabine chemotherapy" in the PROTECHT score is unduly specific, whereas some NSCLC patients with increased VTE risk due to chemotherapy do not necessarily receive such regimen, let alone patients with small cell lung cancer. Accordingly, the efficiency of this risk score in the VTE assessment of lung cancer patients may be undermined in some degree.

The CONKO score performed moderately in Rupa-Matysek's[20], Alexander's[30], as well as the current study. The CONKO score is a modified KRS by replacing BMI with performance status (PS). Despite PS score was confirmed to be associated with an increased risk of VTE in patients with NSCLC [32], the CONKO score was almost the same as the single Khorana score. Consequently, its assessment accuracy for VTE development may be compromised similarly.

The COMPASS-CAT score performed moderately in the current study. Likewise, a large retrospective study among 3814 cancer patients including 1108 ones with lung cancer validated that the VTE assessment accuracy of COMPASS-CAT score was moderate with good negative predictive value, whereas its calibration was poor [33]. The COMPASS-CAT score is a highly comprehensive score that comprises cancer-related risk factors, patient-related predisposing risk factors, and platelets count [16]. Based on its scoring system which totally contains 28 points, many patients with lung cancer can easily reach a score of 7 that is the cutoff value of COMPASS-CAT score. Accordingly, it is a secure score which seldom misses VTE identification or thromboprophylaxis, whereas may generate excessive unnecessary VTE investigations or thromboprophylaxis. A cut-off value more than 7 points may improve its assessment accuracy of VTE development [20, 34]. Besides, the complexity of the score makes it inconvenient for clinicians to use.

The CATS/MICA score that is composed of type of cancer and D-dimer levels is a user-friendly model for the risk evaluation of cancer-associated VTE [34]. Nevertheless, being similar to its disappointing performance in the current study, the CATS/MICA score had no predictive value for VTE in the study of Alexander et al. either [30]. Since the risk for lung cancer is fixed in the CATS/MICA score, the only variable that changes is the D-dimer level. In the CATS/MICA score, the high VTE risk is defined as 6-month cumulative VTE incidence ≥10% that is approximately corresponding to a score of 110. Since patients with lung cancer (high risk tumors) definitely have a score of approximate 50 according to the CATS/MICA score, thereby at least a score of 60 for D-dimer level is required for a total score of 110. Nevertheless, a score of 60 for D-dimer level is approximately corresponding to a D-dimer level > 7 mg/L that is significantly higher than all the cutoff value of D-dimer level in other acknowledged VTE risk assessment scores [12, 21, 22, 35]. As a result, the CATS/MICA score may cause plenty of missed diagnoses due to its simplicity and excessively high cutoff value. In terms of safety, the CATS/MICA score is not a reliable VTE assessment score for patients with lung cancer.

Of note, we did not incorporate the Vienna score and the Tic-Onco score into the current study on account of soluble P-selectin and coagulation genetic variants that are respectively involved in these two scores were not routinely assayed in the hospitals participating the current study. Accordingly, we have no idea of how accurate these two risk scores are for the assessment of VTE development in lung cancer patients, in comparison with other risk scores involved in the current study. Clinical applicability and accurate identification of VTE risk assessment scores are two essential issues highlighted by Khorana [36] and Pabinger et al. [18] To date, since these two risk scores have not been validated in an external cohort, their assessment accuracy for VTE development remain unknown for patients with lung cancer. In terms of clinical applicability, the practical value of these two risk scores are limited to date by the reason that P-selectin and coagulation genetic variants are not universally tested, irrespective of their assessment accuracy for VTE development.

Although the Khorana score was highly recommended in the guidelines, [2, 3] it does not necessarily mean that it can be applied to every occasion. (e.g. lung cancer) [28–30] Fortunately, since the Khorana score was introduced, a multitude of risk assessment models for cancer-associated VTE have sprung up. Although this has led to a blissful annoyance for clinicians to make a choice, concurrently it also provides options to specialist clinicians to select a most appropriate VTE risk assessment score for specific cancer type. Thus the current study was designed and performed to seek the most appropriate one for lung cancer among the authoritative VTE risk assessment scores. Although a single KRS is insufficient to accurately assess the risk of VTE development in patients with lung cancer, a modified KRS can make the difference. Being outstanding in assessment accuracy, clinical applicability and user-friendliness, the ONKOTEV score could be a useful clinical score for clinicians to assess the risk of VTE development among patients with lung cancer in daily clinical practice.

The current study suffers from several limitations. First of all, it was a retrospective study. The prospective validation of the present conclusions among hospitalized and ambulatory lung cancer patients are underway, respectively. Secondly, the time from lung cancer diagnosis to the hospitalization in which data were analyzed among all patients differed from one another, which might introduce the heterogenity of study population. Nevertheless, the median time from lung cancer diagnosis through the hospitalization in which data were analyzed were similar between LC and LC-VTE groups without statistical difference. In addition, since the association between VTE and lung cancer is time-dependent [2], the VTE diagnostic testing approximately one year after lung cancer diagnosis in the present study well reflects the time-dependent VTE prevalence in such patient population. In addition, many of these scores involve the items with respect to cancer therapy. Accordingly, most patients having undergone cancer treatment in the present study suggests that they are suitable candidates of these scores. Thirdly, due to the fragmentary clinical information of ambulatory outpatients with lung cancer in the EMR of participating hospitals, it was intractable to set up a cohort of ambulatory patients as a control group in the present study, albeit it does not affect the results of present study. The last but not least, since the patients being investigated in the current study were all hospitalized medical patients with lung cancer, the results of the current study may not be applicable to ambulatory or surgical patients with lung cancer, or patients with other cancers than lung cancer.

Conclusions

In conclusion, the current study shows that, among the Khorana score, the PROTECHT score, the CONKO score, the ONKOTEV score, the COMPASS-CAT score, and the CATS/MICA score which are approved by authoritative guidelines, the ONKOTEV score is optimal for the assessment of VTE development in hospitalized medical patients with primary lung cancer. This finding could be conducive to the assessment of VTE development and thromboprophylaxis for hospitalized medical patients with lung cancer. Prospective validation of the present conclusions is warranted in the future.

Acknowledgements
Not applicable.

Authors' contributions
WX was in full charge of the design of the study, the analysis and interpretation of the data, and the writing of the manuscript. YFZ, HD, YMW, MX and XJG contributed more or less to the study design, data analysis and interpretation, and the writing of the manuscript. All authors have read and approved the final manuscript.

Author details
[1]Department of Pulmonary and Critical Care Medicine, Xinhua Hospital, Shanghai Jiaotong University School of Medicine,Shanghai, No. 1665, Kongjiang Road, Yangpu District, Shanghai 200092, China. [2]Department of Pulmonary and Critical Care Medicine, Punan Hospital, Pudong New District, Shanghai, China. [3]Department of Medical Oncology, Shanghai Pulmonary Hospital, Tongji University School of Medicine, Shanghai, China. [4]Department of General Medicine, North Bund Community Health Service Center, Hongkou District, Shanghai, China.

References
1. Streiff MB, Holmstrom B, Angelini D, Ashrani A, Bockenstedt PL, Chesney C, et al. NCCN guidelines insights: Cancer-associated venous thromboembolic disease, version 2.2018. J Natl Compr Cancer Netw. 2018;16(11):1289–303. https://doi.org/10.6004/jnccn.2018.0084.
2. Farge D, Frere C, Connors JM, Ay C, Khorana AA, Munoz A, et al. 2019 international clinical practice guidelines for the treatment and prophylaxis of venous thromboembolism in patients with cancer. Lancet Oncol. 2019; 20(10):e566–81. https://doi.org/10.1016/S1470-2045(19)30336-5.
3. Key NS, Khorana AA, Kuderer NM, Bohlke K, Lee AYY, Arcelus JI, et al. Venous thromboembolism prophylaxis and treatment in patients with Cancer: ASCO clinical practice guideline update. J Clin Oncol. 2020;38(5): 496–520. https://doi.org/10.1200/JCO.19.01461.
4. Shimabukuro-Vornhagen A, Böll B, Kochanek M, Azoulay É, von Bergwelt-Baildon MS. Critical care of patients with cancer. CA Cancer J Clin. 2016; 66(6):496–517. https://doi.org/10.3322/caac.21351.
5. Curigliano G, Cardinale D, Dent S, Criscitiello C, Aseyev O, Lenihan D, et al. Cardiotoxicity of anticancer treatments: epidemiology, detection, and management. CA Cancer J Clin. 2016;66(4):309–25. https://doi.org/10.3322/caac.21341.
6. Siegel RL, Miller KD, Fuchs HE, Jemal A. Cancer statistics, 2021. CA Cancer J Clin. 2021;71(1):7–33. https://doi.org/10.3322/caac.21654.
7. Bade BC, Dela Cruz CS. Lung Cancer 2020: epidemiology, etiology, and prevention. Clin Chest Med. 2020;41(1):1–24. https://doi.org/10.1016/j.ccm.2019.10.001.
8. Ay C, Ünal UK. Epidemiology and risk factors for venous thromboembolism in lung cancer. Curr Opin Oncol. 2016;28(2):145–9. https://doi.org/10.1097/CCO.0000000000000262.
9. Huang H, Korn JR, Mallick R, Friedman M, Nichols C, Menzin J. Incidence of venous thromboembolism among chemotherapy-treated patients with lung cancer and its association with mortality: a retrospective database study. J Thromb Thrombolysis. 2012;34(4):446–56. https://doi.org/10.1007/s11239-012-0741-7.
10. Howlett J, Benzenine E, Cottenet J, Foucher P, Fagnoni P, Quantin C. Could venous thromboembolism and major bleeding be indicators of lung cancer mortality? A nationwide database study. BMC Cancer. 2020;20(1):461. https://doi.org/10.1186/s12885-020-06930-1.
11. Khorana AA, Kuderer NM, Culakova E, Lyman GH, Francis CW. Development and validation of a predictive model for chemotherapy-associated thrombosis. Blood. 2008;111(10):4902–7. https://doi.org/10.1182/blood-2007-10-116327.
12. Ay C, Dunkler D, Marosi C, Chiriac AL, Vormittag R, Simanek R, et al. Prediction of venous thromboembolism in cancer patients. Blood. 2010; 116(24):5377–82. https://doi.org/10.1182/blood-2010-02-270116.
13. Verso M, Agnelli G, Barni S, Gasparini G, LaBianca R. A modified Khorana risk assessment score for venous thromboembolism in cancer patients receiving chemotherapy: the Protecht score. Intern Emerg Med. 2012;7(3):291–2. https://doi.org/10.1007/s11739-012-0784-y.
14. Pelzer U, Sinn M, Stieler J, Riess H. Primary pharmacological prevention of thromboembolic events in ambulatory patients with advanced pancreatic cancer treated with chemotherapy. Dtsch Med Wochenschr. 2013;138(41): 2084–8. https://doi.org/10.1055/s-0033-1349608.
15. Cella CA, Di Minno G, Carlomagno C, et al. Preventing venous thromboembolism in ambulatory cancer patients: the ONKOTEV study. Oncologist. 2017;22(5):601–8. https://doi.org/10.1634/theoncologist.2016-0246.
16. Gerotziafas GT, Taher A, Abdel-Razeq H, AboElnazar E, Spyropoulos AC, el Shemmari S, et al. A predictive score for thrombosis associated with breast, colorectal, lung, or ovarian cancer: the prospective COMPASS-cancer-associated thrombosis study. Oncologist. 2017;22(10):1222–31. https://doi.org/10.1634/theoncologist.2016-0414.
17. Munoz Martin AJ, Ortega I, Font C, et al. Multivariable clinical-genetic risk model for predicting venous thromboembolic events in patients with cancer. Br J Cancer. 2018;118(8):1056–61. https://doi.org/10.1038/s41416-018-0027-8.
18. Pabinger I, van Es N, Heinze G, Posch F, Riedl J, Reitter EM, et al. A clinical prediction model for cancer-associated venous thromboembolism: a development and validation study in two independent prospective cohorts. Lancet Haematol. 2018;5(7):e289–98. https://doi.org/10.1016/S2352-3026(18)30063-2.
19. van Es N, Di Nisio M, Cesarman G, et al. Comparison of risk prediction scores for venous thromboembolism in cancer patients: a prospective cohort study. Haematologica. 2017;102(9):1494–501. https://doi.org/10.3324/haematol.2017.169060.
20. Rupa-Matysek J, Lembicz M, Rogowska EK, Gil L, Komarnicki M, Batura-Gabryel H. Evaluation of risk factors and assessment models for predicting venous thromboembolism in lung cancer patients. Med Oncol. 2018;35(5): 63. https://doi.org/10.1007/s12032-018-1120-9.
21. Konstantinides SV, Meyer G, Becattini C, Bueno H, Geersing GJ, Harjola VP, et al. 2019 ESC guidelines for the diagnosis and management of acute pulmonary embolism developed in collaboration with the European Respiratory Society (ERS). Eur Heart J. 2020;41(4):543–603. https://doi.org/10.1093/eurheartj/ehz405.
22. Xiong W, Du H, Xu M, et al. An authoritative algorithm most appropriate for the prediction of pulmonary embolism in patients with AECOPD. Respir Res. 2020;21(1):218. https://doi.org/10.1186/s12931-020-01483-0.
23. Guo J, Deng QF, Xiong W, Pudasaini B, Yuan P, Liu JM, et al. Comparison among different presentations of venous thromboembolism because of lung cancer. Clin Respir J. 2019;13(9):574–82. https://doi.org/10.1111/crj.13060.
24. Xiong W, Zhao Y, Xu M, Guo J, Pudasaini B, Wu X, et al. The relationship between tumor markers and pulmonary embolism in lung cancer. Oncotarget. 2017;8(25):41412–21. https://doi.org/10.18632/oncotarget.17916.
25. Chen W, Zhang Y, Yang Y, Zhai Z, Wang C. Prognostic significance of arterial and venous thrombosis in resected specimens for non-small cell lung cancer. Thromb Res. 2015;136(2):451–5. https://doi.org/10.1016/j.thromres.2015.06.014.
26. Deng C, Wu S, Zhang L, Yang M, Lin Q, Xie Q, et al. Role of monocyte tissue factor on patients with non-small cell lung cancer. Clin Respir J. 2018;12(3): 1125–33. https://doi.org/10.1111/crj.12640.
27. Hicks LK, Cheung MC, Ding K, Hasan B, Seymour L, le MaÃ®tre AÃ©, et al. Venous thromboembolism and nonsmall cell lung cancer: a pooled analysis of National Cancer Institute of Canada clinical trials group trials. Cancer. 2009;115(23):5516–25. https://doi.org/10.1002/cncr.24596.

28. Mansfield AS, Tafur AJ, Wang CE, Kourelis TV, Wysokinska EM, Yang P. Predictors of active cancer thromboembolic outcomes: validation of the Khorana score among patients with lung cancer. J Thromb Haemost. 2016; 14(9):1773–8. https://doi.org/10.1111/jth.13378.
29. Dapkevičiūtė A, Daškevičiūtė A, Zablockis R, Kuzaitė A, Jonušienė G, Diktanas S, et al. Association between the Khorana score and pulmonary embolism risk in patients with advanced stage lung cancer. Clin Respir J. 2020;14(1):3–8. https://doi.org/10.1111/crj.13092.
30. Alexander M, Ball D, Solomon B, MacManus M, Manser R, Riedel B, et al. Dynamic thromboembolic risk modelling to target appropriate preventative strategies for patients with non-small cell lung Cancer. Cancers (Basel). 2019; 11(1):50. https://doi.org/10.3390/cancers11010050.
31. Mellema WW, van der Hoek D, Postmus PE, Smit EF. Retrospective evaluation of thromboembolic events in patients with non-small cell lung cancer treated with platinum-based chemotherapy. Lung Cancer. 2014;86(1): 73–7. https://doi.org/10.1016/j.lungcan.2014.07.017.
32. Dou F, Li H, Zhu M, Liang L, Zhang Y, Yi J, et al. Association between oncogenic status and risk of venous thromboembolism in patients with non-small cell lung cancer. Respir Res. 2018;19(1):88. https://doi.org/10.1186/s12931-018-0791-2.
33. Spyropoulos AC, Eldredge JB, Anand LN, Zhang M, Qiu M, Nourabadi S, et al. External validation of a venous thromboembolic risk score for Cancer outpatients with solid tumors: the COMPASS-CAT venous thromboembolism risk assessment model. Oncologist. 2020;25(7):e1083–90. https://doi.org/10.1634/theoncologist.2019-0482.
34. Gerotziafas GT, Mahé I, Lefkou E, AboElnazar E, Abdel-Razeq H, Taher A, et al. Overview of risk assessment models for venous thromboembolism in ambulatory patients with cancer. Thromb Res. 2020;191(Suppl 1):S50–7. https://doi.org/10.1016/S0049-3848(20)30397-2.
35. Kearon C, de Wit K, Parpia S, Schulman S, Afilalo M, Hirsch A, et al. Diagnosis of pulmonary embolism with d-dimer adjusted to clinical probability. N Engl J Med. 2019;381(22):2125–34. https://doi.org/10.1056/NEJMoa1909159.
36. Khorana AA. Simplicity versus complexity: an existential dilemma as risk tools evolve. Lancet Haematol. 2018;5(7):e273–4. https://doi.org/10.1016/S2352-3026(18)30067-X.

13

Patients with venous thromboembolism after spontaneous intracerebral hemorrhage

Qiyan Cai[1], Xin Zhang[2] and Hong Chen[1]* iD

Abstract

Background: Patients with spontaneous intracerebral hemorrhage (ICH) have a higher risk of venous thromboembolism (VTE) and in-hospital VTE is independently associated with poor outcomes for this patient population.

Methods: A comprehensive literature search about patients with VTE after spontaneous ICH was conducted using databases MEDLINE and PubMed. We searched for the following terms and other related terms (in US and UK spelling) to identify relevant studies: intracerebral hemorrhage, ICH, intraparenchymal hemorrhage, IPH, venous thromboembolism, VTE, deep vein thrombosis, DVT, pulmonary embolism, and PE. The search was restricted to human subjects and limited to articles published in English. Abstracts were screened and data from potentially relevant articles was analyzed.

Results: The prophylaxis and treatment of VTE are of vital importance for patients with spontaneous ICH. Prophylaxis measures can be mainly categorized into mechanical prophylaxis and chemoprophylaxis. Treatment strategies include anticoagulation, vena cava filter, systemic thrombolytic therapy, catheter-based thrombus removal, and surgical embolectomy. We briefly summarized the state of knowledge regarding the prophylaxis measures and treatment strategies of VTE after spontaneous ICH in this review, especially on chemoprophylaxis and anticoagulation therapy. Early mechanical prophylaxis, especially with intermittent pneumatic compression, is recommended by recent guidelines for patients with spontaneous ICH. While decision-making on chemoprophylaxis and anticoagulation therapy evokes debate among clinicians, because of the concern that anticoagulants may increase the risk of recurrent ICH and hematoma expansion. Uncertainty still exists regarding optimal anticoagulants, the timing of initiation, and dosage.

Conclusion: Based on current evidence, we deem that initiating chemoprophylaxis with UFH/LMWH within 24–48 h of ICH onset could be safe; anticoagulation therapy should depend on individual clinical condition; the role of NOACs in this patient population could be promising.

Keywords: Intracerebral hemorrhage, Venous thromboembolism, Pulmonary embolism, Deep venous thrombosis, Anticoagulation

* Correspondence: hopehong2019@126.com
[1]Department of Pulmonary and Critical Care Medicine, the First Affiliated Hospital of Chongqing Medical University, No.1 Youyi Road, Yuzhong District, Chongqing 400016, China
Full list of author information is available at the end of the article

Introduction

Intracerebral hemorrhage (ICH) accounts for approximately 10–30% of all strokes, but is associated with over-proportionally high mortality and enormous health-care costs [1–3]. The most prevalent subtype of ICH is spontaneous ICH, which is principally caused by cerebral small vessel diseases; vascular malformations, tumors, anticoagulants, antiplatelet medication, and vasculitis are among the other reasons [4]. Venous thromboembolism (VTE), including deep venous thrombosis (DVT) and pulmonary embolism (PE), is a common complication in hospitalized patients and is associated with substantial morbidity, mortality, and health-care cost [5]. Patients with ICH have a higher risk of VTE, which can reach 2–4 times that of patients with acute ischemic stroke [6, 7]. In some large database retrospective studies, the incidence of VTE, symptomatic DVT, and clinically evident PE in hospitalized patients with spontaneous ICH has been estimated to be 2–4%, 1–2%, and 0.7–2%, respectively [6–10]. In two prospective studies, the incidence of DVT detected by ultrasonography during hospitalization reached 20–40% [11, 12].

VTE is one of the most common and preventable complications of spontaneous ICH. However, the treatment options of the two are full of contradictions. The focus of VTE treatment is anticoagulation and prevention of recurrent thrombosis, while the treatment of ICH is focused on hemostasis and averting hematoma expansion. For such patients, how should clinicians balance the treatment need of the two conditions and make appropriate treatment strategies is a question worthy of discussion.

In this review, we will briefly summarize the state of knowledge regarding the risk factors, prophylaxis measures, and treatment strategies of VTE after spontaneous ICH.

Risk factors

Virchow's triad

Virchow's triad describes the three key predisposing factors to VTE: abnormal flow, vessel wall abnormalities (endothelial injury), and coagulation state [13]. In patients with spontaneous ICH, there is venous stasis due to immobility and hemiplegia [14, 15], endothelial injury caused by invasive operations, and hypercoagulability as a result of dehydrating, hemostatic and antifibrinolytic agents [16].

Other factors

A large number of studies on the risk factors of VTE in patients with spontaneous ICH were conducted; nevertheless, no independent study on this aspect of PE has been performed. Advanced age, immobility, hemiplegia, high D-Dimer and CRP value, high NIHSS score, and previous VTE history as risk factors of VTE in patients with spontaneous ICH have basically reached a consensus [8, 9, 12, 17].

Melmed et al. [18] conducted a study on 414 patients with ICH to clarify the relationship between infection and VTE. They found that respiratory and bloodstream infections were associated with VTE after primary ICH, while urinary and other infections were not.

Whether gender is a relevant risk factor remains controversial. Retrospective studies published by Kim et al. [8] and Ding et al. [9], and the prospective cohort study published by Ogata et al. [12] all pointed out that gender was not a risk factor of VTE. While the prospective cohort studies published by Kawase et al. [11] for the Japanese population and Cheng et al. [17] for the Chinese population indicated that female sex was a risk factor. The discrepancy in the results could be due to differences in design, sample size and population.

Prophylaxis measures

Patients with spontaneous intracerebral hemorrhage are predisposed to VTE and in-hospital VTE is independently associated with poor outcomes at discharge, 3-month, and 1-year [19]. One study demonstrated that without prophylaxis, up to 75% of patients with residual hemiplegia following ICH developed DVT, and PE-related deaths occurred in approximately 5% of patients with ICH [20]. As a consequence, the prophylaxis of VTE is of vital importance. Prophylaxis measures can be categorized into active limb movement, mechanical prophylaxis, and chemoprophylaxis. Active limb movement, such as ankle pump exercise (APE) which rhythmically contracts and relaxes the calf muscles through the ankle joint movement, and squeezes the venous plexus to promote the venous blood return in lower limbs, is efficient and cost-effective in eliminating venous stasis to contribute to the prophylaxis of DVT [21–23]. We mainly focus on mechanical and chemical prophylaxis in this review.

Mechanical prophylaxis

For some hospitalized medical patients at high risk of thrombosis (e.g. patients with hemorrhagic stroke [7], lower extremity fractures [24], nephrotic syndrome [25], etc.) who are bleeding or at high risk of major bleeding, the guideline from American College of Chest Physicians (ACCP) has suggested the optimal use of mechanical prophylaxis with graduated compression stockings (GCS) or intermittent pneumatic compression (IPC), rather than no mechanical prophylaxis [26].

GCS and IPC

For the prophylaxis of VTE, guidelines published in recent years recommended the use of IPC and/or GCS

Table 1 Recommendations for GCS and IPC in recent guidelines for patients with spontaneous ICH

Years	Organization	GCS	IPC	Timing	Grade
2012	ACCP [26]	√	√	Not mentioned	Weak recommendation, low-quality evidence
2014	ESO [27]	×	√	Not mentioned	Strong recommendation, moderate-quality evidence
2015	AHA/ASA [28]	×	√	At admission	Strong recommendation, high-quality evidence
2016	NCS [29]	√	√	At admission	Strong recommendation, high-quality evidence
2018	NICE [30]	×	√	Within 3 days	Not mentioned
2020	HSFC [31]	×	√	At admission	High-quality evidence

ACCP the American College of Chest Physicians; *ESO* European Stroke Organization; *AHS/ASA* the American Heart Association/American Stroke Association; *NCS* the Neurocritical Care Society; *NICE* National Institute for Health and Care Excellence; *HSFC* Heart and Stroke Foundation of Canada
√ recommended, × not recommended

(Table 1). The Clots in Legs Or sTockings after Stroke (CLOTS) trial 1, a multicenter and randomized controlled trial in stroke patients who were enrolled between 2001 and 2008 (*n* = 2518, 232 with ICH), demonstrated that GCS alone was ineffective in preventing DVT (10.0% vs. 10.5%, OR 0.98, 95%CI 0.76–1.27) and caused more adverse effects, including skin breaks, ulcers, blisters, and necrosis of lower extremities (5.0% vs. 1.0%, OR 4.18, 95%CI 2.40–7.27) [32]. The CLOTS trial 3, which was also a multicenter and randomized controlled trial conducted between 2008 to 2012 in patients who were immobile after stroke (*n* = 2876, 376 with ICH) to assess the effectiveness of IPC in preventing DVT, addressed that the routine application of IPC in patients with ICH was associated with a significantly decreased risk of DVT (6.7% vs. 17.0%, OR 0.36, 95%CI 0.17–0.75) [33]. Therefore, recent guidelines have tended to recommend IPC alone.

Timing of initiation
Regarding the timing of intervention for mechanical prophylaxis in patients with spontaneous ICH, the recommendations of the current guidelines (Table 1) have tended to converge: start at the time of hospital admission and use as early as possible. In 2018, the guideline from NICE added recommendations that mechanical prophylaxis should be initiated within 3 days of ICH [30].

Chemoprophylaxis
The use of chemoprophylaxis with unfractionated heparin (UFH), low molecular weight heparin (LMWH), and direct oral anticoagulants (e.g. warfarin, rivaroxaban, apixaban, dabigatran, etc.) in patients with spontaneous ICH is an area of ongoing debate. Determining appropriate chemoprophylaxis is challenging in the presence of ICH. The concern of hematoma expansion and recurrent ICH limits the use of chemoprophylaxis in clinical practice. A large database retrospective study including 32,690 patients with spontaneous ICH from 2006 to 2010 demonstrated that 5395 patients (16.5%) received chemoprophylaxis [34]. Another multicenter observational cohort study demonstrated

that among 74,283 patients with ICH, only 5929 received chemoprophylaxis while 66,444 received mechanical prophylaxis (7.9% vs. 89.4%) [35].

Timing of initiation
To date, the optimal timing for the initiation of chemoprophylaxis is still uncertain. A large database retrospective study demonstrated 44.8% (2416/5395) of patients with spontaneous ICH received prophylactic anticoagulation with UFH, enoxaparin, or dalteparin by day 2 of onset [34]. Hematoma expansion usually occurs in the early phase of ICH. Results from imaging studies have demonstrated that 70% of patients with spontaneous ICH have hematoma expansion within 24 h of onset and expansion after 24 h seems extremely rare [36, 37]. In contrast, patients with ICH develop DVT as early as the second day without prophylaxis, with the peak incidence occurring between days 2 and 7 [38]. In addition, anticoagulation is associated with recurrent ICH in patients with active bleeding, while no such association has been found in patients who have documentation of hematoma stabilization on neuroimaging [39]. Therefore, we speculate that initiating chemoprophylaxis within 24–48 h of onset, under the circumstance of no signs of hematoma expansion or active bleeding on neuroimaging, could be safe and effective. A number of studies (Table 2) demonstrated that initiating chemoprophylaxis with UFH/LMWH within 24–48 h was safe for being not associated with hematoma expansion or recurrent ICH, but differed in the efficiency. Initiating chemoprophylaxis within 24–48 h seems not to be more effective in reducing the risk of VTE than other timing. Recommendations in relevant guidelines vary as well (Table 3). Hence, more high-quality studies are needed on the timing of initiating chemoprophylaxis among patients with spontaneous ICH.

Anticoagulants
Anticoagulants mostly used in relevant studies are UFH or LMWH. A large database retrospective study on

Table 2 Studies about chemoprophylaxis in patients with spontaneous ICH

First author (year)	Design	N of pts	Timing	Prophylaxis	Risk of VTE	Risk of HE /recurrent ICH
Boeer [40] (1991)	Prospective	68	2 days vs. 4 days vs. 10 days	UFH 5000 U q8h	Reduction in number of PE in 2 days group (1 vs. 5 vs. 9)	No significant difference
Wasay [41] (2008)	Prospective	458	1–6 days	UFH 2500-5000 U bid+GCS vs. GCS alone	No significant difference	No significant difference
Orken [42] (2009)	Randomized trial	75	48 h	Enoxaparin 4000 IU qd vs. GCS	No significant difference	No significant difference
Kiphuth [43] (2009)	Retrospective	97	< 36 h	Enoxaparin 4000 IU qd or dalteparin 2500 IU qd	Not mentioned	0 at day 2
Faust [44] (2017)	Retrospective	400	<48 h vs. ≥48 h	Not mentioned	0.7% vs. 3.1% ($P = 0.17$)	5.6% vs. 5.0% ($P = 0.80$)
Ianosi [45] (2019)	Retrospective	134	<48 h vs. ≥48 h	Enoxaparin 2000 IU/4000 IU qd	Not mentioned	No significant difference
Kananeh [46] (2021)	Retrospective	163	<24 h vs. ≥24 h	UFH 5000 U q8h	Not mentioned	3.4% vs. 6.7% ($P = 0.49$)
Qian [47] (2021)	Randomized trial	139	24 h vs. 72 h	Enoxaparin 2000 IU bid	No significant difference	No significant difference

N of pts number of patients; *UFH* unfractionated heparin; *GCS* graduated compression stockings; *HE* hematoma expansion

patients with spontaneous ICH from 2006 to 2010 ($n =$ 32,690) showed that the most commonly used agents for VTE prophylaxis were heparin (71.1%), enoxaparin (27.5%), and dalteparin(1.4%) [34]. The efficacy and safety of most direct oral anticoagulants (DOACs) in preventing VTE in patients with spontaneous ICH have not been evaluated because they have been excluded from randomized trials on VTE chemoprophylaxis with DOACs. The majority of studies (Table 2) have demonstrated that UFH or LMWH is not associated with recurrent ICH, hematoma expansion, and increased mortality. A meta-analysis, including 9 studies and 4055 patients with spontaneous ICH, also showed that chemoprophylaxis with UFH/LMWH was not associated with a significant increase in hematoma expansion (6.6% vs. 3.2%, $P = 0.14$) or mortality (12.0% vs. 11.8%, $P = 0.29$) in comparison with non-heparin prophylaxis [48]. However, the efficacy of VTE chemoprophylaxis has not reached a consensus (Table 2).

Dosage

The appropriate anticoagulant dosage is still inconclusive. For VTE prophylaxis with UFH, the suggested dosage is 5000 units subcutaneously two or three times daily. No consensus has been established regarding the optimal frequency of dosing (two vs. three times daily). While with LMWH, Tetri et al. retrospectively evaluated the safety and efficacy of enoxaparin in VTE prophylaxis among 407 patients with spontaneous ICH and demonstrated that the appropriate dosage could be 2000 or 4000 IU once daily [49]. Wu et al. [50] also pointed out that subcutaneous administration of 4000 IU of enoxaparin once daily can prevent DVT in patients with ICH without hematoma expansion or recurrent ICH.

In conclusion, controversies exist regarding the efficacy, optimal anticoagulants, timing, and dosage of VTE chemoprophylaxis for patients with spontaneous ICH. Recommendations vary among relevant guidelines (Table 3). We expect more high-quality studies to provide direction for clinical decision-making.

Treatment strategies

The treatment strategies for VTE include anticoagulation, vena cava filter, systemic thrombolytic therapy, catheter-based thrombus removal, and surgical embolectomy. Controversies and uncertainties remain in the

Table 3 Recommendations for chemoprophylaxis in recent guidelines for patients with spontaneous ICH

Years	Organization	LMWH	UFH	Timing	Grade
2012	ACCP [26]	√	√	2–4 days	Weak recommendation, low-quality evidence
2014	ESO [27]	Not mentioned	Not mentioned	Not mentioned	Weak recommendation, low-quality evidence
2015	AHA/ASA [28]	√	√	Not mentioned	Weak recommendation, moderate-quality evidence
2016	NCS [29]	√	√	Within 48 h	Weak recommendation, low-quality evidence
2020	HSFC [31]	√	Not mentioned	After 48 h	Moderate-quality evidence

ACCP the American College of Chest Physicians; *ESO* European Stroke Organization; *AHS/ASA* the American Heart Association/American Stroke Association; *NCS* the Neurocritical Care Society; *HSFC* Heart and Stroke Foundation of Canada; *UFH* unfractionated heparin; *LMWH* low molecular weight heparin
√ recommended, × not recommended

treatment of VTE after spontaneous ICH, especially in the acute phase of ICH (usually within 2 weeks of onset) which has a high risk of hematoma expansion and recurrence [51]. We briefly summarize the evidence of VTE treatment after acute spontaneous ICH as follows.

Anticoagulation

Anticoagulation therapy is the cornerstone of VTE treatment. However, active bleeding is considered a contraindication to anticoagulation therapy. Decision-making on anticoagulation therapy after spontaneous ICH evokes debate among clinicians and the inadequacies in the evidence, for the reason that such patients have been excluded from randomized trials of anticoagulation therapy for VTE, makes the decision-making challenging. The three questions that need to be answered are as follows: first, whether anticoagulation therapy should be applied on such patients; second, when is the appropriate timing to initiate anticoagulation; and third, which anticoagulant is the optimal choice.

Anticoagulation or not

Limited data are available on the pros and cons of anticoagulation therapy for VTE following spontaneous ICH. Whether anticoagulation should be used depends on the individual risk-benefit ratio of anticoagulation therapy, that is, the risk of recurrent ICH and hematoma expansion versus the risk of VTE progression.

No reliable methods have been established to predict the risk of recurrent ICH and hematoma expansion. The pathophysiological mechanism of hematoma expansion remains unclear. A number of studies have demonstrated that previous use of anticoagulants or antiplatelet agents, advanced age, systolic hypertension, hyperglycemia, high NIHSS score or Glasgow Coma Scale score are related clinical risk factors for hematoma expansion [52–61]; CTA spot sign, blend sign, black hole sign, island sign, and iodine sign are the radiological risk factors [62–68]. The annualized rate of recurrent spontaneous ICH is approximately 2% [1, 69]. Spontaneous ICH principally results from small vessel diseases that are mainly composed of hypertensive arteriopathy and cerebral amyloid angiopathy (CAA). Hypertension has been identified as one of the most crucial and modifiable risk factors for recurrent ICH. Lowering blood pressure is associated with a reduced recurrence of ICH [70–72]. Amyloid angiopathy has a predilection for the cortical arteries, hence CAA is a major contributor of spontaneous lobar ICH, which has a significantly higher risk for recurrence compared to deep ICH [73–75]. In addition, a number of studies have demonstrated that older age, cerebral microbleeds (CMB) and cortical superficial siderosis (cSS) on MRI, and Apolipoprotein E (APOE) genotype (ε2 or ε4) are associated with a higher recurrence

risk [76–78]. In conclusion, anticoagulation therapy should be more careful in patients with the risk factors mentioned above. Besides, the modifiable risk factors, such as hypertension and hyperglycemia, should be minimized if anticoagulants are to be used in this patient population.

Patients with spontaneous ICH have been excluded from prospective studies and randomized trials on anticoagulation therapy for VTE. The available literature is almost exclusively case reports. Ajmeri et al. [79] presented a case of a 68-year-old male who suffered from recent ICH and recurrent PE. The anticoagulation therapy was initiated with UFH after a CT scan was done to eliminate active bleeding, and then altered to enoxaparin. The patient was discharged from the hospital in a stable condition without neurological deficits. Similar cases were also reported by Becattini et al. [80] and Lee et al. [81]

A Danish large-database retrospective study (n = 2978) which was focusing on patients with spontaneous ICH, demonstrated that oral anticoagulant (OAC) resumption was associated with decreased risk of thrombotic events and not increasing the risk of recurrent ICH [82]. Current studies on anticoagulation therapy are mostly focused on the OAC resumption after anticoagulation-related ICH. In addition to VTE, the indications for anticoagulation resumption include atrial fibrillation, mechanical valves, myocardial infarction, etc. The majority of studies have tended to reach a consensus that anticoagulation resumption results in a clinical benefit in terms of thromboembolic event reduction without increasing the risk of recurrent ICH or hematoma expansion (Table 4). These results were confirmed by a meta-analysis (8 studies, 5306 patients with ICH) that demonstrated restarting OAC decreased the risk of thrombotic events (6.7% vs. 17.6%, RR 0.34, 95%CI 0.25–0.45) without significantly increased risk of recurrent ICH (8.7% vs. 7.8%, RR 1.01, 95%CI 0.58–1.77) [87]. What is noteworthy is that only the patients with smaller hemorrhage volumes and mild functional changes have been eligible for anticoagulation resumption in many studies, consequently decreasing the risk of recurrent ICH.

Nevertheless, some opposite results exist. A retrospective study with 79 patients who had brain tumors and following anticoagulation-related ICH showed that anticoagulation resumption with LMWH or DOACs was associated with a significantly lower risk of recurrent VTE (8.1% vs. 35.3%, P = 0.003) but a higher risk of recurrent ICH (6.1% vs. 4.2%), especially in patients with primary brain tumors and major ICH [88]. Different study designs and research objects may explain the opposite results. Several retrospective studies and meta-analysis studies have shown that anticoagulation is associated with an increased risk of ICH in patients with

Table 4 Studies on anticoagulation resumption after ICH

First author (year)	Design	ICH type	N of pts	Indications	Timing of resumption	Anticoagulants	Comparator	Risk of TE	Risk of recurrent ICH
Majeed [83] (2010)	Retrospective	Anticoagulation-related	234	AF, MV, VTE	Median 5.6 weeks	Warfarin	Without AC	Not mentioned	8 vs. 10 (HR 5.6, 95%CI 1.8–17.2)
Yung [84] (2012)	Retrospective	Anticoagulation-related	284	AF, MV, VTE	Within a month	Warfarin	Without AC	Not mentioned	15.4% vs. 15.0% (P = 0.94)
Kuramatsu [85] (2015)	Retrospective	Anticoagulation-related	719	AF, MV, VTE	Median 31 days	OAC	Without AC	5.2% vs. 15.0% (P < 0.001)	8.1% vs. 6.6% (P = 0.48)
Witt [86] (2015)	Retrospective	Anticoagulation-related	160	AF, MI, MV, IS, VTE	Median 14 days	Warfarin	Without AC	3.7% vs. 12.3% (P = 0.092)	7.6% vs.3.7% (P = 0.497)
Ottosen [82] (2016)	Retrospective	Spontaneous	2978	AF, IS, MI, MV, PAD, VTE	Not mentioned	OAC	Without AC	Lower (HR 0.58, 95%CI 0.35–0.97)	Not increased (HR 0.90, 95%CI 0.44–1.82)

N of pts number of patients; *AF* atrial fibrillation; *MV* mechanical valves; *MI* myocardial infarction; *IS* ischemic stroke; *PAD* peripheral vascular disease; *OAC* oral anticoagulants; *AC* anticoagulants; *TE* thrombotic events; *HR* hazard ratio

primary brain tumors, however, the association seems not to be found in patients with metastatic brain tumors [89–91]. Hence, anticoagulation resumption in patients with ICH and primary brain tumors must be cautious.

Timing of initiation

No consensus exists on optimal timing for initiation of anticoagulation therapy following spontaneous ICH. The timing ranged from 2.5 days to 18 weeks in retrospective studies on anticoagulation resumption after ICH [92]. No randomized trial data are available to guide the decision. Hence, the timing of initiating anticoagulation therapy should depend on the individual clinical conditions.

Anticoagulant choice

No comparative studies on different anticoagulants in patients with VTE after spontaneous ICH have been published. Existing studies mostly focus on the safety of anticoagulants and ICH is one of the crucial indicators. The relevant studies almost exclusively referred to vitamin-K antagonists used for anticoagulation resumption after ICH. However, the role of novel oral anticoagulants (NOACs), including dabigatran (inhibitor of factor IIa), rivaroxaban, apixaban, and edoxaban (inhibitors of factor Xa), may be more promising than vitamin-K antagonists for the reasons as follows: (1) NOACs are more convenient to use for lack of monitoring requirements and less interaction with food and other drugs; (2) a number of large-scale retrospective studies and randomized trials have proved that NOACs are associated with a reduction in the risk of ICH compared with vitamin K antagonists (Table 5); (3) NOACs-related ICH is less severe than warfarin-related ICH, with smaller hematoma volume, lower rate of hematoma expansion, favorable functional and vital outcomes, and lower

mortality [98–100]; (4) the availability of antidotes (idarucizumab and andexanet) that allow an immediate and complete reversal of the anticoagulant effect of NOACs [101–103]. We expect high-quality and large-scale studies on patients with spontaneous ICH to provide support.

Inferior vena cava filter

The efficacy of inferior vena cava (IVC) filter in preventing formation or aggravation of PE caused by shedding of deep vein thrombosis of lower extremities has been confirmed in general patients. However, none of the studies have focused solely on patients with spontaneous ICH.

A retrospective study included 371 stroke patients (including 105 patients with hemorrhagic stroke) who received IVC filters and demonstrated that IVC filters were effective in preventing life-threatening PE; however, the filter-related complications, including filter migration, filter fracture, and filter thrombosis, were also worthy of attention [104]. Meritxell et al. [105] used the data of the RIETE registry to figure out the association between the use of IVC filters and the outcome of patients presenting with major bleeding during anticoagulation for VTE. Among 1065 patients (including 124 patients with intracranial hemorrhage) in this study, 11% received IVC filters; the result suggested that patients receiving IVC filters had a lower risk for all-cause death (HR 0.55, 95%CI 0.23–1.40) and a similar risk for PE recurrence (HR 1.57, 95%CI 0.38–6.36). However, the study by Kare et al. [106] on 1068 patients with acute brain injury (the proportion of ICH was not mentioned) who received IVC filters demonstrated that IVC filters were ineffective in preventing PE (HR 3.19, 95%CI 1.3–3.3) and reducing mortality (HR 1.0, 95%CI 0.8–1.3). Besides, once IVC filters were placed, few were removed.

Table 5 Studies about NOACs vs. warfarin in patients with VTE

First author (year)	Design	N of pts	Anticoagulant	Comparator	Recurrent VTE and VTE-related death	Risk of ICH
Schulman [93] (2009)	Randomized trial	2564	Dabigatran	Warfarin	2.4% vs. 2.1%, HR 1.10 (0.65–1.84)	0 vs. 3
Buller [94] (2012)	Randomized trial	4832	Rivaroxaban	Enoxaparin, followed by warfarin	2.1% vs. 1.8%, HR 1.12 (0.75–1.68)	3 vs. 12
Agnelli [95] (2013)	Randomized trial	5395	Apixaban	Enoxaparin, followed by warfarin	2.3% vs. 2.7%, HR 0.84 (0.60–1.18)	3 vs. 6
Buller [96] (2013)	Randomized trial	4921	Edoxaban	Warfarin	3.2% vs. 3.5%, HR 0.89 (0.70–1.13)	0 vs. 6
Lamsam [97] (2018)	Retrospective	218,620	NOACs	Warfarin	Not mentioned	1/1000 vs. 3.3/1000 ($P < 0.0001$)

N of pts number of patients; *NOACs* novel oral anticoagulants; *HR* hazard ratio

Jan et al. [107] also supported this result. Among 204 retrievable IVC filters inserted in neurosurgical patients in their study, only 19% were retrieved and 55% converted to permanent devices. We deem that the difference in results is partly due to the different patient groups included in each study. Therefore, whether the IVC filters are beneficial to patients with VTE after spontaneous ICH still needs targeted studies.

Other treatments

The application of systemic thrombolytic therapy, catheter-based thrombus removal, and surgical embolectomy in patients with VTE after spontaneous ICH is only seen in a few case reports and still needs further exploration.

Current guidelines have recommended the immediate administration of thrombolytic therapy in patients with massive PE and without contraindications [26]. Thrombolytic therapy is said to be contraindicated in the presence of ICH. However, some case reports revealed that thrombolysis could be safe and effective in patients with the two conditions. Wendy et al. [108] presented a case of a 60-year-old woman with massive PE (led to cardiac arrest with pulseless electrical activity) and a recent hemorrhagic cerebrovascular accident who was administered tissue plasminogen activator (t-PA). No hematoma expansion occurred, and the patient was eventually discharged from the hospital. In another report, systemic thrombolysis with recombinant tissue plasminogen activator (rt-PA) for massive PE was used with success in a 53-year-old male with acute spontaneous ICH [109]. Therefore, in patients who are at high risk of death from massive pulmonary embolism, contraindications to thrombolysis should be weighed against the potential benefit.

The ACCP guideline recommends catheter-based thrombus removal or surgical embolectomy in patients with acute PE who have hypotension and contraindications to thrombolysis if appropriate expertise and resources are available [26]. No studies or case reports have been reported in the application of catheter-based thrombus removal in patients with VTE after spontaneous ICH as yet. For surgical methods, Endo et al. [110] reported a 69-year-old presented with acute PE 11 days after ICH and underwent surgical embolectomy with cardiopulmonary bypass. No recurrence of ICH was observed in this patient.

Patients with preexisting VTE and ICH

Although this review mainly focuses on the prophylaxis and treatment of VTE after spontaneous ICH, another crucial and overlapping clinical scenario that happens in patients with preexisting VTE and following ICH is also noteworthy. Anticoagulation-related ICH is more common in this patient population due to the need for long-term anticoagulation therapy of VTE. Anticoagulation-related ICH is more severe and associated with a higher risk of hematoma expansion and higher mortality, compared to other spontaneous ICH [56, 85, 111]. Managements of anticoagulation-related ICH include halting anticoagulation and anticoagulants reversal, which has protamine sulfate, vitamin K, fresh frozen plasma (FFP), prothrombin complex concentrate (PCC), rFVIIa, idarucizumab, and andexanet as options for different anticoagulants [112]. In addition, anticoagulation resumption should also be considered in patients with preexisting VTE. Anticoagulation should be restarted when the risk of VTE progression outweighs recurrent ICH or hematoma expansion. However, as the description in Section 4.1, the optimal timing and anticoagulants remain unclear.

Conclusion

(1) Early mechanical prophylaxis with IPC and/or GCS is recommended, having a preference for IPC.

Controversies exist regarding the effectiveness, optimal anticoagulants, timing, and dosage of VTE chemoprophylaxis. Initiating chemoprophylaxis with UFH/LMWH within 24–48 h of spontaneous ICH onset could be safe.

(2) Given the limited evidence and the observational nature of the studies regarding anticoagulation therapy, uncertainty exists regarding anticoagulation, timing, and anticoagulants. Anticoagulation treatment should depend on individual clinical condition. The role of NOACs in this patient population could be promising.

(3) More targeted and high-quality studies on vena cava filter, systemic thrombolytic therapy, catheter-based thrombus removal, and surgical embolectomy are needed.

Abbreviations
ACCP: the American College of Chest Physicians; AF: Atrial fibrillation; AHS/ASA: the American Heart Association/American Stroke Association; DOACs: Direct oral anticoagulants; DVT: Deep venous thrombosis; ESO: European Stroke Organization; GCS: Graduated compression stockings; HE: Hematoma expansion; HR: Hazard ratio; HSFC: Heart and Stroke Foundation of Canada; ICH: Intracerebral hemorrhage; IPC: Intermittent pneumatic compression; IVC: Inferior vena cava; LMWH: Low molecular weight heparin; MI: Myocardial infarction; MV: Mechanical valves; NCS: The Neurocritical Care Society; NICE: National Institute for Health and Care Excellence; OAC: Oral anticoagulants; PAD: Peripheral vascular disease; PE: Pulmonary embolism; UFH: Unfractionated heparin; VTE: Venous thromboembolism

Acknowledgements
Not applicable.

Authors' contributions
QC wrote the manuscript, XZ designed the tables and HC reviewed the manuscript. All authors read and approved the final manuscript.

Author details
[1]Department of Pulmonary and Critical Care Medicine, the First Affiliated Hospital of Chongqing Medical University, No.1 Youyi Road, Yuzhong District, Chongqing 400016, China. [2]Respiratory Disease Department, Xinqiao Hospital, Chongqing, China.

References
1. Poon MTC, Fonville AF, Al-Shahi SR. Long-term prognosis after intracerebral haemorrhage: systematic review and meta-analysis. J Neurol Neurosurg Psychiatry. 2014;85(6):660–7.
2. Feigin VL, Norrving B, Mensah GA. Global burden of stroke. Circ Res. 2017;120(3):439–48.
3. van Asch CJ, Luitse MJ, Rinkel GJ, van der Tweel I, Algra A, Klijn CJ. Incidence, case fatality, and functional outcome of intracerebral haemorrhage over time, according to age, sex, and ethnic origin: a systematic review and meta-analysis. Lancet Neurol. 2010;9(2):167 76.
4. Dastur CK, Yu W. Current management of spontaneous intracerebral haemorrhage. Stroke Vasc Neurol. 2017;2(1):21–9.
5. Di Nisio M, van Es N, Büller HR. Deep vein thrombosis and pulmonary embolism. Lancet. 2016;388(10063):3060–73.
6. Skaf E, Stein PD, Beemath A, Sanchez J, Bustamante MA, Olson RE. Venous thromboembolism in patients with ischemic and hemorrhagic stroke. Am J Cardiol. 2005;96(12):1731–3.
7. Gregory PC, Kuhlemeier KV. Prevalence of venous thromboembolism in acute hemorrhagic and thromboembolic stroke. Am J Phys Med Rehabil. 2003;82(5):364–9.
8. Kim KS, Brophy GM. Symptomatic venous thromboembolism: incidence and risk factors in patients with spontaneous or traumatic intracranial hemorrhage. Neurocrit Care. 2009;11(1):28–33.
9. Ding D, Sekar P, Moomaw CJ, Comeau ME, James ML, Testai F, et al. Venous thromboembolism in patients with spontaneous Intracerebral hemorrhage: a multicenter study. Neurosurgery. 2019;84(6):E304–E10.
10. Goldstein JN, Fazen LE, Wendell L, Chang Y, Rost NS, Snider R, et al. Risk of thromboembolism following acute intracerebral hemorrhage. Neurocrit Care. 2009;10(1):28–34.
11. Kawase K, Okazaki S, Toyoda K, Toratani N, Yoshimura S, Kawano H, et al. Sex difference in the prevalence of deep-vein thrombosis in Japanese patients with acute intracerebral hemorrhage. Cerebrovasc Dis. 2009;27(4):313–9.
12. Ogata T, Yasaka M, Wakugawa Y, Inoue T, Ibayashi S, Okada Y. Deep venous thrombosis after acute intracerebral hemorrhage. J Neurol Sci. 2008;272(1–2):83–6.
13. Malone PC, Agutter PS. The aetiology of deep venous thrombosis. QJM : monthly journal of the Association of Physicians. 2006;99(9):581–93.
14. Sartori M, Favaretto E, Cosmi B. Relevance of immobility as a risk factor for symptomatic proximal and isolated distal deep vein thrombosis in acutely ill medical inpatients. Vascular medicine (London, England). 2021;26(5):542–8.
15. Pottier P, Hardouin JB, Lejeune S, Jolliet P, Gillet B, Planchon B. Immobilization and the risk of venous thromboembolism. A meta-analysis on epidemiological studies. Thromb Res. 2009;124(4):468–76.
16. Kelly J, Hunt BJ, Lewis RR, Swaminathan R, Moody A, Seed PT, et al. Dehydration and venous thromboembolism after acute stroke. QJM. 2004;97(5):293–6.
17. Cheng X, Zhang L, Xie NC, Ma YQ, Lian YJ. High plasma levels of D-dimer are independently associated with a heightened risk of deep vein thrombosis in patients with Intracerebral hemorrhage. Mol Neurobiol. 2016;53(8):5671–8.
18. Melmed KR, Boehme A, Ironside N, Murthy S, Park S, Agarwal S, et al. Respiratory and blood stream infections are associated with subsequent venous thromboembolism after primary Intracerebral hemorrhage. Neurocrit Care. 2020;34(1):85–91.
19. Li J, Wang D, Wang W, Jia J, Kang K, Zhang J, et al. In-hospital venous thromboembolism is associated with poor outcome in patients with spontaneous intracerebral hemorrhage: a multicenter, prospective study. J Stroke Cerebrovasc Dis. 2020;29(8):104958.
20. Wijdicks EF, Scott JP. Pulmonary embolism associated with acute stroke. Mayo Clin Proc. 1997;72(4):297–300.
21. Sochart DH, Hardinge K. The relationship of foot and ankle movements to venous return in the lower limb. J Bone Joint Surg Br. 1999;81(4):700–4.
22. Li Y, Guan X-H, Wang R, Li B, Ning B, Su W, et al. Active ankle movements prevent formation of lower-extremity deep venous thrombosis after orthopedic surgery. Med Sci Monit. 2016;22:3169–76.
23. Palamone J, Brunovsky S, Groth M, Morris L, Kwasny M. "Tap and twist": preventing deep vein thrombosis in neuroscience patients through foot and ankle range-of-motion exercises. J Neurosci Nurs. 2011;43(6).
24. Whiting PS, Jahangir AA. Thromboembolic disease after orthopedic trauma. Orthop Clin North Am. 2016;47(2):335–44.
25. Singhal R, Brimble KS. Thromboembolic complications in the nephrotic syndrome: pathophysiology and clinical management. Thromb Res. 2006;118(3):397–407.

26. Guyatt GH, Akl EA, Crowther M, Gutterman DD, Schuunemann HJ. American College of Chest Physicians Antithrombotic T, et al. executive summary: antithrombotic therapy and prevention of thrombosis, 9th ed: American college of chest physicians evidence-based clinical practice guidelines. Chest. 2012;141(2 Suppl):7S–47S.

27. Steiner T, Al-Shahi Salman R, Beer R, Christensen H, Cordonnier C, Csiba L, et al. European stroke organisation (ESO) guidelines for the management of spontaneous intracerebral hemorrhage. International journal of stroke : official journal of the International Stroke Society. 2014;9(7):840–55.

28. Hemphill JC 3rd, Greenberg SM, Anderson CS, Becker K, Bendok BR, Cushman M, et al. Guidelines for the Management of Spontaneous Intracerebral Hemorrhage: a guideline for healthcare professionals from the American Heart Association/American Stroke Association. Stroke. 2015;46(7):2032–60.

29. Nyquist P, Bautista C, Jichici D, Burns J, Chhangani S, DeFilippis M, et al. Prophylaxis of venous thrombosis in Neurocritical care patients: an evidence-based guideline: a statement for healthcare professionals from the Neurocritical care society. Neurocrit Care. 2015;24(1):47–60.

30. Dawoud D, Lewis S, Glen J, Sharpin C, Committee NG. Venous thromboembolism in over 16s: reducing the risk of hospital-acquired deep vein thrombosis or pulmonary embolism. NICE guideline [NG89]. 2018.

31. Shoamanesh Co-Chair A, Patrice Lindsay M, Castellucci LA, Cayley A, Crowther M, de Wit K, et al. Canadian stroke best practice recommendations: Management of Spontaneous Intracerebral Hemorrhage, 7th edition update 2020. Int J Stroke. 2021;16(3):321–41.

32. Dennis M, Sandercock PAG, Reid J, Graham C, Murray G, Venables G, et al. Effectiveness of thigh-length graduated compression stockings to reduce the risk of deep vein thrombosis after stroke (CLOTS trial 1): a multicentre, randomised controlled trial. Lancet. 2009;373(9679):1958–65.

33. Dennis M, Sandercock P, Reid J, Graham C, Forbes J, Murray G. Effectiveness of intermittent pneumatic compression in reduction of risk of deep vein thrombosis in patients who have had a stroke (CLOTS 3): a multicentre randomised controlled trial. Lancet. 2013;382(9891):516–24.

34. Prabhakaran S, Herbers P, Khoury J, Adeoye O, Khatri P, Ferioli S, et al. Is prophylactic anticoagulation for deep venous thrombosis common practice after intracerebral hemorrhage? Stroke. 2015;46(2):369–75.

35. Cherian LJ, Smith EE, Schwamm LH, Fonarow GC, Schulte PJ, Xian Y, et al. Current practice trends for use of early venous thromboembolism prophylaxis after Intracerebral hemorrhage. Neurosurgery. 2018;82(1):85–92.

36. Brott T, Broderick J, Kothari R, Barsan W, Tomsick T, Sauerbeck L, et al. Early hemorrhage growth in patients with intracerebral hemorrhage. Stroke. 1997;28(1):1–5.

37. Kazui S, Naritomi H, Yamamoto H, Sawada T, Yamaguchi T. Enlargement of spontaneous intracerebral hemorrhage. Incidence and time course. Stroke. 1996;27(10):1783–7.

38. Kelly J, Rudd A, Lewis R, Hunt BJ. Venous thromboembolism after acute stroke. Stroke. 2001;32(1):262–7.

39. Burchell SR, Tang J, Zhang JH. Hematoma expansion following Intracerebral hemorrhage: mechanisms targeting the coagulation Cascade and platelet activation. Curr Drug Targets. 2017;18(12):1329–44.

40. Boeer A, Voth E, Henze T, Prange HW. Early heparin therapy in patients with spontaneous intracerebral haemorrhage. J Neurol Neurosurg Psychiatry. 1991;54(5):466–7.

41. Wasay M, Khan S, Zaki KS, Khealani BA, Kamal A, Azam I, et al. A non-randomized study of safety and efficacy of heparin for DVT prophylaxis in intracerebral haemorrhage. J Pak Med Assoc. 2008;58(7):362–4.

42. Orken DN, Kenangil G, Ozkurt H, Guner C, Gundogdu L, Basak M, et al. Prevention of deep venous thrombosis and pulmonary embolism in patients with acute intracerebral hemorrhage. Neurologist. 2009;15(6):329–31.

43. Kiphuth IC, Staykov D, Köhrmann M, Struffert T, Richter G, Bardutzky J, et al. Early administration of low molecular weight heparin after spontaneous intracerebral hemorrhage. A safety analysis. Cerebrovascular diseases (Basel, Switzerland). 2009;27(2):146–50.

44. Faust AC, Finch CK, Hurdle AC, Elijovich L. Early versus delayed initiation of pharmacological venous thromboembolism prophylaxis after an intracranial hemorrhage. Neurologist. 2017;22(5):166–70.

45. Ianosi B, Gaasch M, Rass V, Huber L, Hackl W, Kofler M, et al. Early thrombosis prophylaxis with enoxaparin is not associated with hematoma expansion in patients with spontaneous intracerebral hemorrhage. Eur J Neurol. 2019;26(2):333–41.

46. Kananeh MF, Fonseca-Paricio MJ, Liang JW, Sullivan LT, Sharma K, Shah SO, et al. Ultra-early venous thromboembolism (VTE) prophylaxis in spontaneous Intracerebral hemorrhage (sICH). J Stroke Cerebrovasc Dis. 2021;30(2):105476.

47. Qian C, Huhtakangas J, Juvela S, Bode MK, Tatlisumak T, Savolainen M, et al. Early vs late enoxaparin for the prevention of venous thromboembolism in patients with ICH: A double blind placebo controlled multicenter study Clin Neurol Neurosurg 2021;202:106534.

48. Pan X, Li J, Xu L, Deng S, Wang Z. Safety of prophylactic heparin in the prevention of venous thromboembolism after spontaneous Intracerebral hemorrhage: a Meta-analysis. J Neurol Surg A Cent Eur Neurosurg. 2020; 81(3):253–60.

49. Tetri S, Hakala J, Juvela S, Saloheimo P, Pyhtinen J, Rusanen H, et al. Safety of low-dose subcutaneous enoxaparin for the prevention of venous thromboembolism after primary intracerebral haemorrhage. Thromb Res. 2008;123(2):206–12.

50. Wu TC, Kasam M, Harun N, Hallevi H, Bektas H, Acosta I, et al. Pharmacological deep vein thrombosis prophylaxis does not lead to hematoma expansion in intracerebral hemorrhage with intraventricular extension. Stroke. 2011;42(3):705–9.

51. Godoy DA, Piñero GR, Koller P, Masotti L, Di Napoli M. Steps to consider in the approach and management of critically ill patient with spontaneous intracerebral hemorrhage. World J Crit Care Med. 2015;4(3):213–29.

52. Ohwaki K, Yano E, Nagashima H, Hirata M, Nakagomi T, Tamura A. Blood pressure management in acute intracerebral hemorrhage: relationship between elevated blood pressure and hematoma enlargement. Stroke. 2004;35(6):1364–7.

53. Rodriguez-Luna D, Piñeiro S, Rubiera M, Ribo M, Coscojuela P, Pagola J, et al. Impact of blood pressure changes and course on hematoma growth in acute intracerebral hemorrhage. Eur J Neurol. 2013;20(9):1277–83.

54. Toyoda K, Okada Y, Minematsu K, Kamouchi M, Fujimoto S, Ibayashi S, et al. Antiplatelet therapy contributes to acute deterioration of intracerebral hemorrhage. Neurology. 2005;65(7):1000–4.

55. Camps-Renom P, Alejaldre-Monforte A, Delgado-Mederos R, Martínez-Domeño A, Prats-Sánchez L, Pascual-Goñi E, et al. Does prior antiplatelet therapy influence hematoma volume and hematoma growth following intracerebral hemorrhage? Results from a prospective study and a meta-analysis. Eur J Neurol. 2017;24(2):302–9.

56. Flibotte JJ, Hagan N, O'Donnell J, Greenberg SM, Rosand J. Warfarin, hematoma expansion, and outcome of intracerebral hemorrhage. Neurology. 2004;63(6):1059–64.

57. Huynh TJ, Aviv RI, Dowlatshahi D, Gladstone DJ, Laupacis A, Kiss A, et al. Validation of the 9-point and 24-point hematoma expansion prediction scores and derivation of the PREDICT a/B scores. Stroke. 2015;46(11):3105–10.

58. Parikh NS, Kamel H, Navi BB, Iadecola C, Merkler AE, Jesudian A, et al. Liver fibrosis indices and outcomes after primary Intracerebral hemorrhage. Stroke. 2020;51(3):830–7.

59. Marini S, Morotti A, Ayres AM, Crawford K, Kourkoulis CE, Lena UK, et al. Sex differences in intracerebral hemorrhage expansion and mortality. J Neurol Sci. 2017;379:112–6.

60. Forti P, Maioli F, Domenico Spampinato M, Barbara C, Nativio V, Coveri M, et al. The Effect of Age on Characteristics and Mortality of Intracerebral Hemorrhage in the Oldest-Old. Cerebrovascular diseases (Basel, Switzerland). 2016;42(5–6):485–92.

61. Sakuta K, Yaguchi H, Sato T, Mukai T, Komatsu T, Sakai K, et al. The NAG scale can screen for hematoma expansion in acute intracerebral hemorrhage-a multi-institutional validation. J Neurol Sci. 2020;414:116834.

62. Fu F, Sun S, Liu L, Gu H, Su Y, Li Y. Iodine sign as a novel predictor of hematoma expansion and poor outcomes in primary Intracerebral hemorrhage patients. Stroke. 2018;49(9):2074–80.

63. Wada R, Aviv RI, Fox AJ, Sahlas DJ, Gladstone DJ, Tomlinson G, et al. CT angiography "spot sign" predicts hematoma expansion in acute intracerebral hemorrhage. Stroke. 2007;38(4):1257–62.

64. Tan CO, Lam S, Kuppens D, Bergmans RHJ, Parameswaran BK, Forghani R, et al. Spot and diffuse signs: quantitative markers of intracranial hematoma expansion at dual-energy CT. Radiology. 2019;290(1):179–86.

65. Zhang M, Chen J, Zhan C, Liu J, Chen Q, Xia T, et al. Blend sign is a strong predictor of the extent of early hematoma expansion in spontaneous Intracerebral hemorrhage. Front Neurol. 2020;11:334.

66. Li Q, Zhang G, Huang Y-J, Dong M-X, Lv F-J, Wei X, et al. Blend sign on computed tomography: novel and reliable predictor for early hematoma growth in patients with Intracerebral hemorrhage. Stroke. 2015;46(8):2119–23.

67. Li Q, Zhang G, Xiong X, Wang X-C, Yang W-S, Li K-W, et al. Black hole sign: novel imaging marker that predicts hematoma growth in patients with Intracerebral hemorrhage. Stroke. 2016;47(7):1777–81.

68. Li Q, Liu Q-J, Yang W-S, Wang X-C, Zhao L-B, Xiong X, et al. Island sign: an imaging predictor for early hematoma expansion and poor outcome in patients with Intracerebral hemorrhage. Stroke. 2017;48(11):3019–25.

69. Vermeer SE, Algra A, Franke CL, Koudstaal PJ, Rinkel GJE. Long-term prognosis after recovery from primary intracerebral hemorrhage. Neurology. 2002;59(2):205–9.

70. Arakawa S, Saku Y, Ibayashi S, Nagao T, Fujishima M. Blood pressure control and recurrence of hypertensive brain hemorrhage. Stroke. 1998;29(9):1806–9.

71. Arima H, Tzourio C, Anderson C, Woodward M, Bousser MG, MacMahon S, et al. Effects of perindopril-based lowering of blood pressure on intracerebral hemorrhage related to amyloid angiopathy: the PROGRESS trial. Stroke. 2010;41(2):394–6.

72. Biffi A, Anderson CD, Battey TWK, Ayres AM, Greenberg SM, Viswanathan A, et al. Association between blood pressure control and risk of recurrent Intracerebral hemorrhage. JAMA. 2015;314(9):904–12.

73. Vinters HV, Gilbert JJ. Cerebral amyloid angiopathy: incidence and complications in the aging brain. II. The distribution of amyloid vascular changes. Stroke. 1983;14(6):924–8.

74. Charidimou A, Imaizumi T, Moulin S, Biffi A, Samarasekera N, Yakushiji Y, et al. Brain hemorrhage recurrence, small vessel disease type, and cerebral microbleeds: a meta-analysis. Neurology. 2017;89(8):820–9.

75. Weimar C, Benemann J, Terborg C, Walter U, Weber R, Diener HC, et al. Recurrent stroke after lobar and deep intracerebral hemorrhage: a hospital-based cohort study. Cerebrovasc Dis. 2011;32(3):283–8.

76. O'Donnell HC, Rosand J, Knudsen KA, Furie KL, Segal AZ, Chiu RI, et al. Apolipoprotein E genotype and the risk of recurrent lobar intracerebral hemorrhage. N Engl J Med. 2000;342(4):240–5.

77. Charidimou A, Boulouis G, Roongpiboonsopit D, Xiong L, Pasi M, Schwab KM, et al. Cortical superficial siderosis and recurrent intracerebral hemorrhage risk in cerebral amyloid angiopathy: large prospective cohort and preliminary meta-analysis. Int J Stroke. 2019;14(7):723–33.

78. Li L, Poon MTC, Samarasekera NE, Perry LA, Moullaali TJ, Rodrigues MA, et al. Risks of recurrent stroke and all serious vascular events after spontaneous intracerebral haemorrhage: pooled analyses of two population-based studies. Lancet Neurol. 2021;20(6):437–47.

79. Ajmeri AN, Zaheer K, McCorkle C, Amro A, Mustafa B. Treating venous thromboembolism post intracranial hemorrhage: a case report. Cureus. 2020;12(1):e6746.

80. Becattini C, Cimini LA, Carrier M. Challenging anticoagulation cases: a case of pulmonary embolism shortly after spontaneous brain bleeding. Thromb Res. 2021;200:41–7.

81. Lee WC, Fang HY. Management of pulmonary embolism after recent intracranial hemorrhage: a case report. Medicine (Baltimore). 2018;97(15):e0479.

82. Ottosen TP, Grijota M, Hansen ML, Brandes A, Damgaard D, Husted SE, et al. Use of antithrombotic therapy and long-term clinical outcome among patients surviving Intracerebral hemorrhage. Stroke. 2016;47(7):1837–43.

83. Majeed A, Kim Y-K, Roberts RS, Holmström M, Schulman S. Optimal timing of resumption of warfarin after intracranial hemorrhage. Stroke. 2010;41(12):2860–6.

84. Yung D, Kapral MK, Asllani E, Fang J, Lee DS. Reinitiation of anticoagulation after warfarin-associated intracranial hemorrhage and mortality risk: the best practice for reinitiating anticoagulation therapy after intracranial bleeding (BRAIN) study. Can J Cardiol. 2012;28(1):33–9.

85. Kuramatsu JB, Gerner ST, Schellinger PD, Glahn J, Endres M, Sobesky J, et al. Anticoagulant Reversal, Blood Pressure Levels, and Anticoagulant Resumption in Patients With Anticoagulation-Related Intracerebral Hemorrhage. Jama. 2015;313(8).

86. Witt DM, Clark NP, Martinez K, Schroeder A, Garcia D, Crowther MA, et al. Risk of thromboembolism, recurrent hemorrhage, and death after warfarin therapy interruption for intracranial hemorrhage. Thromb Res. 2015;136(5):1040–4.

87. Murthy SB, Gupta A, Merkler AE, Navi BB, Mandava P, Iadecola C, et al. Restarting anticoagulant therapy after intracranial hemorrhage: a systematic review and Meta-analysis. Stroke. 2017;48(6):1594–600.

88. Carney BJ, Uhlmann EJ, Puligandla M, Mantia C, Weber GM, Neuberg DS, et al. Anticoagulation after intracranial hemorrhage in brain tumors: risk of recurrent hemorrhage and venous thromboembolism. Res Pract Thromb Haemost. 2020;4(5):860–5.

89. Mantia C, Zwicker JI. Anticoagulation in the setting of primary and metastatic brain tumors. Cancer Treat Res. 2019;179:179–89.

90. Donato J, Campigotto F, Uhlmann EJ, Coletti E, Neuberg D, Weber GM, et al. Intracranial hemorrhage in patients with brain metastases treated with therapeutic enoxaparin: a matched cohort study. Blood. 2015;126(4):494–9.

91. Porfidia A, Giordano M, Sturiale CL, D'Arrigo S, Donadini MP, Olivi A, et al. Risk of intracranial bleeding in patients with primary brain cancer receiving therapeutic anticoagulation for venous thromboembolism: a meta-analysis. Brain Behav. 2020;10(6):e01638.

92. Zhou Z, Yu J, Carcel C, Delcourt C, Shan J, Lindley RI, et al. Resuming anticoagulants after anticoagulation-associated intracranial haemorrhage: systematic review and meta-analysis. BMJ Open. 2018;8(5):e019672.

93. Schulman S, Kearon C, Kakkar AK, Mismetti P, Schellong S, Eriksson H, et al. Dabigatran versus warfarin in the treatment of acute venous thromboembolism. N Engl J Med. 2009;361(24):2342–52.

94. Büller HR, Prins MH, Lensin AWA, Decousus H, Jacobson BF, Minar E, et al. Oral rivaroxaban for the treatment of symptomatic pulmonary embolism. N Engl J Med. 2012;366(14):1287–97.

95. Agnelli G, Buller HR, Cohen A, Curto M, Gallus AS, Johnson M, et al. Oral apixaban for the treatment of acute venous thromboembolism. N Engl J Med. 2013;369(9):799–808.

96. Büller HR, Décousus H, Grosso MA, Mercuri M, Middeldorp S, Prins MH, et al. Edoxaban versus warfarin for the treatment of symptomatic venous thromboembolism. N Engl J Med. 2013;369(15):1406–15.

97. Lamsam L, Sussman ES, Iyer AK, Bhambhvani HP, Han SS, Skirboll S, et al. Intracranial hemorrhage in deep vein thrombosis/pulmonary Embolus patients without atrial fibrillation. Stroke. 2018;49(8):1866–71.

98. Inohara T, Xian Y, Liang L, Matsouaka RA, Saver JL, Smith EE, et al. Association of Intracerebral Hemorrhage among Patients Taking non-Vitamin K Antagonist vs vitamin K antagonist Oral anticoagulants with in-hospital mortality. JAMA. 2018;319(5):463–73.

99. Hagii J, Tomita H, Metoki N, Saito S, Shiroto H, Hitomi H, et al. Characteristics of intracerebral hemorrhage during rivaroxaban treatment: comparison with those during warfarin. Stroke. 2014;45(9):2805–7.

100. Wilson D, Charidimou A, Shakeshaft C, Ambler G, White M, Cohen H, et al. Volume and functional outcome of intracerebral hemorrhage according to oral anticoagulant type. Neurology. 2016;86(4):360–6.

101. Pollack CV, Reilly PA, van Ryn J, Eikelboom JW, Glund S, Bernstein RA, et al. Idarucizumab for Dabigatran reversal - full cohort analysis. N Engl J Med. 2017;377(5):431–41.

102. Connolly SJ, Crowther M, Eikelboom JW, Gibson CM, Curnutte JT, Lawrence JH, et al. Full study report of Andexanet Alfa for bleeding associated with factor Xa inhibitors. N Engl J Med. 2019;380(14):1326–35.

103. Siegal DM, Curnutte JT, Connolly SJ, Lu G, Conley PB, Wiens BL, et al. Andexanet Alfa for the reversal of factor Xa inhibitor activity. N Engl J Med. 2015;373(25):2413–24.

104. Somarouthu B, Yeddula K, Wicky S, Hirsch JA, Kalva SP. Long-term safety and effectiveness of inferior vena cava filters in patients with stroke. J Neurointerv Surg. 2011;3(2):141–6.

105. Mellado M, Trujillo-Santos J, Bikdeli B, Jiménez D, Núñez MJ, Ellis M, et al. Vena cava filters in patients presenting with major bleeding during anticoagulation for venous thromboembolism. Intern Emerg Med. 2019;14(7):1101–12.

106. Melmed K, Chen ML, Al-Kawaz M, Kirsch HL, Bauerschmidt A, Kamel H. Use and removal of inferior vena cava filters in patients with acute brain injury. The Neurohospitalist. 2020;10(3):188–92.

107. Hansmann J, Sheybani A, Minocha J, Bui JT, Lipnik AJ, Shah KY, et al. Retrievable inferior vena cava filters in neurosurgical patients: retrieval rates and clinical outcomes. Clin Neurol Neurosurg. 2019;179:30–4.
108. Bottinor W, Turlington J, Raza S, Roberts CS, Malhotra R, Jovin IS, et al. Life-saving systemic thrombolysis in a patient with massive pulmonary embolism and a recent hemorrhagic cerebrovascular accident. Tex Heart Inst J. 2014;41(2):174–6.
109. Koroneos A, Koutsoukou A, Zervakis D, Politis P, Sourlas S, Pagoni E, et al. Successful resuscitation with thrombolysis of a patient suffering fulminant pulmonary embolism after recent intracerebral haemorrhage. Resuscitation. 2007;72(1):154–7.
110. Endo H, Kubota H, Sato M, Sudo K. Surgical treatment of pulmonary embolism with recent intracranial hemorrhage. Ann Thorac Cardiovasc Surg. 2005;11(4):256–9.
111. Hanger HC, Fletcher VJ, Wilkinson TJ, Brown AJ, Frampton CM, Sainsbury R. Effect of aspirin and warfarin on early survival after intracerebral haemorrhage. J Neurol. 2008;255(3):347–52.
112. Mittal MK, Rabinstein AA. Anticoagulation-related intracranial hemorrhages. Curr Atheroscler Rep. 2012;14(4):351–9.

14

Differences between surviving and non-surviving venous thromboembolism COVID-19 patients

Mauricio Castillo-Perez[1], Carlos Jerjes-Sanchez[1,2,3,4*], Alejandra Castro-Varela[1], Jose Gildardo Paredes-Vazquez[1,3], Eduardo Vazquez-Garza[1,2], Ray Erick Ramos-Cazares[1], Jose Alfredo Salinas-Casanova[1], Abigail Montserrat Molina-Rodriguez[1], Arturo Adrián Martinez-Ibarra[1], Mario Alejandro Fabiani[3], Yoezer Z Flores-Sayavedra[1], Jaime Alberto Guajardo-Lozano[1], Hector Lopez-de la Garza[1], Hector Betancourt-del Campo[1], Daniela Martinez-Magallanes[1] and Jathniel Panneflek[2]

Abstract

Background: To our knowledge, the treatment, outcome, clinical presentation, risk stratification of patients with venous thromboembolism and COVID-19 have not been well characterized.

Methods: We searched for systematic reviews, cohorts, case series, case reports, editor letters, and venous thromboembolism COVID-19 patients' abstracts following PRISMA and PROSPERO statements. We analyzed therapeutic approaches and clinical outcomes of venous thromboembolism COVID-19 patients. Inclusion: COVID-19 patients with venous thromboembolism confirmed by an imaging method (venous doppler ultrasound, ventilation-perfusion lung scan, computed tomography pulmonary angiogram, pulmonary angiography). We assessed and reported the original Pulmonary Embolism Severity Index for each pulmonary embolism patient. In addition, we defined major bleedings according to the International Society of Thrombosis and Haemostasis criteria.

Results: We performed a systematic review from August 9 to August 30, 2020. We collected 1,535 papers from PubMed, Scopus, Web of Science, Wiley, and Opengrey. We extracted data from 89 studies that describe 143 patients. Unfractionated and low-molecular-weight heparin was used as parenteral anticoagulation in 85/143 (59%) cases. The Food and Drug Administration-approved alteplase regimen guided the advanced treatment in 39/143 (27%) patients. The mortality was high (21.6%, CI 95% 15.2-29.3). The incidence of major bleeding complications was 1 (0.9%) in the survival group and 1 (3.2%) in the death group. Pulmonary Embolism Severity Index was class I in 11.6% and II in 22.3% in survivors compared to 0% and 6.5% in non-survivors, respectively. Patients who experienced venous thromboembolism events at home were more likely to live than in-hospital events.

* Correspondence: jerjes@prodigy.net.mx; carlos.jerjes@udicem.org
[1]Tecnologico de Monterrey. Escuela de Medicina y Ciencias de la Salud., Nuevo Leon, San Pedro Garza Garcia, Mexico
[2]Centro de Investigacion Biomedica del Hospital Zambrano Hellion, TecSalud, Escuela de Medicina y Ciencias de la Salud, Tecnologico de Monterrey, Nuevo Leon, San Pedro Garza Garcia, Mexico
Full list of author information is available at the end of the article

Conclusions: We determined a high mortality incidence of pulmonary embolism and a low rate of bleeding. Unfractionated and low-molecular-weight heparin drove parenteral anticoagulation and alteplase the advanced treatment in both groups. The original Pulmonary Embolism Severity Index could be helpful in the risk stratification.

Keywords: SARS-CoV-2, COVID-19, Venous thromboembolism, Pulmonary embolism, Deep vein thrombosis, Thrombolysis, Anticoagulation

Background

The rapidly evolving coronavirus disease 2019 (COVID-19) global pandemic has been one of the most significant public health challenges since the Spanish flu pandemic over 100 years ago [1]. COVID-19, caused by the severe acute respiratory syndrome coronavirus 2 (SARS-CoV-2), is a multifaceted disease characterized by a wide range of clinical presentations and degrees of severity [2]. In the beginning, the target organ seemed to be only the respiratory system, inducing severe pneumonia and acute respiratory distress syndrome. However, an important lesson learned was that SARS-CoV-2 causes a high prothrombotic state, venous and arterial thrombosis [1]. Thus, the clinical presentation eventually resembles a thrombotic storm characterized by higher D-dimer measurements and high von Willebrand factor levels [3]. Additionally, thrombosis mechanisms linking inflammation pathways, coagulation system activity, immunothrombosis, cytokine storm, and renin-angiotensin-aldosterone system dysregulation [4–8] seem to be involved.

Therefore, in severe COVID-19, venous thromboembolism (VTE) emerges as a critical and frequent complication [9, 10], with a high incidence (15.3%, CI 95% 9.8-21.9) and mortality rate (45.1%, CI 95% 22.0-69.4), in pulmonary embolism (PE) patients [11]. Although there is a trend to better survival in patients treated with heparins (anticoagulation and anti-inflammatory effect) [12, 13], we do not have enough data on the best primary prevention doses, therapeutic approaches, and outcomes [9, 14, 15]. Also, there are no advanced treatment recommendations in massive and submassive PE [16, 17]. Therefore, we performed a systematic review using the Preferred Reporting Items for Systematic Reviews and Metanalyses (PRISMA) statement to determine the therapeutic trends and outcomes in VTE COVID-19 patients. Also, we assessed the original Pulmonary Embolism Severity Index (PESI) in PE patients.

Methods

Search strategy

We searched for systematic reviews, cohorts, case series, case reports, editor letters, and VTE COVID-19 patients' abstracts through the PRISMA statement search [18]. We register the protocol in the International Prospective Register protocol of Systematic Reviews (PROSPERO); registration number: CRD42020203688). The patients must have received anticoagulation or thrombolysis. The objective was to assess the therapeutic trends and clinical outcomes of VTE COVID-19 patients.

Additionally, we analyzed the clinical presentation, risk stratification, and diagnostic approach. We included deep vein thrombosis (DVT) and PE confirmed by an imaging method (venous doppler US, ventilation-perfusion lung scan, computed tomography pulmonary angiogram, pulmonary angiography). We assessed the original PESI since it works better than the simplified PESI [19]. We established two groups, survivors and those who died. We performed a systematic review through PubMed, Scopus, Web of Science, Wiley, and OpenGrey and provided the complete search strategies in the e-Appendix. We used snowballing [20], a manual search to avoid lost reports, controlled vocabulary, and no language restriction. We do not contact authors to obtain additional information in cases with critical missing variables.

Study selection and data collection

We identified potentially eligible studies by examining titles and abstracts. We obtained full papers to assess eligibility criteria before the critical appraisal and extracted cases that met the eligibility criteria. All investigators analyzed data extraction of every case report to improve quality data extraction. The corresponding author is a cardiologist with expertise in the field (CJS). We conducted a group discussion daily to assess all the information extracted from the cases included in a database. Disagreements were solved posteriorly by consensus. We performed two meetings to ensure the data's quality through a random review of 20% of the papers. The primary outcomes were therapeutic approaches, in-hospital death, intracranial hemorrhage (ICH), major, and minor.

Additionally, we analyzed the clinical presentation, the PE risk, COVID-19 severity, VTE primary prevention, and the thrombus's location in the pulmonary circulation. According to the International Society of Thrombosis and Haemostasis criteria, we defined major bleedings [21]; we established the presence of right ventricular dysfunction according to the European Society of Cardiology guidelines of PE: right ventricular end-diastolic diameter/left ventricular end-diastolic diameter ratio $\geq 2{:}1$, (b) regional or global right ventricular hypokinesis, (c) McConnell's sign, (d) right ventricular diameter >35 mm, (e) systolic pulmonary arterial pressure ≥50 mm Hg; B-type brain natriuretic peptide (BNP) measurement (>90 pg/mL) or N-terminal proBNP (NT-proBNP) (>300 pg/mL); dynamic electrocardiographic changes (new complete or incomplete right bundle-branch block, anteroseptal ST elevation or depression, or anteroseptal T-wave inversion) [22]; other definitions, including the PESI score, massive PE and intensive care unit (ICU) VTE risk factors, are available in the e-Appendix.

Based on the high SARS-CoV-2 thrombogenicity and to understand its behavior in the venous system, we also analyzed acute cerebral venous sinus thrombosis (CVST), whether associated or not with VTE.

Statistical analysis
We used summary statistics for continuous and categorical variables according to their types and distributions. We report the frequency and percentage (n >20) for categorical variables, and for continuous variables, we report the mean and standard deviation. We used the IBM SPSS® software platform for descriptive statistical analysis.

Results
We carried out the systematic review from August 9 to August 30, 2020. Figure 1 shows the flowchart, including the four phases of PRISMA, and we obtained, eliminated, and excluded duplicated reports. In the identification phase, we collected 1,535 papers from PubMed, Scopus, Web of Science, Wiley, and Opengrey. Next, we carefully reviewed the full text for eligibility criteria and selected 107 reports for the quality assessment. Finally, we extracted the data for this review from 89 studies (references in supplementary material).

Baseline demographics and primary outcomes
Table 1 shows baseline demographics, clinical presentation, VTE and PE risk factors, DVT classification, PESI, and VTE onset. We identified 143 COVID-19 patients with VTE; most were relatively young overweight males with isolated PE with or without proximal DVT. The earliest clinical PE findings were severe oxygen desaturation, sudden dyspnea, and leg pain in DVT survived patients (Table 1). A remarkable characteristic was the lowest oxygen saturation in those who died. Among the usual comorbidities in COVID-19, hypertension had a higher incidence in patients who died. Cardiovascular risk factors (hypertension and diabetes) and those associated with in-hospital and ICU stay were more prevalent in those who died (Table 1). The proportion of low-risk and submassive PE was higher in patients who

survived than those who died, where massive PE was predominant (Table 1). In this group, the detection of proximal or distal DVT was scarce. The original PESI classes II and III identified patients who lived (Table 1). Finally, patients with acute VTE events at home were more likely to live than in-hospital events. We identified reduced thromboprophylaxis use in both groups (Table 2). Initial treatment shows that unfractionated and low-molecular-weight heparin drove parenteral anticoagulation in both groups. Also, direct-acting oral anticoagulant use was rare. Alteplase 100 mg 2-hours infusion was the advanced treatment in both groups (Table 2). The mortality was high (21.6%, CI 95% 15.2-29.3), and there was a low incidence of bleeding complications, including ICH, in those who survived (Table 2).

Table 3 shows characteristics of VTE, including biomarkers, imaging studies, and severity, laboratories. Imagin and previous anticoagulation use related to COVID-19. Patients who died had a higher D dimer expression and right ventricular dysfunction (Table 3), and the use of biomarkers was low. [22] (Table 3). The computed tomography pulmonary angiography (CTPA) demonstrated a wide distribution of thrombus locations in surviving patients (Table 3). The variables mainly related to mortality were acute respiratory distress syndrome, mechanical ventilation, ICU stay, and higher C reactive protein measurements in patients with PE associated with severe COCID-19 patients.

Cerebral venous sinus thrombosis
We identified 15 young patients with a similar gender proportion practically without a history of contraceptives (Table 4). CVST clinical presentation included neurologic alterations at home, abnormal D dimer measurements, and only one case associated with a submassive PE. Most patients were asymptomatic or had COVID-19 pneumonia. Despite in-hospital primary prevention, five patients had CVST. We identified a remarkably high prevalence of ICH (10/15 patients) (66.7% CI95 38.4-88.2) and increased mortality (3/15 patients) (20% CI954.3-48.1) (Table 4).

Discussion
This systematic review highlights the therapeutic trends and outcomes of VTE survivors compared with those who died. The main observations were: First, unfractionated and low-molecular-weight heparin was the cornerstone in the VTE treatment. Also, 2-hours alteplase infusion was the most frequent advanced treatment in PE patients. Second, we identified high mortality in the

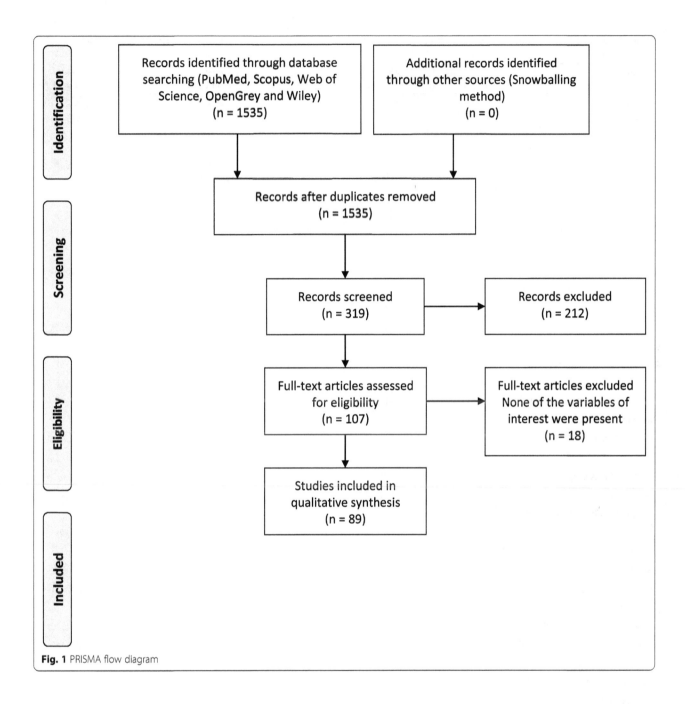

Fig. 1 PRISMA flow diagram

ICU associated with severe COVID-19 with a low incidence of bleeding complications in massive PE. Third, the original PESI score II-III recognized patients who survived, suggesting its usefulness in the risk stratification in COVID-19 patients. Fourth, elevated C reactive protein and D dimer measurements and right ventricular dysfunction identified poor in-hospital outcomes. Finally, the exploratory analysis showed the same high ICH incidence in CVST mild COVID-19 patients than non-COVID-19 patients [23].

Recent systematic reviews and meta-analyses focused on the incidence, primary and secondary VTE prevention, bleeding complications [24–27], and the association of D-dimer with mortality [28, 29]. Therefore, therapeutic approaches, outcomes, clinical presentation, risk stratification, and patient characteristics are unclear.

Although still under debate, recent evidence from a small sample suggests that patients with severe COVID-19 disease are at high risk for thromboinflammation since they have SARS-CoV-2 infection, risk factors, cardiovascular, renal, or chronic pulmonary inflammatory comorbidities [2]. An increased frequency of arterial and venous thrombosis at the beginning of the pandemic was remarkable [30]. VTE is now recognized as among

Table 1 Baseline demographics, clinical presentation, VTE risk factors, PE risk stratification, VTE classification, DVT classification, PESI, and VTE onset

Variables	All patients N = 143 (%)	Survival N = 112 (%)	Death N = 31 (%)
Age (years), mean ± SD	58.5 ± 12.7	58.1 ± 13.6	60.0 ± 8.8
Gender (male)	91 (63.6)	70 (62.5)	21 (67.7)
BMI (kg/m2), mean ± SD	30.9 ± 5.6	30.3 ± 5.6	31.6 ± 5.6
VTE Clinical presentation			
O2 saturation (%), mean ± SD	87.9 ± 7.6	88.3 ± 7.4	85 ± 9.4
Sudden dyspnea	31 (21.7)	29 (25.9)	2 (6.5)
Progressive dyspnea	26 (18.2)	23 (20.5)	3 (9.7)
Pleuritic chest pain	20 (14)	19 (17)	1 (3.2)
Ischemic chest pain	2 (1.4)	2 (1.8)	0 (0)
Leg pain	13 (9.1)	11 (9.8)	2 (6.5)
Medical history and risk factors			
Hypertension	50 (35)	34 (30.4)	16 (51.6)
Diabetes	33 (23.1)	25 (22.3)	8 (25.8)
Lung disease	16 (11.2)	15 (13.4)	1 (3.2)
Medical history of cancer	7 (4.9)	5 (4.5)	2 (6.5)
Active cancer	5 (3.5)	3 (2.7)	2 (6.5)
Previous venous thromboembolism	2 (1.4)	2 (1.8)	0 (0)
In-hospital and ICU risk factors			
Immobilization	88 (61.5)	63 (56.3)	25 (80.6)
Sedation	51 (35.7)	27 (24.1)	24 (77.4)
Central venous lines	52 (36.4)	28 (25)	24 (77.4)
Vasopressors	15 (10.5)	4 (3.6)	11 (35.5)
PE risk stratification (ACC/AHA)			
Low risk	24 (18.3)	23 (20.5)	1 (3.2)
Submassive	31 (23.7)	29 (25.9)	2 (6.5)
Massive	39 (29.8)	21 (18.8)	18 (58)
Unable to classify	37 (28.2)	29 (25.9)	8 (25.8)
VTE classification			
Isolated pulmonary embolism	112 (78.3)	85 (75.9)	27 (87.1)
Isolated deep venous thrombosis	12 (8.4)	10 (8.9)	2 (6.5)
Pulmonary embolism plus DVT	18 (12.6)	16 (14.3)	2 (6.5)
Pulmonary embolism plus CVT	1 (0.7)	1 (0.9)	0 (0)
DVT classification			
Proximal DVT	14 (9.8)	11 (9.8)	3 (9.7)
Distal DVT	5 (3.5)	5 (4.5)	0 (0)
Proximal plus distal DVT	5 (3.5)	5 (4.5)	0 (0)
Upper limb DVT	6 (4.2)	4 (3.6)	2 (6.5)
Original PESI			
I (Very low risk)	13 (9.1)	13 (11.6)	0 (0)
II (Low risk)	27 (18.9)	25 (22.3)	2 (6.5)
III (Intermediate risk)	45 (31.5)	37 (33)	8 (25.8)
IV (High risk)	11 (7.7)	11 (9.8)	0 (0)
V (Very high risk)	35 (24.5)	19 (17)	16 (51.6)

Table 1 Baseline demographics, clinical presentation, VTE risk factors, PE risk stratification, VTE classification, DVT classification, PESI, and VTE onset *(Continued)*

Variables	All patients N = 143 (%)	Survival N = 112 (%)	Death N = 31 (%)
VTE onset			
Home	53 (37.1)	48 (42.9)	5 (16.1)
In-hospital	90 (62.9)	64 (57.1)	26 (83.9)

BMI body mass index, *ICU* intensive care unit, *PESI* Pulmonary Embolism Severity Index, *VTE* venous thromboembolism, *DVT* deep venous thrombosis, *CVT* cerebral venous thrombosis, *PE* pulmonary embolism, *ACC/AHA* American College of Cardiology/American Heart Association

the predominant cardiovascular hazards [30], with the highest incidence in the intensive care unit setting (25%), increasing to 69% after surveillance venous ultrasonography [30]. Also, thromboprophylaxis, the foundation to prevent in-hospital VTE, fails in a subset of COVID-19 patients [30]. Additionally, quantifying the risk of thrombosis and cardiovascular complications is complicated in this heterogeneous population by reports of limited sample size, restriction of assessments to the

ICU setting, outcome definitions, and differing thromboprophylaxis strategies [30].

Our findings suggest that intravenous or subcutaneous anticoagulation remains the cornerstone of therapy in deep venous thrombosis and PE COVID-19 patients. Strategies for reperfusion therapy included the thrombolysis regimen recommended for international guidelines [22] or "safe dose" in PE patients [31–33]. The rationale for advanced treatment in PE is to avert or improve

Table 2 Therapeutic approaches and outcomes

Variables	All patients N = 143 (%)	Survival N = 112 (%)	Death N = 31 (%)
Thromboprophylaxis			
Unfractionated heparin	17 (11.9)	11 (9.8)	6 (19.4)
Low-molecular weight heparin	31 (21.7)	20 (17.9)	11 (35.5)
Unspecified	3 (2.1)	2 (1.8)	1 (3.2)
Not received	89 (62.2)	77 (68.8)	12 (38.7)
Treatment			
Unfractionated heparin	28 (19.6)	22 (19.6)	6 (19.4)
Low-molecular-weight-heparin	57 (39.9)	49 (43.8)	8 (25.8)
Warfarin	0 (0)	0 (0)	0 (0)
Fondaparinoux	3 (2.1)	3 (2.7)	0 (0)
Direct-acting oral anticoagulants	8 (5.6)	8 (7.1)	0 (0)
Apixaban	4 (2.8)	4 (3.6)	0 (0)
Rivaroxaban	2 (1.4)	2 (1.8)	0 (0)
Unspecified DOACs	2 (1.4)	2 (1.8)	0 (0)
Alteplase 100 mg	33 (23.1)	20 (17.9)	13 (41.9)
Alteplase 50 mg	6 (4.2)	4 (3.6)	2 (6.5)
Tenecteplase	1 (0.7)	0 (0)	1 (3.2)
Catheter-directed thrombolysis	1 (0.7)	1 (0.9)	0 (0)
Ultrasound-facilitated catheter-directed thrombolysis	3 (2.1)	3 (2.7)	0 (0)
Mechanical thrombectomy	3 (2.1)	3 (2.7)	0 (0)
Surgical thrombectomy	4 (2.8)	3 (2.7)	1 (3.2)
Outcomes			
Death	31 (21.6)	112 (78.39)	31 (21.6)
Intracranial hemorrhage	2 (1.4)	1 (0.9)	1 (3.2)
Major bleeding	2 (1.4)	1 (0.9)	1 (3.2)
Minor bleeding	2 (1.4)	1 (0.9)	1 (3.2)

DOACs direct-acting oral anticoagulants

Table 3 Characteristics of venous thromboembolism in COVID-19 patients

Variables	All patients N = 143 (%)	Survival N = 112 (%)	Death N = 31 (%)
Biomarkers			
D-dimer (mcg/mL), median (IQR)	7794 (3320 – 17,460)	7700 (3200 – 16,125)	8897 (4352 – 33,175)
Hs-cTn (ng/mL), median (IQR)	57 (14.5 – 191)	-	-
Ferritin (ng/mL), median (IQR)	765 (402 – 1456)	-	-
Imaging studies			
Right ventricular dysfunction (TTE)	56 (39.2)	35 (31.3)	21 (67.8)
CTPA			
Saddle PE	10 (7)	9 (8)	1 (3.2)
Main branches	38 (26.6)	34 (30.4)	4 (12.9)
Lobar branches	22 (15.4)	19 (17)	3 (9.7)
Segmental branches	27 (18.9)	23 (20.5)	4 (12.9)
Subsegmental branches	7 (4.9)	7 (6.3)	0 (0)
Doppler US and DVT	30 (20.9)	25 (22.3)	5 (16.1)
COVID-19 severity			
Asymptomatic	14 (9.8)	12 (10.7)	2 (6.5)
Mild symptoms	9 (6.3)	8 (7.1)	1 (3.2)
Fever	27 (18.9)	23 (20.5)	4 (12.9)
Pneumonia	62 (43.4)	55 (49.1)	7 (22.6)
ARDS	58 (40.6)	37 (33)	21 (67.7)
Mechanical ventilation	56 (39.2)	32 (28.6)	24 (77.4)
ICU	69 (48.3)	40 (35.7)	29 (93.5)
Laboratories			
Leukocytes (10(9) u/L), median (IQR)	11.9 (9.7 – 15.4)	11.4 (9.4 – 13.6)	13.8 (10.8 – 20.3)
Lymphocytes (10(3) u/L), mean ± SD	928.3 ± 448.5	994.1 ± 461.5	731.1 ± 360.1
Platelets (10(3) u/L), mean ± SD	246.8 ± 129.8	254.4 ± 122.9	233.7 ± 143.7
LDH (U/L), median (IQR)	575 (391.8 – 739.3)	-	-
CRP (mg/L), median (IQR)	113.1 (50.6 – 222.5)	92.9 (50 – 160)	244.9 (154 – 345.4)
RT-PCR SARS-CoV-2 (+)	142 (99.3)	111 (99.1)	31 (100)
Imagen studies			
Bilateral infiltrates (chest X-ray)	49 (34.3)	37 (33)	12 (38.7)
CT with CO-RADS 5	49 (34.3)	43 (38.4)	6 (19.4)
Previous anticoagulation treatment			
Direct-acting oral anticoagulants	1 (0.7)	1 (0.9)	0 (0)
Vitamin K antagonists	2 (1.4)	1 (0.9)	1 (3.2)

TTE transthoracic echocardiogram, *CTPA* computed tomographic pulmonary angiography, *PE* pulmonary embolism, *US* ultrasound, *DVT* deep vein thrombosis, *ARDS* acute respiratory distress syndrome, *ICU* intensive care unit, *LDH* lactate dehydrogenase, *CRP* C-reactive protein, *RT-PCR* reverse transcription-polymerase chain reaction, *CO-RADS 5* COVID-19 Reporting and Data System with typical imaging for COVID-19

impending clinical instability secondary to right ventricular dysfunction to improve the outcome. The presence of several pulmonary hypertension mechanisms (PE, hypoxic vasoconstriction, pulmonary microthrombi, ACE2 dysregulation, and cytokine storm) inducing right ventricular dysfunction suggests the possibility to obtain a CTPA before clinical decision-making in this population [34]. In the presence of high clinical suspicion and clinical instability, systemic thrombolysis use has evidence level IC [22]. Despite systemic thrombolysis, bleeding complication incidence was lower (0.9% vs. 3.2%) than recent evidence (21.4%) using intermediate- or full-heparin dose without advanced treatment and bleeding definitions according to the individual studies

Table 4 Cerebral venous sinus thrombosis

Variables	N = 15
Age	56 ± 14.3
Gender (male)	7
Risk factors	
Comorbidities (≥1)	2
Oral contraceptives	2
D-dimer (mcg/mL), mean ± SD	3698.4 ± 2017.3
Submassive pulmonary embolism	1
CVT presentation	
Altered mental status	6
Headache	8
Aphasia	6
Hemiparesis	7
Seizures	4
At home	9
COVID-19 clinical presentation	
Fever	3
Progressive dyspnea	3
Asymptomatic	3
Mild symptoms	1
Pneumonia	6
Computed tomography with CO-RADS 5	6
Thromboprophylaxis	5
Treatment and outcomes	
Unfractionated heparin	3
Low-molecular-weight-heparin	12
Intracranial hemorrhage	7
Death	3

CO-RADS 5 COVID-19 Reporting and Data System with typical imaging for COVID-19

[27]. This difference in the incidence of bleeding complications is unclear because relevant clinical or significant bleedings are usually reported. We showed high mortality (46% in massive PE in severe COVID-19 patients. It is higher than observed in massive PE non-COVID-19 patients (33%) [35]; the mortality rates observed are also related to severe COVID-19 and higher than previous other viral pandemics experienced in the past [36]. Additionally, mortality appears to be multifactorial and driven by adult respiratory distress syndrome (ARDS) and massive PE. In the absence of a validated risk score for patients with severe COVID-19 and PE, current risk stratification in PE [22] could lose accuracy and explain the high percentage of unclassified PE patients.

The original PESI score is a helpful tool for immediate and bedside risk stratification [22]; if this score helps to stratify bedside high clinical suspicion PE in COVID-19 patients is unanswered. The original PESI risk score had greater precision in identifying low and intermediate PE risks and identified a high proportion of high-risk patients with very high risk [19]. In addition, COVID-19 in the health systems usually conditions a delay recommended diagnostic approaches in high clinical suspicion PE patients [22]; thus, the original PESI score could be helpful in high clinical suspicion COVID-19 patients. However, clinicians should also consider that the simplified PESI score may fail [37], and a multimodal approach improves risk stratification accuracy. (PESI score definition is available in the e-Appendix).

Another remarkable finding shows VTE events despite thromboprophylaxis. Recent evidence indicates that thrombotic events occur primarily within the first ten days after admission [38]. In addition, Hardy et al. [39] observed an increase in thrombin generation associated with a decrease in overall fibrinolytic capacity during the first week of hospitalization, resulting in a strong procoagulant state. Thus, current evidence suggests administering heparin at standard doses in non-critically ill patients without risk factors for thrombosis or at a high dose for critically ill patients (intermediate or therapeutic dose) [40].

Additionally, high-dose thromboprophylaxis might be adjusted according to inflammation's progression without increasing bleeding Risk in critically ill COVID-19 patients [38]. Randomized controlled trials comparing different thromboprophylaxis doses are needed to establish the best therapeutic approach [38]. The most consistent biomarker abnormalities related to mortality were higher C-reactive protein and D-dimer measurement levels, both associated with ICU admission and death [15]. Additionally, several plausible reasons for elevated D-dimer in patients with SARS-CoV-2: severe infection, VTE, pulmonary and coronary microthrombus, acute kidney, cardiac injury, and pro-inflammatory cytokines [29].

Overlapping severe COVID-19 pneumonia and PE is a challenge, and any pneumonia increases VTE risk [34, 41, 42]. A higher D-dimer measurement and severe oxygen desaturation are possible clinical markers to establish high clinical suspicion and PE severity. Recently, in a case series, the clinical presentation was similar: persistent or worsening respiratory symptoms increased oxygen requirements and DD levels several-fold higher [43]. We suggest that physicians in charge consider these clinical variables and never ignore abnormal or significantly elevated D-dimer because it is an expression of the coagulation system and secondary fibrinolysis activity, suggesting a high risk of acute thrombosis [34]. Sudden hypotension could be another clinical element for PE suspicion in the setting of pneumonia COVID-19 [34]. In the group with CVST, only two patients had a history of oral contraceptives and no history of hereditary prothrombotic factors. These findings suggest an essential role of SARS-CoV-2 in pathogenicity as a trigger of thrombosis. Although early ICH (present at the time of diagnosis) is a frequent complication (40%) [44, 45], current evidence demonstrates a low incidence of new ICH after initiating treatment with anticoagulation [23, 44–46]. Our findings identified a high ICH incidence, probably secondary to CVST. Although anticoagulation is the standard of care in CVST patients (avoid thrombus growth, prevent VTE), the high prevalence of ICH suggests that physicians in charge have to be warning for early detection of this feared complication [45].

Study limitations

The significant limitations of the study included a potential loss of case reports from search engines. There is a trend not to report patients with poor in-hospital outcomes or serious adverse events. In addition, it was not possible to obtain information on the timing of the D-dimer measurements and other biomarkers and bleeding complications outcome in the follow-up. We got the most information from case reports, and we did not contact any author. Additionally, the results should be analyzed with caution as most papers are case reports or case series. Despite a large number of published studies in Covid VTE, the number of studies that report outcomes based on treatments is unacceptably small to draw new conclusions, given the different stages of the pandemic, Covid-19 treatments, and international differences. The usable studies had in common and why the other studies were rejected; could this be the basis of reporting standards for the pandemic to help a unified assessment. The impact of VTE on critically ill patients seems no different from other diseases - so is it just that we cannot cure the underlying disease, or is there something unique about COVID-19 thrombosis.

Conclusions

This systematic review analyzes 143 survivors and non-survivors VTE COVI-19 patients. We determined a high mortality incidence of pulmonary embolism (21.6%) and a low rate of bleeding. Unfractionated and low-molecular-weight heparin drove parenteral anticoagulation and alteplase the advanced treatment in both groups. The original PESI could be helpful in risk stratification. However, the minuscule number of evaluated patients cannot possibly be representative, and therefore, the international community should urgently agree on reporting standards to answer the remaining questions in Covid-19. Prospective clinical trials are mandatory to elucidate the optimal primary or secondary prevention and advanced treatment in this population of patients.

Abbreviations
COVID-19: Coronavirus disease 2019; SARS-CoV-2: Severe acute respiratory syndrome coronavirus 2; VTE: Venous thromboembolism; PE: Pulmonary embolism; PESI: Original Pulmonary Embolism Severity Index; PROSPERO: The International Prospective Register protocol of Systematic Reviews; PRISMA: The Preferred Reporting Items for Systematic Reviews and Metanalyses; DVT: Deep vein thrombosis; PESI: Simplified Pulmonary Embolism Severity Index; BNP: B-type brain natriuretic peptide; NT-proBNP: N-terminal proBNP; CVT: Cerebral vein thrombosis; ICU: Intensive care unit; ICH: Intracranial hemorrhage; CTPA: Computed tomography pulmonary angiography

Acknowledgements
Not applicable.

Authors' contributions
MCP: Substantial contributions to the conception, design of the work; research idea development; database; the acquisition, analysis, interpretation of data; have drafted the work and substantively revised it. CJS: Leaded the research team, research idea development, revising and approving the project design, and moderating group discussions. Also, he elaborated the project's protocol and final tables and manuscripts. ACV: The data acquisition, have drafted the work and substantively revised it. He contributed to revising the database and the elaboration and revision of the tables and final manuscript. JGPV: The data acquisition database; have drafted the work and substantively revised it. EVG: Acquisition and analysis of the database and interpretation of initial data. Have drafted the work and substantively revised it. RERC: Managed the systematic search alongside MCP, created the database, collected and interpreted data. JASC: Acquisition and analysis of the database and interpretation of initial data. Have drafted the work and substantively revised it. AMMR: Acquisition and analysis of the database and interpretation of initial data. Have drafted the work and substantively revised it. AAMI: Acquisition and analysis of the database and interpretation of initial data. Have drafted the work and substantively revised it. MAF: The design of the work, data acquisition, and revision of the manuscript. YZFS: Acquisition and analysis of the database and interpretation of initial data. Have drafted the work and substantively revised it. JAGL: Acquisition and analysis of the database and interpretation of initial data. Have drafted the work and substantively revised it. HLG: data acquisition, analysis, and interpretation; Have drafted the work and substantively revised it. HBC: Acquisition and analysis of the database and interpretation of initial data. Have drafted the work and substantively revised it. DMM: contributions to the design, data interpretation, interpretation of initial data. Have drafted the work and substantively revised it. JP: Acquisition and analysis of the database and interpretation of initial data. Have drafted the work and substantively revised it. The author(s) read and approved the final manuscript.

Author details
[1]Tecnologico de Monterrey. Escuela de Medicina y Ciencias de la Salud., Nuevo Leon, San Pedro Garza Garcia, Mexico. [2]Centro de Investigacion Biomedica del Hospital Zambrano Hellion, TecSalud, Escuela de Medicina y Ciencias de la Salud, Tecnologico de Monterrey, Nuevo Leon, San Pedro Garza Garcia, Mexico. [3]Instituto de Cardiologia y Medicina Vascular, TecSalud, Escuela de Medicina y Ciencias de la Salud, Tecnologico de Monterrey, Batallón San Patricio 112, Real de San Agustin, Nuevo Leon 66278 San Pedro Garza Garcia, Mexico. [4]Tecnologico de Monterrey, Escuela de Medicina y Ciencias de la Salud, Av. Ignacio Morones Prieto 3000, N.L. CP, 64718 Monterrey, Mexico.

References

1. McFadyen JD, Stevens H, Peter K. The emerging threat of (Micro)thrombosis in COVID-19 and its therapeutic implications. Circ Res. 2020;127(4):571–87.
2. Chen T, Wu D, Chen H, Yan W, Yang D, Chen G, et al. Clinical characteristics of 113 deceased patients with coronavirus disease 2019: retrospective study. BMJ. 2020;368:m1091.
3. Becker RC. COVID-19 update: Covid-19-associated coagulopathy. J Thromb Thrombolysis. 2020;50(1):54–67.
4. Vazquez-Garza E, Jerjes-Sanchez C, Navarrete A, Joya-Harrison J, Rodriguez D. Venous thromboembolism: thrombosis, inflammation, and immunothrombosis for clinicians. J Thromb Thrombolysis. 2017;44(3):377–85.
5. Archer SL, Sharp WW, Weir EK. Differentiating COVID-19 pneumonia from Acute Respiratory Distress Syndrome (ARDS) and High Altitude Pulmonary Edema (HAPE): therapeutic implications. Circulation. 2020. https://doi.org/10.1161/CIRCULATIONAHA.120.047915.
6. Fox SE, Akmatbekov A, Harbert JL, Li G, Brown JQ, Vander Heide RS. Pulmonary and cardiac pathology in Covid-19: the first autopsy series from New Orleans. Pathology. 2020. [citado el 14 de abril de 2020]. Disponible en: https://doi.org/medrxiv.org/lookup/doi/10.1101/2020.04.06.20050575.
7. Vaduganathan M, Vardeny O, Michel T, McMurray JJV, Pfeffer MA, Solomon SD. Renin–angiotensin–aldosterone system inhibitors in patients with Covid-19. N Engl J Med. 2020;382(17):1653–9.
8. Poor HD, Ventetuolo CE, Tolbert T, Chun G, Serrao G, Zeidman A, et al. COVID-19 critical illness pathophysiology driven by diffuse pulmonary thrombi and pulmonary endothelial dysfunction responsive to thrombolysis. Respir Med. 2020. [citado el 2 de mayo de 2020]. Disponible en: https://doi.org/medrxiv.org/lookup/doi/10.1101/2020.04.17.20057125.
9. Atri D, Siddiqi HK, Lang J, Nauffal V, Morrow DA, Bohula EA. COVID-19 for the cardiologist: a current review of the virology, clinical epidemiology, cardiac and other clinical manifestations and potential therapeutic strategies. JACC Basic Transl Sci. 2020;5(5):518–536.
10. Poissy J, Goutay J, Caplan M, Parmentier E, Duburcq T, Lassalle F, et al. Pulmonary embolism in COVID-19 patients: awareness of an increased prevalence. Circulation. 2020:CIRCULATIONAHA.120.047430.
11. Liao S-C, Shao S-C, Chen Y-T, Chen Y-C, Hung M-J. Incidence and mortality of pulmonary embolism in COVID-19: a systematic review and meta-analysis. Crit Care. 2020;24(1):464.
12. Tang N, Bai H, Chen X, Gong J, Li D, Sun Z. Anticoagulant treatment is associated with decreased mortality in severe coronavirus disease 2019 patients with coagulopathy. J Thromb Haemost. 2020. [citado el 14 de abril de 2020]. Disponible en: https://doi.org/doi.wiley.com/10.1111/jth.14817.
13. Thachil J. The versatile heparin in COVID-19. J Thromb Haemost. 2020. [citado el 14 de abril de 2020]. Disponible en: http://doi.wiley.com/https://doi.org/10.1111/jth.14821.
14. Liu PP, Blet A, Smyth D, Li H. The science underlying COVID-19: implications for the cardiovascular system. Circulation. 2020:CIRCULATIONAHA.120.047549.
15. Bikdeli B, Madhavan MV, Jimenez D, Chuich T, Dreyfus I, Driggin E, et al. COVID-19 and thrombotic or thromboembolic disease: implications for prevention, antithrombotic therapy, and follow-up. J Am Coll Cardiol. 2020:S0735109720350087.
16. Wang J, Hajizadeh N, Moore EE, McIntyre RC, Moore PK, Veress LA, et al. Tissue Plasminogen Activator (tPA) treatment for COVID-19 Associated Acute Respiratory Distress Syndrome (ARDS): a case series. J Thromb Haemost. 2020. [citado el 14 de abril de 2020]. Disponible en: https://doi.org/doi.wiley.com/10.1111/jth.14828.
17. Oudkerk M, Büller HR, Kuijpers D, van Es N, Oudkerk SF, McLoud TC, et al. Diagnosis, prevention, and treatment of thromboembolic complications in COVID-19: report of the national institute for public health of the Netherlands. Radiology. 2020:201629.
18. Moher D, Liberati A, Tetzlaff J, Altman DG, The PRISMA Group. Preferred reporting items for systematic reviews and meta-analyses: the PRISMA statement. PLoS Med. 2009;6(7):e1000097.
19. Vinson DR, Ballard DW, Mark DG, Huang J, Reed ME, Rauchwerger AS, et al. Risk stratifying emergency department patients with acute pulmonary embolism: does the simplified Pulmonary Embolism Severity Index perform as well as the original? Thromb Res. 2016;148:1–8.
20. Greenhalgh T, Peacock R. Effectiveness and efficiency of search methods in systematic reviews of complex evidence: audit of primary sources. BMJ. 2005;331(7524):1064–5.
21. Schulman S, Kearon C, the SUBCOMMITTEE ON CONTROL OF ANTICOAGULATION OF THE SCIENTIFIC AND STANDARDIZATION COMMITTEE OF THE INTERNATIONAL SOCIETY ON THROMBOSIS AND HAEMOSTASIS. Definition of major bleeding in clinical investigations of antihemostatic medicinal products in non-surgical patients: definitions of major bleeding in clinical studies. J Thromb Haemost. 2005;3(4):692–4.
22. Konstantinides SV, Meyer G, Becattini C, Bueno H, Geersing G-J, Harjola V-P, et al. 2019 ESC Guidelines for the diagnosis and management of acute pulmonary embolism developed in collaboration with the European Respiratory Society (ERS). Eur Heart J. 2019:ehz405.
23. de Bruijn SFTM, Stam J, Randomized. Placebo-controlled trial of anticoagulant treatment with low-molecular-weight heparin for cerebral sinus thrombosis. Stroke. 1999;30(3):484–8.
24. Lu Y, Pan L, Zhang W-W, Cheng F, Hu S-S, Zhang X, et al. A meta-analysis of the incidence of venous thromboembolic events and impact of anticoagulation on mortality in patients with COVID-19. Int J Infect Dis. 2020;100:34–41.
25. Porfidia A, Valeriani E, Pola R, Porreca E, Rutjes AWS, Di Nisio M. Venous thromboembolism in patients with COVID-19: systematic review and meta-analysis. Thromb Res. 2020;196:67–74.
26. Zhang C, Shen L, Le K-J, Pan M-M, Kong L-C, Gu Z-C, et al. Incidence of venous thromboembolism in hospitalized coronavirus disease 2019 patients: a systematic review and meta-analysis. Front Cardiovasc Med. 2020;7:151.
27. Jiménez D, García-Sanchez A, Rali P, Muriel A, Bikdeli B, Ruiz-Artacho P, et al. Incidence of venous thromboembolism and bleeding among hospitalized patients with COVID-19: a systematic review and meta-analysis. Chest. 2020:S0012369220351461.
28. Chi G, Lee JJ, Jamil A, Gunnam V, Najafi H, Memar Montazerin S, et al. Venous thromboembolism among hospitalized patients with COVID-19 undergoing thromboprophylaxis: a systematic review and meta-analysis. J Clin Med. 2020;9(8):2489.
29. Bansal A, Singh AD, Jain V, Aggarwal M, Gupta S, Padappayil RP, et al. The association of D-dimers with mortality, intensive care unit admission or acute respiratory distress syndrome in patients hospitalized with coronavirus disease 2019 (COVID-19): a systematic review and meta-analysis. Heart Lung. 2020:S0147956320303800.
30. Piazza G, Campia U, Hurwitz S, Snyder JE, Rizzo SM, Pfeferman MB, et al. Registry of arterial and venous thromboembolic complications in patients with COVID-19. J Am Coll Cardiol. 2020;76(18):2060–72.
31. Sharifi M, Larijani F, Wycliffe R, Loggins B, Schroeder B, Monteros DDL, et al. Low dose systemic thrombolysis and new oral anticoagulants in the treatment of large thrombi in the right heart. J Am Coll Cardiol. 2017;69(11):2079.
32. Sharifi M, Vajo Z, Freeman W, Bay C, Sharifi M, Schwartz F. Transforming and simplifying the treatment of pulmonary embolism: "safe dose" thrombolysis plus new oral anticoagulants. Lung. 2015;193(3):369–74.
33. Sharifi M, Bay C, Schwartz F, Skrocki L. Safe-dose thrombolysis plus rivaroxaban for moderate and severe pulmonary embolism: drip, drug, and discharge: thrombolysis plus rivaroxaban in PE. Clin Cardiol. 2014;37(2):78–82.
34. Betancourt-del Campo H, Jerjes-Sanchez C, Castillo-Perez M, López-de la Garza H, Paredes-Vázquez JG, Flores-Sayavedra YZ, et al. Systemic thrombolysis and anticoagulation improved biomarker measurements in massive-like pulmonary embolism and severe COVID-19 pneumonia: a case report. Brown RA, Bouzas-Mosquera A, Cankovic MZ, Rampat R, Sayers M, Thomson R, editores. Eur Heart J - Case Rep. 2020:ytaa448.
35. Piazza G. Advanced management of intermediate- and high-risk pulmonary embolism. J Am Coll Cardiol. 2020;76(18):2117–27.
36. Malas MB, Naazie IN, Elsayed N, Mathlouthi A, Marmor R, Clary B. Thromboembolism risk of COVID-19 is high and associated with a higher risk of mortality: a systematic review and meta-analysis. EClinicalMedicine. 2020;29–30:100639.
37. Trevino AR, Perez L, Jerjes-Sanchez C, Rodriguez D, Panneflek J, Ortiz-Ledesma C, et al. Factor Xa inhibition and sPESI failure in intermediate-high-risk pulmonary embolism. Am J Emerg Med. 2018;36(10):1925.e3-1925.e4.
38. Tacquard C, Mansour A, Godon A, Godet J, Poissy J, Garrigue D, et al. Impact of high dose prophylactic anticoagulation in critically ill patients with COVID-19 pneumonia. Chest. 2021:S0012369221000477.
39. Hardy M, Michaux I, Lessire S, Douxfils J, Dogné J-M, Bareille M, et al. Prothrombotic disturbances of hemostasis of patients with severe COVID-19: a prospective longitudinal observational study. Thromb Res. 2021;197:20–3.

40. Susen S, Tacquard CA, Godon A, Mansour A, Garrigue D, Nguyen P, et al. Prevention of thrombotic risk in hospitalized patients with COVID-19 and hemostasis monitoring. Crit Care. 2020;24(1):364.

41. The RIETE, Investigators, Frasson S, Gussoni G, Di Micco P, Barba R, Bertoletti L, et al. Infection as cause of immobility and occurrence of venous thromboembolism: analysis of 1635 medical cases from the RIETE registry. J Thromb Thrombolysis. 2016;41(3):404–12.

42. Zhang Y, Zhou Q, Zou Y, Song X, Xie S, Tan M, et al. Risk factors for pulmonary embolism in patients preliminarily diagnosed with community-acquired pneumonia: a prospective cohort study. J Thromb Thrombolysis. 2016;41(4):619–27.

43. Faggiano P, Bonelli A, Paris S, Milesi G, Bisegna S, Bernardi N, et al. Acute pulmonary embolism in COVID-19 disease: preliminary report on seven patients. Int J Cardiol. 2020;313:129–31.

44. Girot M, Ferro JM, Canhão P, Stam J, Bousser M-G, Barinagarrementeria F, et al. Predictors of outcome in patients with cerebral venous thrombosis and intracerebral hemorrhage. Stroke. 2007;38(2):337–42.

45. Saposnik G, Barinagarrementeria F, Brown RD, Bushnell CD, Cucchiara B, Cushman M, et al. Diagnosis and management of cerebral venous thrombosis: a statement for healthcare professionals from the American Heart Association/American Stroke Association. Stroke. 2011;42(4):1158–92.

46. Ferro JM, Coutinho JM, Dentali F, Kobayashi A, Alasheev A, Canhão P, et al. Safety and efficacy of dabigatran etexilate vs dose-adjusted warfarin in patients with cerebral venous thrombosis: a randomized clinical trial. JAMA Neurol. 2019;76(12):1457.

15

Deep venous thrombosis in an individual with statin-exposed anti-SRP myopathy

Jiali Li[1], Mingming Yan[2], Jiao Qin[1], Lingyan He[1], Cao Dai[1] and Rui Wen[1*]

Abstract

Background: Immune-mediated necrotizing myopathy (IMNM) is characterized by proximal muscle weakness, elvated serum muscle enzyme levels, myopathic electromyography findings, and necrotic muscle fiber with few inflammatory cell infiltration in muscle biopsies. Statins, the first line drug to lower triglyceride and cholesterol level in blood, have been reported to be associated with statins-induced necrotizing autoimmune myopathy (SINAM). Although anti-3-hydroxy-3-methylglutarylcoenzyme-A reductase (anti-HMGCR) myopathy is considered as the leading myopathy related to the statins medication, anti-signal recognition particle (SRP) myopathy were also identified in several cases with statin exposure. The risk of deep venous thrombosis (DVT) is substantially high in individuals with autoimmune inflammatory diseases. But few studies have reported the occurrence and recommendation for treatment of DVT in patients with anti-SRP myopathy. Here, we reported a statin-exposed anti-SRP myopathy individual developed DVT who was successfully treated with catheter-directed thrombolysis (CDT) and systemic anticoagulants therapy.

Case presentation: A 56-year-old Chinese female came to the outpatient room with gradually progressive bilateral lower-extremity weakness. Magnetic resonance imaging revealed myopathy in bilateral thighs. Serum anti-SRP antibody was positive. She was diagnosed with anti-SRP myopathy. When treated with corticosteroids and immunosuppressants, the patient developed mild edema and pain of left lower extremity. Angiography and ultrasound revealed diffuse venous thrombosis of left lower extremity. Therapy was initiated with CDT and lower molecular weight heparin, then switched to once daily oral rivaroxaban. Meanwhile, steroids combined with tacrolimus were also carried on while simvastatin was discontinued. One month later, patient's symptoms were resolved and only partial thrombosis in left femoral vein was remained.

Conclusion: The prevalence of DVT in patient with anti-SRP myopathy was rare. No well-established treatment strategy is available to manage the IMNM and DVT at the same time. The systemic anticoagulants therapy combined CDT can be an effective therapeutic approach to address extensive DVT in patient with anti-SRP myopathy.

Keywords: Immune-mediated necrotizing myopathy, Anti-signal recognition particle myopathy, Deep venous thrombosis, Statins

* Correspondence: lijiali32838@163.com
[1]Department of Rheumatology and Immunology, University of South China Affiliated Changsha Central Hospital, 161 South Shaoshan Road, Changsha 410008, Hunan, China
Full list of author information is available at the end of the article

Background

Immune-mediated necrotizing myopathy (IMNM) is a group of inflammatory myopathies, which is clinically characterized with proximal muscle weakness, elvated serum muscle enzyme levels, myopathic electromyography findings, and necrotic muscle fiber with few inflammatory cell infiltration in muscle biopsies [1]. Multiple causes including autoantibodies, statins administration, paraneoplastic, and viral infection are strongly associated with the IMNM [2]. As the first line drug to lower triglyceride and cholesterol level in blood, statins could cause statins-induced necrotizing autoimmune myopathy (SINAM), which is the mainly side effect responsible for the discontinuation of statins medication [3]. Although anti-3-hydroxy-3-methylglutarylcoenzyme-A reductase (anti-HMGCR) antibody is the most common autoantibodies identified in SINAM, the present of anti-signal recognition particle (SRP) was also confirmed by RNA immunoprecipitation in SINAM [4]. Moreover, it has been showed that anti-SRP antibodies levels correlate with disease activity of SINAM [5]. Therefore, this anti-SRP antibodies can be considered as a specific biomarker to classify the category of SINAM.

As the hallmark feature of SINAM is significant muscle fiber necrosis or regeneration with few lymphocytic infiltration, the prevalence of thrombosis in SINAM is rare compared to other autoimmune diseases such as Churg-Strass syndrome and systemic lupus erythematosus [6, 7]. In addition, the management of DVT in SINAM has not yet been well established. Here, we firstly reported that a patient diagnosed with anti-SRP myopathy developed a severe DVT in left lower extremity. She got a clinical remission after the induction therapy with corticosteroids, immunosuppressants, systemic anticoagulants, and CDT.

Case presentation

A 56-year-old female with a history of hypertension and hyperlipidemia presented to outpatient room with gradually progressive bilateral lower-extremity weakness more than five weeks and exaggeration for one week.

She had difficulty in getting up from the bed and lifting the feet off the floor but denied fever, rash, dysphagia, headache, sialorrhea, diplopia, muscle pain, and sensory changes. There was no family history of genetic myopathies or rheumatologic. She had been taking the amlodipine, metoprolol tartrate, and atorvastatin for 6 years.

A scrotal examination revealed the power in her both upper and lower bilateral proximal extremities was 2/5, and that in both upper and lower bilateral distal extremities was 3/5. Her muscle tone in lower extremities was decreased but deep tendon reflexes were normal.

Laboratory tests showed normal complete blood count and C-reactive protein. Sedimentation rate was slightly elevated to 28 mm/h. There was an increase in creatine kinase (CK) 7892 IU/L, myohemoglobin (MYO) 2315 IU/L, and lactic dehydrogenase 1244 IU/L. AST and ALT were increased to 159 IU/L and 171 IU/L, respectively. Serum magnesium were elevated to 1 mg/dL. Her antinuclear antibody and anti-neutrophil cytoplasmic antibody were normal. Serum immunological studies demonstrated postivie antibodies of anti-SRP and Ro-52. Magnetic resonance imaging of thigh revealed extensive edema, suggestive of diffuse myositis (Fig. 1A). Electromyography showed myogenic lesion. A biopsy of muscle of right thigh revealed necrotic muscle clustered intermingled with few lymphocytes (Fig. 1B and C).

She was diagnosed with anti-SRP myopathy. Statin was discontinued. The patient was started on intravenous immune globulin (IVIG) 0.5 g/kg divided over five-day course. Simultaneously, high-dose methylprednisolone (500 mg/d) was administered for three days, followed by solumedorl 80 mg daily. Following the commencement of tacrolimus (3 mg/day), serum CK and MYO levels decreased to 3603 U/L and 2066 U/L, respectively. Muscle weakness gradually recovered. The oral solumedrol upon discharge was slowly tapered down to maintenance dose of 0.8 mg/kg/day.

The steroid was slowly tapped down over one month. She was readmitted to our intervention department due to mild edema and pain of left lower extremity. Laboratory tests

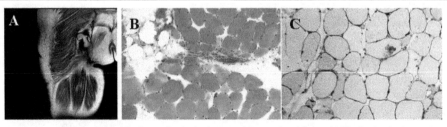

Fig. 1 Magnetic resonance image and histological findings of right thigh. **A** Axial T1-weighted femoral MRI of right thigh on admission showed femoral muscle atrophy with fat replacement. **B** Hematoxylin and eosin staining from muscle biopsy sections of right quadriceps showed necrotic muscle occasionally clustered intermingled with small lymphocytes (**C**)

showed serum CK level decreased to 1241 U/L and serum MYO level decreased to 787 U/L, while D-dimer increased to 22.7 μg/mL. Severe and diffuse venous thrombosis of left lower extremity was confirmed by angiography and ultrasound (Fig. 2A and B). The catheter-directed thrombolysis was performed for revascularization. A self-expandable inferior vena cava filter was deployed and a catheter was percutaneous placed into iliac vein. For thrombolysis, 200,000 U of urokinase (UK) was directly infused twice through catheter within 1 h. After surgery, 400,000 U/day of UK was continuously administrated through catheter for 4 days. Lower weight molecular heparin (5000 U, Q12h) was also injected subcutaneously for five days, followed by orally rivaroxaban 15 mg BID and simvastatin 20 mg qn. To evaluate the efficacy of thrombolysis, percutaneous transluminal angioplasty (PTA) was performed one month after CDT. Angiography revealed partial thrombus removal and good blood flow (Fig. 2C). However, serum CK and MYO levels increased to 4408 U/L and 3681 U/L, respectively. Steroid combined with tacrolimus were carried on while simvastatin was immediately discontinued. With a good response, the power of affected muscle groups was gradually recovered and serum CK level decreased to nearly normal range. After myopathic management, discontinuation of simvastatin, and anticoagulant treatment ultrasonography revealed only partial thrombosis in left femoral vein (Fig. 2D).

Discussion and conclusions

Autoantibodies recognizing the SRP were first identified in the 1980s, which was reported to be highly associated with disease activity of IMNM [8]. Patients with positive anti-SRP myopathy have more severe proximal muscle weakness, higher number of necrotic muscle fibers, more common interstitial lung disease compared to anti-HMGCR myopathy [9]. Statins are associated with a number of myalgia and myopathy including IMNM. Statin-associated myopathy is mainly related with anti-HMGCR antibodies [10]. However, about 20% anti-SRP

myopathy patients have been reported to have statin exposure [11]. After 5 years of atorvastatin medication, our patient developed anti-SRP myopathy with severe proximal muscle damage. With a good response to the immunosuppressive treatment, she had a clinical remission. However, serum CK levels sharply rose when simvastatin was prescribed to treat DVT, which further supported that the occurrence of anti-SRP myopathy was not limited to specific category of statins administration.

This is the first case to report DVT in patients with anti-SRP myopathy. The risk of DVT is substantially high in patients with autoimmune inflammatory diseases. According to Virchow's triad, three main plausible existing mechanisms including venous stasis, increased coagulability of blood and vessel wall damage contribute to the high risk of DVT [12], which is also applied to patients with anti-SRP myopathy. First of all, the patients with anti-SRP myopathy suffer from serious muscle weakness which may lead to venous stasis due to decreased mobility [13]. Moreover, inflammation is able to modulate thrombotic responses by upregulating procoagulants and damaging vessel wall. However, as anti-SRP myopathy is characterized by myofiber necrosis over inflammation [1], venous stasis should be the primary risk factor of DVT. In addition, the use of steroid, which helps to slow the progression of the disease, could be the another driver of the increased risk of DVT [14].

Given the presumptive mechanisms discussed above, the primary recommendation for DVT should be myopathic treatment. At present, there are no clinical trials to guide therapeutic decision in anti-SRP myopathy. The recommendation derived from most recent European Neuromuscular Center criteria for IMNM suggests that corticosteroids plus immunosuppressant is considered to be an initial treatment [15]. High-dose corticosteroids or IVIG could achieve an excellent response in the most severely affected individuals. In this case, a combination of immunosuppressive therapy (eg., high-dose solumedorl,

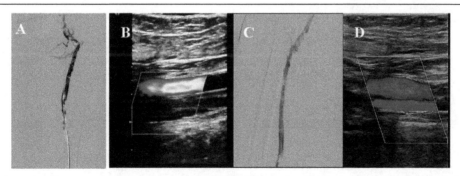

Fig. 2 Arterial duplex scan and computed tomography angiography showed the venous thrombosis of left lower extremity before and after anti-thrombosis management. Severe and diffuse venous thrombosis of left lower extremity was confirmed by admission computed tomography angiography ultrasound (**A**) and arterial duplex (**B**). One month after PTA, computed tomography angiography showed a good blood flow with a markedly decrease in length of thrombosis (**C**). Ultrasonography revealed only partial thrombosis in left femoral vein after half year (**D**)

tacrolimus, and IVIG) achieved a satisfactory clinical outcome. However, she had an acute proximal DVT of the leg on the second admission, which was likely due to simvastatin-induced anti-SRP myopathy. The recommendation for DVT management revealed that anticoagulant therapy plus CDT to restore venous patency is much more effective than anticoagulation alone [15] . Due to the efficacy of selective thrombolysis and reduced hemorrhagic complication compared with systemic infusion, CDT has been an appearing management for DVT [16]. Therefore, we applied CDT combined with both heparin infusion and oral rivaroxaban to counter DVT, which contributed to a full thrombosis remission. In the absence of other studies on management of anti-SRP myopathy and DVT at the same time, this report provide a substantial value for physicians to improve clinical outcome of similar cases.

Abbreviations
IMNM: Immune-mediated necrotizing myopathy; SINAM: statin-induced necrotizing autoimmune myopathy; HMGCR: 3-hydroxy-3-methylglutarylcoenzyme-A reductase; SRP: signal recognition particle; DVT: deep venous thrombosis; CDT: catheter-directed thrombolysis; CK: creatine kinase; MYO: myohemoglobin; IVIG: intravenous immune globulin; PTA: percutaneous transluminal angioplasty

Acknowledgements
Not applicable.

Authors' contributions
JLL and MMY wrote the initial draft of the manuscript. JJL, HGH and CD collected the data. JQ assisted with the literature review for this manuscript. RW supervised the project from initiation and revised the manuscript. The author(s) read and approved the final manuscript.

Author details
[1]Department of Rheumatology and Immunology, University of South China Affiliated Changsha Central Hospital, 161 South Shaoshan Road, Changsha 410008, Hunan, China. [2]Department of Orthopaedic Surgery, The Second Xiangya Hospital of Central South University, Changsha, Hunan, China.

References
1. Selva-O'Callaghan A, Pinal-Fernandez I, Trallero-Araguas E, Milisenda JC, Grau-Junyent JM, Mammen AL. Classification and management of adult inflammatory myopathies. Lancet Neurol. 2018;17(9):816–28. https://doi.org/10.1016/S1474-4422(18)30254-0.
2. Allenbach Y, Keraen J, Bouvier AM, Jooste V, Champtiaux N, Hervier B, et al. High risk of cancer in autoimmune necrotizing myopathies: usefulness of myositis specific antibody. Brain. 2016;139(8):2131–5. https://doi.org/10.1093/brain/aww054.
3. Mammen AL. Statin-associated autoimmune myopathy. N Engl J Med. 2016;374(7):664–9. https://doi.org/10.1056/NEJMra1515161.
4. Suzuki S, Nishikawa A, Kuwana M, Nishimura H, Watanabe Y, Nakahara J, et al. Inflammatory myopathy with anti-signal recognition particle antibodies: case series of 100 patients. Orphanet J Rare Dis. 2015;10(1):61. https://doi.org/10.1186/s13023-015-0277-y.
5. Benveniste O, Drouot L, Jouen F, Charuel JL, Bloch-Queyrat C, Behin A, et al. Correlation of anti-signal recognition particle autoantibody levels with creatine kinase activity in patients with necrotizing myopathy. Arthritis Rheum. 2011;63(7):1961–71. https://doi.org/10.1002/art.30344.
6. Li J, Yan M, Qin J, Ren L, Wen R. Testicular infarction and pulmonary embolism secondary to nonasthmatic eosinophilic granulomatosis with Polyangiitis: a case report. J Investig Allergol Clin Immunol. 2020;30(5):380–1. https://doi.org/10.18176/jiaci.0566.
7. de Groot PG, de Laat B. Mechanisms of thrombosis in systemic lupus erythematosus and antiphospholipid syndrome. Best Pract Res Clin Rheumatol. 2017;31(3):334–41. https://doi.org/10.1016/j.berh.2017.09.008.
8. Reeves WH, Nigam SK, Blobel G. Human autoantibodies reactive with the signal-recognition particle. Proc Natl Acad Sci U S A. 1986;83(24):9507–11. https://doi.org/10.1073/pnas.83.24.9507.
9. Watanabe Y, Uruha A, Suzuki S, Nakahara J, Hamanaka K, Takayama K, et al. Clinical features and prognosis in anti-SRP and anti-HMGCR necrotising myopathy. J Neurol Neurosurg Psychiatry. 2016;87(10):1038–44. https://doi.org/10.1136/jnnp-2016-313166.
10. Christopher-Stine L, Casciola-Rosen LA, Hong G, Chung T, Corse AM, Mammen AL. A novel autoantibody recognizing 200-kd and 100-kd proteins is associated with an immune-mediated necrotizing myopathy. Arthritis Rheum. 2010;62(9):2757–66. https://doi.org/10.1002/art.27572.
11. Pinal-Fernandez I, Casal-Dominguez M, Mammen AL. Immune-mediated necrotizing myopathy. Curr Rheumatol Rep. 2018;20(4):21. https://doi.org/10.1007/s11926-018-0732-6.
12. Malone PC, Agutter PS. The aetiology of deep venous thrombosis. QJM. 2006;99(9):581–93. https://doi.org/10.1093/qjmed/hcl070.
13. Nowak M, Krolak-Nowak K, Sobolewska-Wlodarczyk A, Fichna J, Wlodarczyk M. Elevated risk of venous thromboembolic events in patients with inflammatory myopathies. Vasc Health Risk Manag. 2016;12:233–8. https://doi.org/10.2147/VHRM.S75308.
14. Allenbach Y, Mammen AL, Benveniste O, Stenzel W, Immune-Mediated Necrotizing Myopathies Working G. 224th ENMC International Workshop:: Clinico-sero-pathological classification of immune-mediated necrotizing myopathies Zandvoort, The Netherlands, 14–16 October 2016. Neuromuscul Disord. 2018;28:87–99.
15. Fleck D, Albadawi H, Shamoun F, Knuttinen G, Naidu S, Oklu R. Catheter-directed thrombolysis of deep vein thrombosis: literature review and practice considerations. Cardiovasc Diagn Ther. 2017;7(S3):S228–S37. https://doi.org/10.21037/cdt.2017.09.15.
16. Mewissen MW, Seabrook GR, Meissner MH, Cynamon J, Labropoulos N, Haughton SH. Catheter-directed thrombolysis for lower extremity deep venous thrombosis: report of a national multicenter registry. Radiology. 1999;211(1):39–49. https://doi.org/10.1148/radiology.211.1.r99ap4739.

16

Potential value of the calibrated automated thrombogram in patients after a cerebral venous sinus thrombosis

Myrthe M. van der Bruggen[1], Bram Kremers[1,2], Rene van Oerle[2,3], Robert J. van Oostenbrugge[4] and Hugo ten Cate[1,2*] ⓘ

Abstract

Background: Cerebral venous sinus thrombosis (CVST) is a relatively rare, but potentially lethal condition. In approximately 15% of the patients, the cause of CVST remains unclear. Conventional clotting tests such as prothrombin time and activated partial thromboplastin time are not sensitive enough to detect prothrombotic conditions nor mild haemostatic abnormalities. The calibrated automated thrombogram (CAT) is a physiological function test that might be able to detect minor aberrations in haemostasis. Therefore, we aimed to detect the presence of a prothrombotic state in patients who endured idiopathic CVST with the CAT assay.

Methods: *Five adult patients* with an idiopathic, radiologically proven CVST that had been admitted during the past 3 years were included in this study. The control group consisted of *five* age/gender matched healthy volunteers. Exclusion criteria were known haematological disorders, malignancy (current/past) or hormonal and anticoagulant therapy recipients. We obtained venous blood samples from all participants following cessation of anticoagulation. Using the CAT assay, we determined lag time, normalized endogenous thrombin potential (ETP), ETP reduction and normalized peak height. In addition, prothrombin concentrations were determined.

Results: We found no significant differences in lag time (4.7 min [4.5–4.9] vs 5.3 min [3.7–5.7], $p = 0.691$), normalized ETP (142% [124–148] vs 124% [88–138], $p = 0.222$), ETP reduction (29% [26–35] vs 28% [24–58], $p > 0.999$), and normalized peak height (155% [153–175] vs 137 [94–154], $p = 0.056$) between patients and their age/gender matched controls. In addition, prothrombin concentrations did not significantly differ between patients and controls (120% [105–132] vs 127% [87–139], $p > 0.999$).

Conclusion: Reasons for absent overt hypercoagulability within this study population may be the small patient sample, long time since the event (e.g. 3 years) and avoidance of acquired risk factors like oral contraception. Given the fact that CVST is a serious condition with a more than negligible risk of venous thrombosis event recurrence, exclusion of clinically relevant hypercoagulability remains a challenging topic to further study at the acute and later time points, particularly in patients with idiopathic CVST.

* Correspondence: h.tencate@maastrichtuniversity.nl
[1]Department of Internal Medicine, Maastricht University Medical Centre, Maastricht, the Netherlands
[2]Department of Biochemistry, Cardiovascular Research Institute Maastricht, Maastricht, the Netherlands
Full list of author information is available at the end of the article

Introduction

Cerebral venous sinus thrombosis (CVST) is a relatively rare subtype of stroke. The incidence of this disease reported in the literature is approximately 3 per 100.000 per year, affecting more women than men [1, 2]. Because of its rare occurrence the incidence of this disease might be underestimated, due to unawareness of its diagnosis. In addition, CVST is difficult to diagnose as it has a variable clinical presentation and may be challenging to confirm radiologically [3]. Complications include subarachnoid haemorrhage, cranial nerve palsy, epilepsy and transient ischemic attacks [4–6]. Taken together, the consequences of CVST can be severely incapacitating, and potentially life threatening [4]. This is illustrated by a case from a 19-year old female who visited the emergency room with acute headache in the last 24 h. The pain was progressive, the patient experienced nausea and vertigo, and she had vomited several times. In addition, she was both phono- and photophobic. Her medical history did not show any peculiarities and the family history was negative for thrombotic diseases. She did not suffer head trauma or infections, nor did she use any hormonal/contraceptive therapy. Magnetic resonance imaging showed a thrombosis of the jugular vein, sigmoid sinus, right transverse sinus and the distal part of the sagittal sinus. Thrombophilia analysis did not show any of the common traits including factor V Leiden, prothrombin 20210 or inhibitor deficiencies. Despite adequate treatment with anticoagulants, the patient still regularly experienced loss of vision and headache years after the event. This case illustrates how severe CVST can influence a (young) patient's life.

Recent occurrences of CVST in the setting of Covid-19 vaccination, triggered interest for this disorder [7]. There are several risk factors that contribute to the development of CVST. Examples are prothrombotic conditions such as protein C -, protein S -, and antithrombin deficiency. Furthermore, tumours, haematological disorders and the use of oral hormonal contraception are associated with CVST [1, 8, 9]. The risk factors that contribute to the development of CVST can be identified in most patients. However, in approximately 15–20% of patients no cause or risk factor is identified [1, 10]. Subsequently, monitoring this patient group and estimating the risk for recurrence is rather difficult [11].

In general, hypercoagulability is a key element in venous thrombosis and in addition to the mentioned thrombophilic traits, acquired factors like oral contraceptives have an important impact on coagulation through an acquired resistance against activated protein C [12]. The intrinsic coagulation properties can be assessed through the calibrated automated thrombogram (CAT). The CAT, developed by Hemker and coworkers, is a semi-automated thrombin generation technique, which provides the ability to monitor thrombin concentrations in time, as the substrate for thrombin is fluorescently labeled [13, 14]. The CAT method is currently well-accepted as a research tool and has proven to be useful in several different domains such as platelet-plasma interactions, detection and quantification of thrombotic/bleeding tendency, and control of pro-coagulant and antithrombotic therapy [12, 15–17]. During a curiosity driven exploration of the CAT data in consecutive patients referred to the vascular outpatient clinic, we observed three patients who suffered from idiopathic CVST and had substantial elevations in thrombin generation (i.e. mean endogenous thrombin potential (ETP) 190%, mean normalized peak 352%) without any reasonable explanation.

Based on this unpublished observation we designed the present study to investigate whether abnormal CAT responses would indeed be a consistent finding in patients who suffered a CVST.

Methods

Adult patients who endured CVST without known cause or risk factors were included in this patient study. We searched hospital records for CVST patients between January 1st 2012 and May 24th 2017 using the Dutch financial coding system for hospital care (DBC-codes). There is no specific code for CVST or for cerebral venous thrombosis. Therefore, all records of patients assigned to the code "ischemic stroke", "haemorrhagic stroke", "headache" and "not other specified" were screened. Based on this search strategy we identified 29 CVST patients. Next, patients under 18 years of age, patients with known coagulation disorders, malignancy (in the past), using hormonal contraception or other hormonal therapy, or anticoagulants and patients who are mentally disabled, were excluded from this study.

Blood plasma from healthy age and gender matched volunteers was used as reference material. Healthy volunteers were recruited through advertisements at the faculty of health, medicine and life sciences at Maastricht University. The same exclusion criteria as with patients applied.

All subjects who were eligible for inclusion in this study underwent a venepuncture and filled in a questionnaire with regard to thrombotic risk factors. This was done to place outcome measures in a clinical perspective.

All subjects were informed and provided written consent.

The study was performed at Maastricht University Medical Centre (MUMC+) and approved by the local medical ethical committee (Medical ethical committee MUMC, approval number; NL 63775.068.17).

Blood collection and storage

Four 9 mL tubes with 3.2% trisodium citrate were collected through antecubital venipuncture. The blood was processed to platelet poor plasma (PPP) within 1 h after collection via previously described methods [18, 19]. PPP was stored at -80 °C until analysis [20]. All samples were analyzed at one time point to prevent repeated freeze-thaw cycles. Plasma from healthy volunteers was processed and stored in the same manner, with the same number of freeze-thaw cycles as plasma from patients.

Markers of coagulation

Thrombin generation

The coagulation potential in plasma was assessed using the CAT assay (Thrombinoscope BV, Maastricht, the Netherlands). Within this method, low-affinity fluorogenic substrate for thrombin (Z-Gly-Gly-Arg-AMC; Bachem, Bubendorf, Switzerland) is added to allow continuous monitoring of thrombin formation. For each measurement, 80 μL of human PPP was added to 20 μL of fluorogenic substrate, 20 μL of trigger reagent and calcium chloride, as previous reported [19, 21]. The CAT assay was performed with and without the presence of soluble thrombomodulin (TM; Asahi Kasei Pharma Corporation, Tagata, Japan), to enable protein C depend testing [12]. TG curves were calculated using Thrombinoscope software (Thrombinoscope, Maastricht, The Netherlands). Analysis resulted in four main outcome parameters: 1. Lag time; the time until clotting occurs. 2. ETP; the total amount of thrombin formed during the measurement, i.e. the area under the curve. 3. Peak height; maximum amount of thrombin generation. 4. Peak reduction; time needed for clot degradation [19].

Prothrombin levels

Being an important determinant of the CAT, prothrombin was measured with a one stage FII assay on a Siemens BCSxp instrument according to the manufacturer's instructions.

Statistical analysis

Baseline characteristics were collected and tabulated. Differences in thrombin generation outcome measures between patients and controls were analyzed using the Mann-Whitney U test (nonparametric) because of the small sample size. Results are shown as the median and 25th–75th percentile.

P-values < 0.05 were considered statistically significant. All analyses were performed using GraphPad Prism version 7 for Windows, GraphPad Software, La Jolla California USA, www.graphpad.com.

Results

Baseline characteristics

Eleven patients were eligible for participation in the study. Four patients were not interested in participating. From the remaining seven patients, one patient did not appear at the appointment and one patient used anticoagulant drugs despite the screening efforts. Consequently, 5 patients and 5 controls were enrolled in the study. A flow-chart of the inclusion- and exclusion process can be found in Fig. 1.

At the time of the event, there was no relevant medical history or use of medication that was expected to provoke CVST. Medical history of the five patients at the time of the event included: polyarticular juvenile idiopathic arthritis (1 patient), exertional headaches (1 patient), and hypertension (1 patient). Medication use included TNF-α blocker (1 patient), metoprolol (1 patient), ibuprofen and paracetamol (1 patient). Patient characteristics of all study participants at the time of inclusion are shown in Table 1. No differences in key risk factors and relevant medication between patients and controls were observed.

Markers of coagulation

1.1 No significant differences in thrombin generation were observed

The CAT thrombin generation assay was performed and lag time, ETP, ETP reduction and peak height were assessed [Table 2]. There was no significant difference in lag time between patients and controls ($p = 0.691$) [Fig. 2A]. Although normalized peak height and ETP were both higher in patients than controls, neither difference was statistically significant ($p = 0.056$, $p = 0.222$ respectively) (Table 2 and Fig. 2B/C). ETP reduction, which is the difference in ETP determined with and without presence of TM, was similar between the groups [Table 2 and Fig. 2D].

1.2 No significant differences in prothrombin concentration were observed

Prothrombin was tested as it is known to be a main determinant of peak height and ETP [22–24]. No significant difference in prothrombin concentration was observed [Table 2/Fig. 2E].

Discussion

The present study assessed the presence of unexplained hypercoagulability in patients well beyond the acute phase of a CVST. We analysed thrombin generation by CAT based on a previous finding of elevated TG levels in 3 patients with CVST seen at the outpatient clinic. Two of the original 3 patients were included in the present study, the third patient was on rivaroxaban and could for that reason not be studied.

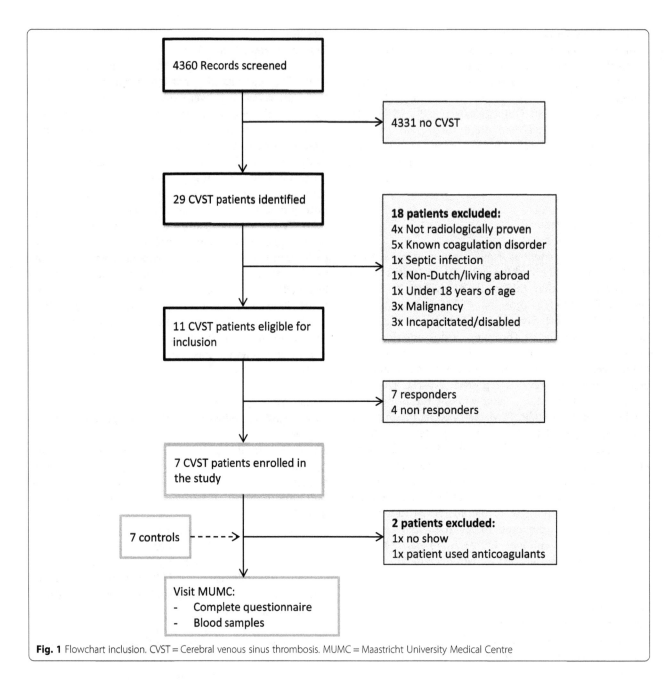

Fig. 1 Flowchart inclusion. CVST = Cerebral venous sinus thrombosis. MUMC = Maastricht University Medical Centre

Table 1 Baseline characteristics

	Patients	Controls
Female gender (%)	100%	100%
Age in years (mean)	42 (±12)	46 (±13)
Years after event (mean)	2,5	
Antiplatelet medication	0	0
Anti-inflammatory drugs	0	1
Alcohol consumption (U/week)	1	2
Smoking	0	0

Thrombin generation via the CAT method was performed in order to assess hypercoagulability. The first outcome parameter we considered was lag time. As expected, lag time did not significantly differ between patients and controls, as idiopathic hypercoagulability is mainly reflected by an increase in ETP and peak height [23, 25].

Subsequently we determined ETP, ETP reduction and peak height. ETP did not significantly differ between patients and controls. We tested ETP reduction by adding TM. Binding of thrombin to TM activates Protein C, a potent anticoagulant factor [13, 26]. We did not observe a significant difference in ETP reduction.

Table 2 Thrombin generation outcome measures shown as median [25–75 percentiles]. No significant differences were observed. ETP = endogenous thrombin potential

	Patients	Controls	P-value
Lag time (min)	4.7 [4.5–4.9]	5.3 [3.7–5.7]	0.691
Normalized ETP (%)	142 [124–148]	124 [88–138]	0.222
ETP reduction (%)	29 [26–35]	28 [24–58]	> 0.999
Normalized Peak Height (%)	155 [153–175]	137.4 [94–154]	0.056
Prothrombin concentration (%)	120 [105–132]	127 [87–139]	> 0.999

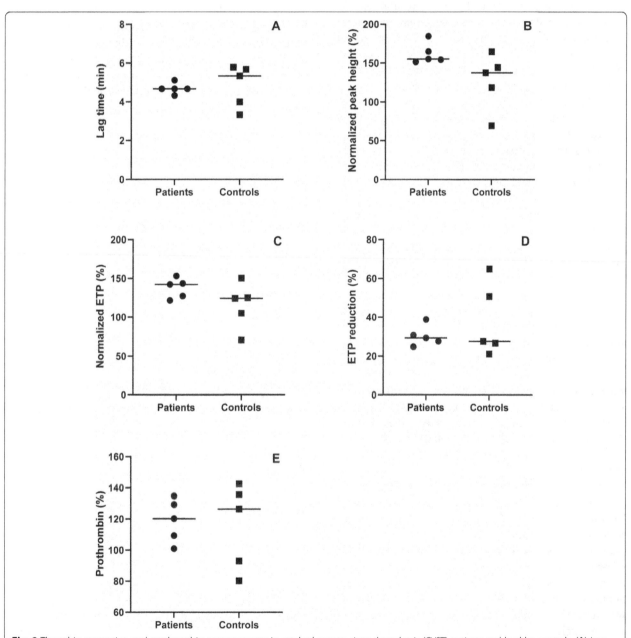

Fig. 2 Thrombin generation and prothrombin measurements in cerebral venous sinus thrombosis (CVST) patients and healthy controls. (**A**) Lag time (**B**) Normalized peak height. (**C**) Normalized endogenous thrombin potential (ETP). (**D**) ETP reduction (**E**) Prothrombin concentration

In addition, peak height of the thrombin generation curve was determined. Although there is a visual difference between the two groups (Fig. 2B), this did not reach statistical significance, probably due to the small sample size.

Based on a previous study which showed increased ETP and peak height in patients after deep venous thrombosis up till 2 years after the event [24], we expected to detect a similar difference in our study population. Other studies do support the findings of increased ETP and peak height after a thrombotic event [24]. The clinical relevance would be found in the ability to predict recurrent thrombotic events. However, results regarding the predictive value of the thrombin generation assay on development of a secondary event (venous thrombotic event) vary widely [20, 27–31]. It should be mentioned that some studies used whole blood, others used PPP or platelet rich plasma, which makes it difficult to compare the outcomes. Nevertheless, we can conclude that the role of thrombin generation as a predictor is still uncertain.

Patients with a first episode of CVST, a potentially devastating condition, are usually treated with anticoagulation for a limited time period, ranging from 3 to 6 months. This time is defined, considering the risk of recurrent disease after cessation of anticoagulation as low. However, this risk is not negligible and incidences ranging from 3 to 18% – depending on the risk factors – for development of recurrence CVST and/or other venous thrombotic events (VTE) have been reported [1, 10, 11]. Literature suggests that the risk of recurrence is highest up till one till 2 year(s) after the event [11, 32]. Therefore, characterizing thrombosis risk after stopping anticoagulation may be useful.

In all patients with CVST, avoidable risk factors like oral contraceptives are typically recorded and eliminated, whereas in younger individual's variable thrombophilia screening is done. Since thrombin generation might have been a convenient single test for detecting thrombophilia, we focused on its use in this population.

Study limitations

Limitations of this study include the small number of participants remaining after an extensive search and selection process. CVST is a relatively rare disease and we selected an even smaller group by only including idiopathic CVST patients. The direction of some of the TG comparisons showed a trend towards hypercoagulability in the patients and it may be assumed that in a larger population true differences may emerge. Furthermore, we excluded patients with a severe course of the disease, as we excluded disabled/incapacitated subjects. This might have led to selection bias in the current population. Finally, the time after the event might be too long

to be able to detect hypercoagulability and in case of risk factors like oral contraceptives, these were eliminated after the first event. We included patients after 3 years on average. It might simply be that the hypercoagulable state tends to normalize after this time interval.

Conclusions

In this pilot study we did not find any significant aberration in haemostasis between patients that suffered from CVST in the past, and age/gender machted controls. This is potentially due to a small sample size and relatively long follow-up time. Given the fact that CVST is a serious condition with a more than negligible risk of (VTE) recurrence, exclusion of clinically relevant hypercoagulability remains a challenging topic to further study at the acute and later time points, particularly in patients with idiopathic CVST.

Abbreviations
CAT: Calibrated automated thrombogram; CVST: Cerebral venous sinus thrombosis; DBC: Diagnosis-treatment combinations; ETP: Endogenous thrombin potential; MUMC: Maastricht university medical centre; PPP: Platelet poor plasma; TM: Thrombomodulin; VTE: Venous thrombotic event

Acknowledgements
Not applicable.

Authors' contributions
MB, RO, RJO, and HT conceived and designed the study. MB, BK and RO performed the measurements. MB, RO and HT analysed the data and interpreted the results. MB drafted the work. MB, BK, RO, RJO, and HT critically edited and revised the manuscript. MB, BK, RO, RJO, and HT have approved the final version of the manuscript and agree to be accountable for their contributions.

Authors' information
Not applicable.

Author details
[1]Department of Internal Medicine, Maastricht University Medical Centre, Maastricht, the Netherlands. [2]Department of Biochemistry, Cardiovascular Research Institute Maastricht, Maastricht, the Netherlands. [3]Clinical Diagnostic Laboratory, Maastricht University Medical Center, Maastricht, the Netherlands. [4]Department of Neurology, Maastricht University Medical Centre, Maastricht, the Netherlands.

References

1. Weimar C. Diagnosis and treatment of cerebral venous and sinus thrombosis. Curr Neurol Neurosci Rep. 2014;14(1):417.
2. Silvis SM, de Sousa DA, Ferro JM, Coutinho JM. Cerebral venous thrombosis. Nat Rev Neurol. 2017;13(9):555–65.
3. Gao L, Xu W, Li T, Yu X, Cao S, Xu H, et al. Accuracy of magnetic resonance venography in diagnosing cerebral venous sinus thrombosis. Thromb Res. 2018;167:64–73.
4. Ferro JM, Canhao P, Stam J, Bousser MG, Barinagarrementeria F, Investigators I. Prognosis of cerebral vein and dural sinus thrombosis: results of the international study on cerebral vein and Dural sinus thrombosis (ISCV T). Stroke. 2004;35(3):664–70.
5. Breteau G, Mounier-Vehier F, Godefroy O, Gauvrit JY, Mackowiak-Cordoliani MA, Girot M, et al. Cerebral venous thrombosis 3-year clinical outcome in 55 consecutive patients. J Neurol. 2003;250(1):29–35.
6. Gameiro J, Ferro JM, Canhao P, Stam J, Barinagarrementeria F, Lindgren A, et al. Prognosis of cerebral vein thrombosis presenting as isolated headache: early vs. late diagnosis. Cephalalgia. 2012;32(5):407–12.
7. Franchini M, Liumbruno GM, Pezzo M. COVID-19 vaccine-associated immune thrombosis and thrombocytopenia (VITT): Diagnostic and therapeutic recommendations for a new syndrome. Eur J Haematol. n/a(n/a).
8. Dentali F, Crowther M, Ageno W. Thrombophilic abnormalities, oral contraceptives, and risk of cerebral vein thrombosis: a meta-analysis. Blood. 2006;107(7):2766–73.
9. Luo Y, Tian X, Wang X. Diagnosis and treatment of cerebral venous sinus thrombosis: a review. Front Aging Neurosci. 2018;10:2.
10. Coutinho JM, Stam J. How to treat cerebral venous and sinus thrombosis. J Thromb Haemost. 2010;8(5):877–83.
11. Palazzo P, Agius P, Ingrand P, Ciron J, Lamy M, Berthomet A, et al. Venous thrombotic recurrence after cerebral venous thrombosis: a long-term follow-up study. Stroke. 2017;48(2):321–6.
12. Dielis AWJHCE, Spronk HMH, van Oerle R, Hamulya'k K, Cate t, Rosing J. Coagulation factors and the protein C system as determinants of thrombin generation in a normal population. Thromb Haemost. 2008;6(1):125–31.
13. Duarte RCF, Ferreira CN, Rios DRA, Reis HJD, Carvalho MDG. Thrombin generation assays for global evaluation of the hemostatic system: perspectives and limitations. Rev Bras Hematol Hemoter. 2017;39(3):259–65.
14. Hemker HC, Giesen P. AR, Regnault V, de Smed E, Lecompte T, Béguin S. the calibrated automated Thrombogram (CAT) a universal routine test for hyper- and hypocoagulability. Pathophysiol Haemost Thromb. 2002;32(5–6):249–53.
15. Bloemen S, Zwaveling S, Ten Cate H, Ten Cate-Hoek A, de Laat B. Prediction of bleeding risk in patients taking vitamin K antagonists using thrombin generation testing. PLoS One. 2017;12(5):e0176967.
16. Hemker HC, Al Dieri R, Beguin S. Thrombin generation assays: accruing clinical relevance. Curr Opin Hematol. 2004;11(3):170–5.
17. Ten Cate H. Thrombin generation in clinical conditions. Thromb Res. 2012;129(3):367–70.
18. Loeffen R, Kleinegris MC, Loubele ST, Pluijmen PH, Fens D, van Oerle R, et al. Preanalytic variables of thrombin generation: towards a standard procedure and validation of the method. J Thromb Haemost. 2012;10(12):2544–54.
19. Spronk HM, Dielis AW, De Smedt E, van Oerle R, Fens D, Prins MH, et al. Assessment of thrombin generation II: validation of the calibrated automated Thrombogram in platelet-poor plasma in a clinical laboratory. Thromb Haemost. 2008;100(2):362–4.
20. Wexels F, Dahl OE, Pripp AH, Seljeflot I. Thrombin generation in patients with suspected venous thromboembolism. Clin Appl Thromb Hemost. 2017;23(5):416–21.
21. Kremers BMM, Birocchi S, van Oerle R, Zeerleder S, Spronk HMH, Mees BME, et al. Searching for a Common Thrombo-Inflammatory Basis in Patients With Deep Vein Thrombosis or Peripheral Artery Disease. Front Cardiovasc Med. 2019;6(33).
22. Butenas S, van't Veer C, Mann KG. "Normal" thrombin generation. Blood. 1999;94(7):2169–78.
23. Hemker HC, Beguin S. Thrombin generation in plasma: its assessment via the endogenous thrombin potential. Thromb Haemost. 1995;74(1):134–8.
24. ten Cate-Hoek AJ, Dielis AW, Spronk HM, van Oerle R, Hamulyak K, Prins MH, et al. Thrombin generation in patients after acute deep-vein thrombosis. Thromb Haemost. 2008;100(2):240–5.
25. Lutsey PL, Folsom AR, Heckbert SR, Cushman M. Peak thrombin generation and subsequent venous thromboembolism: the longitudinal investigation of thromboembolism etiology (LITE) study. Thromb Haemost. 2009;7(10):1639–48.
26. Machlus KR, Colby EA, Wu JR, Koch GG, Key NS, Wolberg AS. Effects of tissue factor, thrombomodulin and elevated clotting factor levels on thrombin generation in the calibrated automated thrombogram. Thromb Haemost. 2009;102(5):936–44.
27. Joly BS, Sudrie-Arnaud B, Barbay V, Borg JY, Le Cam Duchez V. Thrombin generation test as a marker for high risk venous thrombosis pregnancies. J Thromb Thrombolysis. 2018;45(1):114–21.
28. Park MS, Spears GM, Bailey KR, Xue A, Ferrara MJ, Headlee A, et al. Thrombin generation profiles as predictors of symptomatic venous thromboembolism after trauma: a prospective cohort study. J Trauma Acute Care Surg. 2017;83(3):381–7.
29. Riva N, Vella K, Hickey K, Bertu L, Zammit D, Spiteri S, et al. Biomarkers for the diagnosis of venous thromboembolism: D-dimer, thrombin generation, procoagulant phospholipid and soluble P-selectin. J Clin Pathol. 2018;71(11):1015–22.
30. Voils SA, Lemon SJ, Jordan J, Riley P, Frye R. Early thrombin formation capacity in trauma patients and association with venous thromboembolism. Thromb Res. 2016;147:13–5.
31. Lippi G, Danese E, Favaloro EJ, Montagnana M, Franchini M. Diagnostics in venous thromboembolism: from origin to future prospects. Semin Thromb Hemost. 2015;41(4):374–81.
32. Miranda B, Ferro JM, Canhao P, Stam J, Bousser MG, Barinagarrementeria F, et al. Venous thromboembolic events after cerebral vein thrombosis. Stroke. 2010;41(9):1901–6.

17

Implementation of an acute DVT ambulatory care pathway in a large urban centre: Current challenges and future opportunities

Sarah Kelliher[1]*[iD], Patricia Hall[2], Barry Kevane[1,3], Daniela Dinu[1,2], Karl Ewins[1], Peter MacMahon[4], Fionnuala Ní Áinle[1,3,5,6] and Tomás Breslin[2]

Abstract

Background: Ambulatory management of isolated acute deep venous thrombosis (DVT) is the recommended standard of care in selected populations. However, in practice a significant number of patients continue to be managed as in-patients.

Objectives: In this study we aimed to evaluate acute DVT treatment pathways in our emergency department (ED) in practice and to identify barriers to outpatient management.

Methods: This study was a cross-sectional analysis of prospectively collected data pertaining to consecutive patients presenting to the ED of a large, city center, academic teaching hospital over a 46 week period who were diagnosed with DVT.

Results: Implementation of an outpatient care pathway led to the majority of patients presenting with DVT in our institution being treated without hospital admission. Forty percent (31/78) of patients with DVT were treated with a direct oral anticoagulant (DOAC) as an outpatient in line with international best practice guidelines.

Conclusion: The study provides a clear picture of the clinical profile and management of patients in clinical practice. Due to the lack of resources and supported infrastructure it is difficult to effectively implement outpatient venous thromboembolism (VTE) management to its full potential. Directing resources towards strategies which facilitate outpatient DVT treatment among vulnerable patient groups could represent a means of reducing hospital admissions for DVT in urban centers. Our study highlights the success and clinical limitations of the outpatient treatment model, which should become standard as part of wider VTE care.

Keywords: Venous thromboembolism, Deep venous thrombosis, Anticoagulation, Direct oral anticoagulant, Ambulatory care pathway, Intravenous drug use

Introduction

Venous thromboembolism (VTE) comprises deep vein thrombosis (DVT) and pulmonary embolism (PE) and is a major contributor to global disease burden, affecting millions of individuals worldwide every year [1, 2]. The incidence of DVT in Europe has recently been reported as 70–149 cases/100000 person-years [3]. The majority of cases are diagnosed and initial treatment is commenced in the emergency department (ED) [4, 5]. It has been established that ambulatory management of isolated DVT, without inpatient admission, is safe and feasible in appropriately selected populations [6–9]. Currently published data suggests that ambulatory care with low molecular weight heparin (LMWH) is safe for selected patients with acute DVT [7]. In recent years, direct oral anticoagulants (DOACs) have been compared with warfarin in randomized phase 3 trials and are now suggested as first-line treatment for VTE over vitamin K antagonists for most

* Correspondence: sarah.kelliher@ucdconnect.ie
[1]Department of Haematology, Mater Misericordiae University Hospital, Eccles St, Dublin 7, Ireland
Full list of author information is available at the end of the article

patients [10]. Moreover, DOACs are associated with additional benefits in particular for patient management in the outpatient setting, including lack of requirement for monitoring of anticoagulant effect and a lower risk of major haemorrhage including intracranial haemorrhage [11, 12]. International guidelines from the European Society of Cardiology recommend the application of specific clinical criteria to identify patients with DVT suitable for outpatient or ambulatory management [13]. However despite this available evidence, in practice a significant number of patients (> 50%) continue to be managed as inpatients, including those potentially suitable for out of hospital management [4, 12, 14]. In this study we aimed to evaluate acute DVT treatment pathways in our ED, to examine the implementation of these guidelines in practice and to identify barriers to outpatient management.

Methods

This study was a cross-sectional analysis of prospectively collected data pertaining to consecutive patients presenting to the emergency department (ED) of a large, city centre, academic teaching hospital in Dublin City Centre (Mater Misericordiae University Hospital; MMUH) between October 2014 and September 2015 who were diagnosed with DVT. Patients presenting to the MMUH ED and diagnosed with DVT are managed according to a structured care pathway (under the governance of the multidisciplinary MMUH VTE Working Group). This pathway provides guidance for selection of patients suitable for outpatient DVT management. Clinical pre-test probability was assessed using the two level modified Wells Score. The Wells Score assigns points to clinical variables including active cancer treatment, paralysis, recent surgery, calf swelling and tenderness in order to predict likelihood of DVT [13]. In cases where DVT was unlikely (modified Wells score ≤ 1), D-dimer testing was carried out and a negative result out ruled DVT. In patients with 'likely' DVT (modified Wells score > 1) patients proceeded directly to imaging with compression ultrasonography (CUS). Patients with a confirmed diagnosis of DVT were managed as outpatients providing they did not meet the exclusion criteria listed in local guidelines: alcohol dependence, signs or symptoms suggestive of pulmonary embolus (PE) or confirmed PE, age < 18, patients already on anticoagulation at time of diagnosis, pregnancy, significant issues with compliance, cognition, mobility or communication, active or significant risk of bleeding, or comorbidities requiring medical or surgical admission (which at the time of the study included active malignancy, severe liver and renal impairment, bleeding disorder). Suitable patients preferring a long-term once daily option rather than twice daily therapy were prescribed rivaroxaban 15 mg twice daily for three weeks, followed by 20 mg once daily for three

months total duration unless an indication to continue therapy existed upon review, including patients with unprovoked DVT or a persisting provoking factor. All other patients were prescribed therapeutic dose LMWH. Tinzaparin 175 units/kilogram once daily was the LMWH of choice at our centre. Patients were reviewed by the VTE clinical nurse specialist on the same day where possible. Patients for whom a clear date of discontinuation after three months was not suitable were followed up in the MMUH thrombosis clinic.

In this study, data were prospectively recorded at the time of diagnosis via the ED in a local hospital database. Variables recorded were age, Wells pre-test probability score, D-dimer, compression ultrasound result, treatment prescribed, presence of provoking factors, computed tomography pulmonary angiogram (CTPA) result (if also requested based upon symptomatology), previous VTE history, co-medications, early bleeding complications (specifically evaluated at 3 weeks post-diagnosis) and whether outpatient management was feasible. Follow up for sonographic evidence of residual thrombosis was not documented as part of this study.

Patients treated as per the outpatient VTE pathway were contacted by telephone by the VTE clinical nurse specialist at three days and three weeks post DVT to assess for early bleeding complications. This group of patients were scheduled for follow up at the coagulation outpatient clinic with the consultant haematologist three months post DVT at which time they were specifically asked about bleeding. There was no standardised methodology for data collection regarding early bleeding complications for patients that were admitted to hospital for treatment. The study relied on patients self-reporting episodes of bleeding in this cohort during the three month follow up.

We used Microsoft Excel for data entry. We used descriptive statistics to analyse our data. The categorical variables were reported in counts and percentages for our groups of interest; inpatients, outpatients and the total group. For the continuous variables, we calculated the mean accompanied by the standard deviation (SD) and the median accompanied by the interquartile range (IQR) for each group.

Results

Fifty-one thousand five hundred forty-four patients presented to the MMUH ED during the study time period. Of these, 400 patients were investigated for DVT by the VTE clinical nurse specialist, and 78 (19%) had a confirmed diagnosis of DVT on ultrasound. Of the total number of those investigated, the diagnosis was ruled out with Wells Score and D-dimer in 63 (16%), while 259 (65%) had negative sonography.

Patient characteristics are outlined in Table 1. The majority of patients diagnosed with DVT were male (59%; 46/78). The mean age of the total cohort of patients was 47.7 years (SD 18.5). Most DVT events were associated with a provoking factor (63%; 49/78), in individuals without a previous history of VTE (64%; 50/78). Intravenous drug use was the provoking factor for 40% (31/78) of total patients and 63% (31/49) of provoked cases. Other provoking factors included immobilisation (20%; 10/49), oral contraceptive pill (6%; 3/49), post-partum (6%; 3/49) and cancer/active inflammation (4%; 2/49).

In 54% (42/78) of cases, there was documentation of the clinical pre-test probability using the two level modified Wells score. In cases with documentation of Wells Score 19% (8/42) and 81% (34/42) had an unlikely probability and a likely probability of DVT respectively. Wells score was not documented in 46% of patients at

presentation (36/78). For 58% (21/36) of these patients this was an appropriate omission of the score as individuals were post-partum or persons who inject drugs (PWID). 58% (45/78) of patients had a D-dimer level measured in the ED. In 51% (17/33) of patients without recorded D-dimer, the test was not indicated due to intravenous drug use. A D-dimer was ordered erroneously in three patients who presented post-partum.

Two (3%; 2/78) patients presented with upper limb DVT with the remainder of DVTs presenting at the level of the external iliac vein and below. 19% (15/78) of patients with DVTs had a coexisting PE at the time of presentation.

Sixty-eight percent (53/78) of patients were managed as outpatients while 32% (25/78) were admitted for treatment. 58% (31/53) of those treated as outpatients were treated with rivaroxaban while the remaining 42%

Table 1 Characteristics of Patients Presenting to the Emergency Department with DVT between 16/10/2014 and 02/09/2015

Patient Characteristics	Inpatient (n = 25)	Outpatient (n = 53)	Total (total n = 78)
Age			
Mean (SD)	48.1 (21.2)	47.8 (17.6)	47.7 (18.5)
Median (IQR)	40 (34.5)	43 (32)	41 (32.3)
Gender			
Male	13 (52%)	33 (62%)	46 (59%)
Female	12 (48%)	20 (38%)	32 (41%)
Wells Score:			
Unlikely	2 (8%)	6 (11%)	8 (10%)
Likely	10 (40%)	24 (45%)	34 (44%)
Not assessed	13 (52%)	23 (44%)	36 (46%)
D-dimer:			
Raised	12 (48%)	31 (58%)	43 (55%)
Normal Range	0 (0%)	2 (4%)	2 (3%)
Not measured	13 (52%)	20 (38%)	33 (42%)
History of VTE	9 (36%)	19 (36%)	28 (36%)
Provoking factor	17 (68%)	32 (60%)	49 (63%)
Associated PE	12 (48%)	3 (5%)	15 (19%)
Location:			
Upper limb	1 (4%)	1 (2%)	2 (3%)
Lower limb	24 (96%)	52 (98%)	76 (97%)
Treatment:			
Rivaroxaban	4 (16%)	31 (58%)	35 (45%)
LMWH	18 (72%)	22 (42%)	40 (51%)
Not recorded	3 (12%)	0 (0%)	3 (4%)
Medical Comorbidities	5 (25%)	17 (32%)	23 (55%)
IVDU	10 (40%)	21 (42%)	31 (39%)
Bleeding Complications	1 (4%)	5 (9%)	6 (8%)
Not recorded	23 (92%)	29 (54%)	52 (66%)
Post Partum	1 (4%)	2 (4%)	3 (4%)

(22/53) were treated with LMWH. 77% (17/22) of patients commenced on LMWH in the community in preference to rivaroxaban had a history of intravenous drug use. This treatment regimen is in accordance with the MMUH guidelines for outpatient DVT management. 70% (21/30) of PWID were managed with ambulatory care in the community. Of the total number of patients that were admitted to hospital 40% (10/25) were PWID. The documented reason for admission were as follows; 48% (12/25) had co existing pulmonary embolus, 12% (3/25) were admitted for thrombectomy, 16% (4/25) had psychosocial issues and 20% (5/25) had medical comorbidities requiring admission.

Bleeding complications were recorded in 9% (5/53) of those treated as outpatients versus 4% (1/25) of patients initially treated as inpatients. Reported bleeding complications included positive faecal occult blood, haemoptysis, haematuria, menorrhagia and bleeding from a groin abscess. There were a total of six cases of clinically relevant non major bleeding with no episodes of major bleeding recorded in either group assessed according to the International Society of Thrombosis and Haemostasis definitions [15]. In accordance with the outpatient DVT protocol, patients enrolled in the outpatient pathway and commenced on rivaroxaban received a follow up phone call at three days and three weeks from the VTE clinical nurse specialist (CNS) to assess bleeding complications. 47% (37/78) of patients in our study were followed up in this way. There were insufficient resources to formally follow up every patient included in the study with CNS led phone calls. Patients admitted to hospital for initial therapy were followed up by the admitting medical team, the outcomes of which were outside the scope of our data collection in certain cases. Patients anticoagulated with LMWH had contact with healthcare professionals in the majority of cases therefore follow up phone calls were not prioritised for this group for pragmatic reasons.

Discussion

Implementation of an outpatient care pathway led to the majority of patients presenting with DVT in our institution being treated without hospital admission. Sixty-eight percent of all patients were treated as outpatients during the study period. Forty percent of patients with DVT were treated with a DOAC as an outpatient in line with international best practice guidelines. A further 28% were treated in the community with LMWH, 77% of those were PWID. There is a high prevalence of intravenous drug use among patients within the catchment of our inner city, urban centre. LMWH is currently recommended for pragmatic reasons for these patients, as most Dublin drug treatment centres are familiar with and most comfortable with direct administration of

LMWH for these clients. With the development of pathways and infrastructure in inclusion health in Dublin city centre, this may change in the future. Inpatients were treated with LMWH (72%) or a DOAC (16%), with the remaining three cases undocumented. The most prominent barrier to ambulatory management in our cohort appears to be DVT with associated PE. Consequently, development of safe pathways for outpatient management of PE has been prioritised by the hospital VTE Committee. The implementation of validated risk assessment tools in the ED may identify low risk patients with PE suitable for outpatient management. The introduction of eligibility criteria and coordination with the outpatient department to ensure appropriate interval follow up for this cohort, could facilitate safe outpatient management of specific patients presenting with PE [16]. Almost 20% of patients presented with DVT and associated PE. This is similar to figures cited in international literature [11]. While the prevalence of intravenous drug use was stable between the inpatient and outpatient group (40% versus 42%) concomitant medical and psychosocial issues were documented in the group for admission. Development of inclusion health pathways in collaboration with medical social workers dedicated to the care and management of patients with social challenges including homelessness and drug and alcohol addictions has been prioritized as a key outcome of this study. In order to meet this objective, the Hospital VTE Committee will also work closely with colleagues in primary care who provide dedicated support to these vulnerable patients and with colleagues in other Dublin City Centre Hospitals, as patients with inclusion health needs frequently attend several hospitals due to their circumstances [17, 18].

In 34% of cases presenting to the ED where Wells Score was indicated (excluding PWID and post-partum cases), record of the score was inappropriately omitted from the patient documents. This is a crucial step in the evaluation of clinically suspected DVT and guides further investigation. This revealed non-compliance with the recommended structured care pathway for DVT in the ED and is not in line with best practice as outlined by international guidelines [13]. Patients with complete DVT work up including documentation of Wells Score were more likely to be treated as an outpatient. While D-dimer was measured in 58% of cases, deviation from clinical practice guidelines occurred in only one case when the test was inappropriately requested with a documented high clinical probability of DVT as established by the Wells Score [13]. The presence of a provoking factor and unusual site of DVT, such as upper limb thrombi, were both factors associated with admission to hospital.

The data in this study was collected consecutively and prospectively. All radiologically proven cases of DVT were recorded in the data set by the research team. This approach aimed to minimise bias due to low response and to prevent misclassification due to recall bias as can be seen in cross-sectional studies. The main limitation of the study was its observational design. Physicians in the ED were unaware that the data collection was taking place and therefore did not clearly document the clinical criteria supporting admission. Patients with suspected DVT were seen directly by the VTE CNS during office hours under the supervision of the Emergency Medicine (EM) consultant staff, but outside of these hours patients were assessed by junior and senior EM doctors, which likely accounts for variance in assessment and documentation. Contraindications to outpatient management were inferred from studying the patient's clinical data in the context of the structured care pathway. This study reports the prevalence of DVT presenting to the ED and describes the subsequent management pathway, however it is not possible to fully elucidate the patient factors impacting clinical decision making and treatment choice. Cause and effect relationships and associations are be difficult to interpret. There were missing data in our study. Incomplete data entry was noted most particularly when recording early bleeding complications. Accurate records of follow up complications are not available to us for all cases. This study did not set out to primarily assess bleeding complications. We are limited in our ability to comment on bleeding complications between the two treatment pathways and between the different anticoagulant agents due to the lack of standardisation in our methods for assessing bleeding complications between the two groups. However, despite limitations, the study provides a clear picture of the clinical profile and management of patients in clinical practice.

Conclusion

The results of this study are relevant throughout the world today. Clinical trials have long since established that outpatient DVT management is a safe and effective treatment. There is now an emerging evidence base for the outpatient treatment of pulmonary embolism [19]. However despite the progress in the field of research, it is clear from this data that there is scope for further development of the outpatient DVT pathway in clinical practice. The findings of this study are consistent when compared with international data [4, 12, 14]. Directing resources towards strategies which facilitate outpatient DVT treatment among vulnerable patient groups could represent a means of reducing hospital admissions for DVT in urban centres and, ultimately, lead to health care savings. The majority of hospitals in Ireland do not have a permanent VTE CNS in the ED. Due to the lack of resources and supported infrastructure it is difficult to effectively implement outpatient VTE management to its full potential. Our study

highlights the success of this model, which should become standard as part of wider VTE care in Ireland.

Abbreviations
CNS: Clinical nurse specialist; CTPA: Computed tomography pulmonary angiogram; DOAC: Direct oral anticoagulant; DVT: Deep venous thrombosis; ED: Emergency Department; LMWH: Low molecular weight heparin; MMUH: Mater Misericordiae University Hospital; PE: Pulmonary embolism; PWID: Person who injects drugs; SD: Standard deviation; VTE: Venous thromboembolism

Acknowledgements
Not applicable

Authors' contributions
SK interpreted the data and wrote the manuscript. PH, DD and KE collected the data. BK collected data and contributed to writing the manuscript. PMacM interpreted the radiology. TB and FNíÁ implemented the pathway and contributed to writing the manuscript. All authors read and approved the final manuscript.

Author details
[1]Department of Haematology, Mater Misericordiae University Hospital, Eccles St, Dublin 7, Ireland. [2]Department of Emergency Medicine, Mater Misericordiae University Hospital, Eccles St, Dublin 7, Ireland. [3]Department of Haematology, Rotunda Hospital, Dublin 1, Ireland. [4]Department of Radiology, Mater Misericordiae University Hospital, Eccles St, Dublin 7, Ireland. [5]School of Medicine, University College Dublin (UCD), Dublin 4, Ireland. [6]UCD Conway Institute SPHERE Research Group, UCD, Dublin 4, Ireland.

References
1. Thrombosis: a major contributor to the global disease burden. Isth Steering Committee for World Thrombosis Day. J Thromb Haemost. 2014;12(10):1580–90.
2. Schulman S, Ageno W, Konstantinides SV. Venous thromboembolism: past, Present and Future. Thromb Haemost. 2017;117(7):1219–29.
3. Raskob GE, Angchaisuksiri P, Blanco AN, Buller H, Gallus A, Hunt BJ, Hylek EM, Kakkar A, Konstantinides SV, McCumber M, Ozaki Y, Wendelboe A, Weitz JI. Day ISCfWT. Thrombosis: a major contributor to global disease burden. Arterioscler Thromb Vasc Biol. 2014;34:2363–71.
4. Jimenez S, Ruiz-Artacho P, Merlo M, Suero C, Antolin A, Sanchex M, Ortega-Duarte A, Genis M, Pinera P. Risk profile, management, and outcomes of patients with venos thromboembolism attended in Spanish emergency departments; the ESPHERIA registry. Medicine. 2017;96(48):8796.
5. Vinson D, Berman D. Outpatient treatement of deepvenous thrombosis: a clinical care pathway managed by the emergency department. Ann Emerg Med. 2001;37(3):251–8.
6. Othieno R, Okpo E, Forster R. Home versus in-patient treatment for deepvenous thrmobosis. Cochrane Database Syst Rev. 2018;9:1.

7. Harrison L, et al. Assessment of outpatient treatment of deep-vein thrombosis with low molecular weight heparin. Arch Intern Med. 1998; 158(18):2001–3.

8. Dunn AS, Schechter C, Gotlin A, Vomvolakis D, Jacobs E, Sacks HS, Coller B. Outpatient treatment of deep venous thrombosis in diverse inner-city patients. Am J Med. 2001;110(6):458–62.

9. Condliffe R. Pathways for outpatient management of venous thromboembolism in a UK centre. Thromb J. 2016;14:47.

10. Kearon C, et al. Antithrombotic Therapy for VTE Disease: CHEST Guideline and Expert Panel Report. Chest. 2016;149(2):315–52.

11. Bauersachs R, Berkowitz SD, Brenner B. Oral rivaroxaban for symptomatic venous thromboembolism. N Engl J Med. 2010;363(26):2499–510.

12. Imberti D, Barillari G. Real life Management of Venous Thromboembolsim with rivaroxaban: results from experience VTE, an Italian epidemiological survey. Clinical and Applied Thrombosis/Haemostasis. 2017;24(2):241–7.

13. Mazzolai L, et al. Diagnosis and management of acute deep vein thrombosis: a joint consensus document from the European society of cardiology working groups of aorta and peripheral circulation and pulmonary circulation and right ventricular function. Eur Heart J. 2018; 39(47):4208–18.

14. Douce D, et al. Outpatient Tretament of DeepVein thrombosis in the United States: the reasons for Geogrphical and racial differences in stroke study. J Hosp Med. 2017;12(10):826–30.

15. Kaatz S, Ahmad D, Spyropoulos AC, Schulman S. Subcommittee on control of anticoagulation.. Definition of clinically relevant non-major bleeding in studies of anticoagulants in atrial fibrillation and venous thromboembolic disease in non-surgical patients: communication from the SSC of the ISTH. J Thromb Haemost. 2015 Nov;13(11):2119–26.

16. Roy P, Moumneh T, Penaloza A, Sanchez O. Outpatient management of pulmonary embolism. Thromb Res. 2017 Jul;155:92–100.

17. Our Health Service - Inclusion Health Service At St James's Hospital. Health Servicec Executive. URL: https://www.hse.ie/eng/about/our-health-service/making-it-better/inclusion-health-service-at-st-james-hospital.html . Accessed at: 5 May 2018.

18. Safety net primary care. URL: https://www.primarycaresafetynet.ie/ . Acccessed 5 May 2018.

19. Bledsoe JR, Woller SC, Stevens SM, Aston V, Patten R, Allen T, Horne BD, Dong L, Lloyd J, Snow G, Madsen T, Elliott CG. Management of low-Risk Pulmonary Embolism Patients without Hospitalization: the low-risk pulmonary embolism prospective management study. Chest. 2018; (18)30231–9.

Prevalence, risk and outcome of deep vein thrombosis in acute respiratory distress syndrome

Na Cui[1,2], Chunguo Jiang[1,2], Hairong Chen[3], Liming Zhang[1,2]* and Xiaokai Feng[1,2]* ⓘ

Abstract

Background: Few data exist on deep vein thrombosis (DVT) in patients with acute respiratory distress syndrome (ARDS), a group of heterogeneous diseases characterized by acute hypoxemia.

Study design and methods: We retrospectively enrolled 225 adults with ARDS admitted to the Beijing Chao-Yang Hospital and the First Affiliated Hospital of Shandong First Medical University between 1 January 2015 and 30 June 2020. We analyzed clinical, laboratory, and echocardiography data for groups with and without DVT and for direct (pulmonary) and indirect (extrapulmonary) ARDS subgroups.

Results: Ninety (40.0%) patients developed DVT. Compared with the non-DVT group, patients with DVT were older, had lower serum creatinine levels, lower partial pressure of arterial oxygen/fraction of inspired oxygen, higher serum procalcitonin levels, higher Padua prediction scores, and higher proportions of sedation and invasive mechanical ventilation (IMV). Multivariate analysis showed an association between age, serum creatinine level, IMV, and DVT in the ARDS cohort. The sensitivity and specificity of corresponding receiver operating characteristic curves were not inferior to those of the Padua prediction score and the Caprini score for screening for DVT in the three ARDS cohorts. Patients with DVT had a significantly lower survival rate than those without DVT in the overall ARDS cohort and in the groups with direct and indirect ARDS.

Conclusions: The prevalence of DVT is high in patients with ARDS. The risk factors for DVT are age, serum creatinine level, and IMV. DVT is associated with decreased survival in patients with ARDS.

Keywords: Acute respiratory distress syndrome, Caprini score, Deep vein thrombosis, Invasive mechanical ventilation, Padua prediction score

Introduction

Deep vein thrombosis (DVT) and pulmonary embolism (PE), collectively referred to as venous thromboembolism (VTE), constitute a major global burden of disease [1]. Some studies demonstrated an increased risk of VTE in patients in the intensive care unit (ICU) [2–4]. Patients with acute respiratory distress syndrome (ARDS)

are at high risk for DVT because they are susceptible both to general risk factors for VTE and to those specific to the critically ill, such as advanced age, sedation, immobilization, insertion of a central venous catheter, and mechanical ventilation (MV), combined with a severe inflammatory response and hypercoagulable states [2–6]. ARDS remains under-recognized clinically; however, therapies are limited, complications are frequent, and mortality remains significantly high [7–11]. Patients with ARDS are a heterogeneous group with significant variability in clinical presentation and outcomes. One

* Correspondence: zhangliming@bjcyh.com; fengxiaokai2020@163.com
[1]Department of Pulmonary and Critical Care Medicine, Beijing Chao-Yang Hospital, Capital Medical University, No. 8, Gongti South Road, Chaoyang District, Beijing 100020, People's Republic of China
Full list of author information is available at the end of the article

approach to reducing these heterogeneities is to subclassify patients with ARDS as having direct (pulmonary) or indirect (extrapulmonary) ARDS based on variabilities in the pathological, radiological, and respiratory mechanical responses to different management strategies [12–19].

The incidence of DVT in patients with direct and indirect ARDS has not been investigated.

We performed a multi-institutional study to identify the prevalence, risk factors, and prognosis of DVT and to determine whether the predictors of DVT differed between direct and indirect ARDS in a cohort of patients identified with ARDS.

Methods
Study design and population
We retrospectively enrolled adult patients (≥ 18 years old) with ARDS (according to the Berlin definition) [8] who were admitted to the Department of Pulmonary and Critical Care Medicine, Beijing Chao-Yang Hospital and the Intensive Care Unit, the First Affiliated Hospital of Shandong First Medical University, from 1 January 2015 to 30 June 2020. All patients were included consecutively. Patients with ARDS were classified as having direct ARDS or indirect ARDS based on the underlying risk factors for ARDS recorded by study personnel. Patients with pneumonia and aspiration as risk factors and those with pulmonary sepsis were assigned to the direct ARDS group, whereas those with pancreatitis or non-pulmonary sepsis were assigned to the indirect ARDS group. Patients who could not be classified as uniquely direct or indirect ARDS and patients with both pneumonia and non-pulmonary sepsis were excluded. Other

exclusion criteria include: active malignant tumor, cerebral stroke, acute myocardial infarction, serious trauma, major operation lasting longer than 45 min, fracture of lower limb, joint replacement for hip or knee, and lack of lower extremity venous compression ultrasound data. The first ultrasound examination was performed within 1–3 days after the diagnosis of ARDS, and then the ultrasound scan was reexamined again according to the patient's condition. After intensive treatment, if the patient remained unstable because of conditions such as unexplained hypoxemia or cardiac insufficiency, he or she should be reexamined by ultrasound. If there was more than one ultrasound scan for a single patient, all the results were recorded. Patients were divided into a DVT and a non-DVT group according to the results of the venous ultrasound scans. The flow chart is shown in Fig. 1 (A, B).

The study was approved by the ethics committees of the Beijing Chao-Yang Hospital (2020-ke-429) and the First Affiliated Hospital of Shandong First Medical University (S003) and was conducted in accordance with the 1964 Helsinki Declaration and its later amendments or comparable ethical standards.

Clinical data
We analyzed the medical records of the enrolled patients. Data, which included demographic information, clinical history, vital signs, laboratory findings, treatments, complications, and outcomes of the patients during hospitalization, were collected and analyzed. We analyzed the survival rates of all patients within 28 days after a diagnosis of ARDS. For the patients discharged

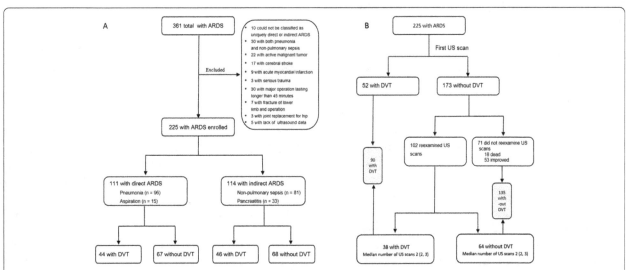

Fig. 1 A, B, Study flow chart. **A,** flow chart for including patients; **B,** flow chart for screening for DVT. The interval from the diagnosis of ARDS to the occurrence of DVT in the DVT group was 5 (2, 9) days, and the interval from the diagnosis of ARDS to the last ultrasound examination in the non-DVT group was 5 (2, 11) days. There were no differences between the two groups (P = 0.784). Abbreviations: ARDS, acute respiratory distress syndrome; DVT, deep vein thrombosis; US, ultrasound

within 28 days, we followed up by telephone concerning their survival status after discharge.

Ultrasound assessment

Bedside ultrasound examinations were performed using a portable color ultrasound scanner (CX50, Philips Medical Systems, the Netherlands, equipped with an L12–3/ S5–1 probe). The lower extremity venous compression ultrasound and echocardiographic data were obtained from the institution's Picture Archiving and Communication System. The levels of DVT included the bilateral common femoral, deep and superficial femoral veins, the popliteal veins, and the anterior tibial, posterior tibial, peroneal, and calf muscle veins. Left ventricular and right ventricular function parameters were captured. The presence of pulmonary artery hypertension was evaluated by adding a tricuspid regurgitation pressure gradient to the estimated right atrial pressure [20].

Definitions

ARDS was defined according to the Berlin definition [8]. Sepsis was defined according to the Third International Consensus Definitions for Sepsis and Septic Shock [21]. A distal thrombosis was defined as a thrombosis in the veins of the calf muscle or in at least 1 branch of the 3 pairs of deep calf veins (anterior tibial vein, posterior tibial vein, or peroneal vein); a proximal thrombosis was defined as a thrombosis in the popliteal vein or above. The Caprini score was defined according to the updated Caprini Risk Assessment Model (2013 Version) [22]. The Padua prediction score was defined according to the Barbar model [23]. We applied the Acute Physiology and Chronic Health Evaluation (APACHE) II score and the Sequential Organ Failure Assessment (SOFA) score to assess the severity of disease [21, 24, 25].

Statistical analyses

Categorical variables were described as number and percentage (%) and continuous variables, as mean, standard deviation, median, and interquartile range. The Shapiro-Wilk test was used to verify normality. Differences between the DVT and the non-DVT groups were assessed by a two-sample t-test for normally distributed continuous variables, the Mann-Whitney U test for non-normally distributed continuous variables, and the χ^2 or Fisher exact test for categorical variables. To determine risk factors for DVT, multivariable logistic regression analysis which was based on the factors with significant differences between DVT and non-DVT groups in univariate analysis and the factors that may be related to dependent variables from the perspective of professional knowledge was performed on the direct and the indirect ARDS subgroups. The adjusted odds ratio (OR) with 95% confidence intervals (CI) was reported. To further

evaluate the observed differences in risk factors for DVT between direct and indirect ARDS, we utilized interaction terms between ARDS type and each risk factor. A receiver operating characteristic (ROC) analysis was performed to calculate the sensitivity and specificity of risk factors for screening for DVT. The comparison methods of diagnostic accuracy for screening for DVT of different ROCs in three ARDS cohorts are as follows: Patients were split by generating random numbers to produce a training data set (n*0.7) and a validation data set (n*0.3) in the overall, direct, and indirect groups respectively. The area under receiver operating characteristic curves (ROC-AUCs) for different risk factors were compared using the method of DeLong et al. [26]. Survival curves were plotted using the Kaplan-Meier method and compared between patients with or without DVT using the log-rank test. To further explore the incidence rate of DVT in patients with ARDS in ICU, we selected non-ARDS patients in ICU consecutively during the same period as controls. And then, we took death as the competitive risk and plotted 28-day cumulative incidence curves (and points estimates with 95% CI) for ARDS and non-ARDS patients. Fine-Gray test was used to compare the incidence rate of DVT between the two groups. All statistical analyses were performed using the Statistical Analysis System, version 9.4 (SAS Institute, Cary, NC, USA). All tests were two-tailed; $P < 0.05$ was considered statistically significant.

Results

A total of 225 patients with ARDS were enrolled in this study; 111 patients were considered to belong in the direct ARDS group and 114 patients in the indirect ARDS group. The flow chart is shown in Fig. 1 (A, B).

Ultrasound scan for screening for DVT

Lower extremity venous ultrasound scanning was performed whenever feasible for 225 patients regardless of clinical symptoms of the lower limbs (Fig. 1B), and the median number of ultrasound examinations was 1 (range, 1–5). Fifty-two (52/225) developed DVT was found and the other 173 was a negative result at the first ultrasound scan. Subsequently, 102 patients underwent more than one ultrasound scan, for whom 38 developed DVT and 64 had no DVT with 2 (range, 2–5) ultrasound examinations. The interval from the diagnosis of ARDS to the occurrence of DVT in the 38 developed DVT group was 7 (4, 14) days, and the interval from the diagnosis of ARDS to the last ultrasound examination in the 64 non-DVT group was 10 (4, 16) days. There was no difference between the two groups ($P = 0.542$). Finally, of the 225 patients, 90 (40.0%) developed DVT, including 7 with proximal DVT and 83 with distal DVT, 73 of whom had muscular calf vein thrombosis only. The incidence of asymptomatic DVT was 75 (33.3%) including 2 (0.9%) proximal DVT and 73 (32.4%) distal DVT, of whom muscular calf vein thrombosis accounted for 70 (31.1%). For all the 225 patients, the interval from the diagnosis of ARDS to the occurrence of DVT in DVT group was 5 (2, 9) days, and the interval from the diagnosis of ARDS to the last ultrasound examination in non-DVT group was 5 (2, 11) days. There was no difference between the two groups ($P = 0.784$). Five patients were clinically suspected of having PE; three were further confirmed by computed tomography pulmonary angiography (CTPA) examination. There was no difference in the prevalence of DVT in patients with direct and indirect ARDS (39.6% [44/111] vs 40.4% [46/114], respectively; $P = 0.913$; Table 1).

Demographic and clinical characteristics of patients with direct and indirect ARDS
Compared with the direct ARDS group (Table 1), patients with indirect ARDS had higher APACHE II scores ($P = 0.010$), higher SOFA scores ($P < 0.001$), higher white blood cell counts ($P < 0.001$), higher neutrophil counts ($P < 0.001$), higher levels of procalcitonin ($P = 0.008$), higher levels of serum creatinine ($P = 0.019$), and higher levels of D-dimer ($P < 0.001$). There were more men in the direct ARDS group ($P < 0.001$). Patients with direct ARDS had lower PaO_2/FiO_2 than those with indirect ARDS ($P < 0.001$).

Demographic and clinical characteristics of DVT vs non-DVT patients in overall ARDS cohort
Compared with the non-DVT group (Table 2), patients with DVT were older ($P < 0.001$) and had lower levels of serum creatinine ($P = 0.007$), lower levels of partial pressure of arterial oxygen/fraction of inspired oxygen (PaO_2/FiO_2; $P = 0.002$), higher levels of serum procalcitonin (PCT; $P < 0.001$), higher Padua prediction scores ($P = 0.023$), and a higher proportion of patients given sedative therapy ($P = 0.001$) and invasive mechanical

Table 1 Demographic and Clinical Characteristics of Patients with Direct and Indirect ARDS

Characteristic	Total (N = 225)	Direct ARDS (N = 111)	Indirect ARDS (N = 114)	P value
Age (years)	66 ± 17	64 ± 15	67 ± 18	0.192
Male, n (%)	144 (64.0)	84 (75.7)	60 (52.6)	< 0.001
BMI	24.1 (21.6, 26.8)	24.0 (21.0, 26.2)	24.4 (21.9, 27.0)	0.274
Bedridden time (days)	8 (4, 15)	9 (5, 15)	8 (4, 16)	0.400
APACHE II score	23 (19, 28)	22 (17, 27)	25 (19, 31)	0.010
SOFA score	8 (5, 10)	6 (4, 6)	9 (6, 11)	< 0.001
Laboratory data				
White blood cells (×10⁹/L)	16.9 (12.0, 21.5)	14.3 (10.1, 20.3)	18.2 (14.4, 23.5)	< 0.001
Neutrophils (×10⁹/L)	14.5 (10.4, 19.7)	12.8 (9.0, 17.7)	16.1 (12.6, 20.8)	< 0.001
Platelets (×10⁹/L)	183.0 (101.0, 253.5)	190.0 (120.0, 270.0)	167.0 (73.8, 238.0)	0.094
C-reactive protein (mg/L)	120.0 (89.4, 120.0)	120.0 (85.0, 120.0)	120.0 (92.2, 120.0)	0.391
Procalcitonin (ng/mL)	5.6 (2.0, 16.2)	4.1 (1.5, 13.5)	7.3 (3.0, 21.2)	0.008
Serum creatinine (μmol/L)	116.7 (66.6, 209.5)	90.5 (65.0, 193.0)	136.9 (67.9, 248.8)	0.019
D-dimer (μg/ml)	1.9 (0.9, 3.8)	1.3 (0.6, 2.5)	2.4 (1.3, 5.3)	< 0.001
PaO_2/FiO_2	158 (103, 199)	136 (80, 186)	170 (130, 208)	< 0.001*
Mild, n (%)	54 (24.0)	22 (19.8)	32 (28.1)	< 0.001#
Moderate, n (%)	116 (51.6)	49 (44.1)	67 (58.8)	
Severe, n (%)	55 (24.4)	40 (36.0)	15 (13.2)	
DVT, n (%)	90 (40.0%)	44 (39.6)	46 (40.4)	0.913
ICU length of stay (days)	11 (6, 24)	13 (7, 25)	10 (5, 24)	0.103
Hospital length of stay (days)	19 (12, 32)	17 (10, 29)	22 (13, 34)	0.055
Mortality, n (%)	77 (34.2)	36 (32.4)	41 (36.0)	0.577

Data are mean ± SD, median (IQR) or n (%). P values comparing Direct and Indirect ARDS groups were from a two-sample t-test, Mann- Whitney U test, or χ² test. P < 0.05 was considered statistically significant
*χ² test comparing Direct and Indirect ARDS groups
#χ² test comparing all subcategories
Abbreviations: APACHE Acute Physiology and Chronic Health Evaluation, ARDS acute respiratory distress syndrome, BMI body mass index, DVT deep venous thrombosis, FiO₂, fraction of inspired oxygen, ICU intensive care unit, IQR interquartile range, mild 200 mmHg<PaO₂/FiO₂ ≤ 300 mmHg, moderate 100 mmHg<PaO₂/FiO₂ ≤ 200 mmHg, PaO₂ partial pressure of arterial oxygen, SD standard deviation, severe PaO₂/FiO₂ ≤ 100 mmHg, SOFA Sequential Organ Failure Assessment

Table 2 Demographic and Clinical Characteristics of DVT Vs Non-DVT Patients in Overall ARDS Cohort

Characteristic	Total (N = 225)	DVT (N = 90)	Non-DVT (N = 135)	P value
Age (years)	66 ± 17	70 ± 13	63 ± 18	< 0.001
Male, n (%)	144 (64.0)	52 (57.8)	92 (68.1)	0.112
BMI	24.1 (21.6, 26.8)	24.0 (20.8, 26.0)	24.2 (22.0, 27.2)	0.146
Direct ARDS				
Pneumonia	96 (86.5)	40 (90.9)	56 (83.6)	0.412
Aspiration	15 (13.5)	4 (9.1)	11 (16.4)	
Indirect ARDS				
Non-pulmonary sepsis	81 (71.1)	33 (71.7)	48 (70.6)	0.894
Pancreatitis	33 (28.9)	13 (28.3)	20 (29.4)	
Bedridden time (days)	8 (4, 15)	10 (5, 18)	7 (4, 15)	0.216
Caprini score	7 (5, 9)	7 (5, 10)	7 (5, 9)	0.135
Padua prediction score	6 (5, 6)	6 (5, 8)	5 (5, 6)	0.023
APACHE II score	23 (19, 28)	24 (20, 28)	23 (18, 29)	0.596
SOFA score	8 (5, 10)	7 (5, 9)	8 (5, 11)	0.622
Laboratory data				
White blood cells ($\times 10^9$/L)	16.9 (12.0, 21.4)	16.5 (13.4, 21.0)	17.1 (11.6, 22.6)	0.733
Neutrophils ($\times 10^9$/L)	14.5 (10.4, 19.7)	14.7 (11.4, 19.3)	14.4 (9.9, 20.1)	0.709
Platelets ($\times 10^9$/L)	183.0 (101.0, 253.5)	196.5 (124.3, 263.3)	172.0 (84.0, 253.0)	0.141
C-reactive protein (mg/L)	120.0 (89.4, 120.0)	120.0 (82.0, 120.0)	120.0 (92.5, 120.0)	0.471
Procalcitonin (ng/mL)	5.6 (2.0, 16.2)	12.7 (3.4, 21.5)	3.5 (1.5, 10.3)	< 0.001
Serum creatinine (μmol/L)	116.7 (66.6, 209.5)	95.1 (58.8, 165.5)	125.6 (70.6, 250.3)	0.007
D-dimer (μg/ml)	1.9 (0.9, 3.8)	2.1 (0.9, 5.0)	1.8 (0.9, 3.3)	0.070
PaO$_2$/FiO$_2$	158 (103, 199)	137 (87, 179)	172 (116, 209)	0.002[*]
Mild, n (%)	54 (24.0)	14 (15.6)	40 (29.6)	0.026[#]
Moderate, n (%)	116 (51.6)	48 (53.3)	68 (50.4)	
Severe, n (%)	55 (24.4)	28 (31.1)	27 (20.0)	
Treatments				
Glucocorticoid therapy, n (%)	51 (22.7)	22 (24.4)	29 (21.5)	0.603
Immunoglobulin, n (%)	5 (2.2)	2 (2.2)	3 (2.2)	1.000
Sedative therapy, n (%)	96 (42.7)	50 (55.6)	46 (34.1)	0.001
Vasoactive agent therapy, n (%)	55 (24.4)	25 (27.8)	30 (22.2)	0.342
CRRT, n (%)	33 (14.7)	10 (11.1)	23 (17.0)	0.218
CVC, n (%)	125 (55.6)	55 (61.1)	70 (51.9)	0.171
IMV, n (%)	122 (54.2)	66 (73.3)	56 (41.5)	< 0.001
Length of IMV (days)	3 (2, 7)	3 (2, 6)	3 (2, 8)	0.543
Length of IMV ≥ 3 days, n (%)	80 (65.6)	43 (65.2)	37 (66.1)	0.915
VTE prophylaxis, n (%)	135 (60.0)	50 (55.6)	85 (63.0)	0.267
LMWH, n (%)	108 (48.0)	39 (43.3)	69 (51.1)	0.253
LMWH + physical prophylaxis, n (%)	75 (33.5)	29 (32.6)	46 (34.1)	0.817
Physical prophylaxis only, n (%)	23 (10.3)	9 (10.1)	14 (10.4)	0.950
ICU length of stay (days)	11 (6, 24)	12 (5, 24)	11 (6, 26)	0.563
Hospital length of stay (days)	19 (12, 32)	20 (11, 32)	19 (12, 31)	0.816
Mortality, n (%)	77 (34.2)	45 (50.0)	32 (23.7)	< 0.001

Data are presented as mean ± SD, median (IQR), or n (%). P values comparing DVT and non-DVT groups were from a two-sample t-test, Mann-Whitney U test, χ^2 test, or Fisher exact test. P < 0.05 was considered statistically significant

*χ^2 test comparing DVT and non-DVT groups

#χ^2 test comparing all subcategories

Abbreviations: APACHE Acute Physiology and Chronic Health Evaluation, ARDS acute respiratory distress syndrome, BMI body mass index, CRRT continuous renal replacement therapy, CVC central venous catheterization, DVT deep venous thrombosis, FiO$_2$ fraction of inspired oxygen, ICU intensive care unit, IMV invasive mechanical ventilation, IQR interquartile range, LMWH low molecular weight heparin, mild 200 mmHg<PaO$_2$/FiO$_2$ ≤ 300 mmHg, moderate 100 mmHg<PaO$_2$/FiO$_2$ ≤ 200 mmHg, PaO$_2$ partial pressure of arterial oxygen, SD standard deviation, severe PaO$_2$/FiO$_2$ ≤ 100 mmHg, SOFA Sequential Organ Failure Assessment, VTE venous thromboembolism

ventilation (IMV; P< 0.001). Patients with DVT had more deaths within 28 days after ARDS than those without DVT (P< 0.001). There were no differences in co-morbidities (P> 0.05 for all; data are not shown) between the DVT and the non-DVT groups. All patients were bedridden for more than 3 days with no difference between the DVT and the non-DVT groups (P = 0.216). For the 135 (60.0%) patients who received VTE prophylaxis, the incidence of DVT was 37.0% (50/135); however, for the patients who did not receive VTE prophylaxis, it was 44.4% (40/90), and there was no significant difference between the two groups (P = 0.271). For the 108 (48.0%) patients who received low molecular weight heparin (LMWH), the incidence of DVT was 36.1% (39/108), and for the 75 (33.5%) patients who received combined treatment with LMWH and physical prevention, it was 37.3% (28/75). There was no significant difference between the two groups (P = 0.866). Among the 90 patients who did not receive VTE prophylaxis, 32 had anticoagulant therapy contraindications, such as stress ulcers and gastrointestinal bleeding (17 patients), platelet counts less than 50×10^9/L (13 patients), and haemoptysis (2 patients). The remaining 58 (25.8%) patients had no clear high-risk factors for bleeding but did not receive VTE prophylaxis due to patient preference of non-adherence to guidelines at that time

in this retrospective observational study. All the 90 patients with DVT were treated with LMWH (66 received dalteparin 5000 IU once per 12 h, 24 received nadroparin 0.1 ml/10 kg once per 12 h).

Echocardiographic findings of DVT vs non-DVT patients in overall ARDS cohort

A total of 215 (95.6%) patients received echocardiographic examinations, with 86 patients in the DVT group and 129 patients in the non-DVT group (Table 3). Compared with the non-DVT group, patients with DVT had a lower left ventricular end-systolic volume index (P = 0.041) and higher pulmonary artery systolic pressure (P = 0.007).

Demographic and clinical characteristics of DVT vs non-DVT patients in direct and indirect ARDS cohorts

In the direct and indirect ARDS cohorts (Table 4), patients with DVT were older, had a lower PaO$_2$/FiO$_2$, a higher level of PCT, and a higher proportion who were given sedative therapy and IMV than patients without DVT (P< 0.05 for all). Patients with DVT had lower serum creatinine levels (P = 0.003) in the direct ARDS cohort and higher Caprini scores (P = 0.021) and higher Padua prediction scores (P = 0.008) in the indirect ARDS cohort. More patients with DVT died within 28 days

Table 3 Echocardiographic Findings of DVT Vs Non-DVT Patients in Overall ARDS Cohort

Variables	Total	DVT	Non-DVT	P value
LA diameter (mm)	48 (43, 53)	47 (42, 53)	48 (43, 52)	0.764
LVESVI (mL/m²)	46 (43, 49)	46 (42, 48)	47 (44, 49)	0.041
LVEDVI (mL/m²)	29 (27, 32)	29 (26, 31)	30 (27, 32)	0.107
Simpson biplane EF (%)	66 (62, 70)	67 (62, 70)	66 (61, 70)	0.513
RA diameter (mm)	45 (41, 48)	45 (41, 48)	44 (40, 48)	0.236
RV diameter (mm)	30 (26, 32)	30 (27, 32)	29 (26, 32)	0.839
PA diameter (mm)	23 (21, 25)	23 (22, 25)	23 (21, 25)	0.933
PASP (mmHg)	40 (36, 48)	43 (38, 60)	38 (35, 46)	0.007
PAH, n (%)	55 (25.6)	25 (29.1)	30 (23.3)	0.338
Pericardial effusion, n (%)	12 (5.6)	4 (4.7)	8 (6.2)	0.628
Tricuspid regurgitation, n (%)	86 (40.0)	38 (44.2)	48 (37.2)	0.306

Data are presented as median (IQR) or n (%). P values comparing DVT and non-DVT were from Mann-Whitney U test, or χ^2 test. P < 0.05 was considered statistically significant

Abbreviations: ARDS acute respiratory distress syndrome, DVT deep vein thrombosis, EF ejection fraction, LA left atrial, LVEDVI left ventricular end-diastolic volume index, LVESVI left ventricular end-systolic volume index, PA pulmonary artery, PAH pulmonary artery hypertension, PASP pulmonary artery systolic pressure, RA right atrial, RV right ventricular

Table 4 Demographic and Clinical Characteristics of DVT Vs Non-DVT Patients in Direct and Indirect ARDS Cohorts

Characteristics	Direct ARDS (n = 111)			Indirect ARDS (n = 114)		
	DVT (n = 44)	Non-DVT (n = 67)	P Value	DVT (n = 46)	Non-DVT (n = 68)	P value
Age (years)	68 ± 11	62 ± 17	0.015	72 ± 15	64 ± 19	0.009
Male, n (%)	32 (72.7)	52 (77.6)	0.557	20 (43.5)	40 (58.8)	0.107
BMI	23.5 (20.6, 25.2)	24.2 (22.2, 27.2)	0.076	24.5 (21.3, 26.8)	24.0 (22.0, 27.3)	0.716
Bedridden time (days)	9 (6, 17)	9 (5, 15)	0.431	10 (4, 19)	7 (4, 14)	0.356
Caprini score	7 (5, 8)	7 (5, 9)	0.891	9 (6, 11)	7 (5,10)	0.021
Padua prediction score	5 (5, 6)	5 (5, 6)	0.689	7 (5, 8)	6 (4, 7)	0.008
APACHE II score	22 (17, 26)	21 (16, 27)	0.568	25 (21, 30)	25 (19, 32)	0.913
SOFA score	6 (5, 9)	6 (4, 10)	0.780	9 (7, 10)	9 (6,11)	0.772
Laboratory data						
White blood cells (×10^9/L)	14.5 (10.0, 18.3)	14.1 (10.2, 20.7)	0.921	18.4 (15.0, 21.5)	18.1 (13.1, 24.2)	0.630
Neutrophils (×10^9/L)	12.8 (9.1, 16.8)	12.8 (8.9, 18.0)	0.935	16.1 (13.3, 19.8)	16.1 (11.0, 21.8)	0.669
Platelets (× 10^9/L)	193.5 (155.3, 279.0)	181.0 (108.0, 257.0)	0.301	202.0 (84.3, 246.5)	148.5 (70.8, 234.0)	0.267
C-reactive protein (mg/L)	120.0 (82, 120.0)	120.0 (89.0,120.0)	0.490	120.0 (86.8, 120.0)	120.0 (94.4, 120.0)	0.758
Procalcitonin (ng/mL)	8.3 (2.6, 17.6)	2.6 (1.1, 9.6)	0.002	15.0 (4.9, 25.0)	4.9 (2.6, 13.5)	0.001
Serum creatinine (μmol/L)	77.3 (56.2, 122.4)	119.0 (70.6, 225.1)	0.003	135.5 (67.3, 208.8)	140.7 (70.0, 275.7)	0.377
D-dimer (μg/ml)	1.8 (0.7, 3.2)	1.2 (0.6, 2.1)	0.211	3.2 (1.6, 7.3)	2.1 (1.3, 4.7)	0.123
PaO2/FiO2	111 (71, 176)	150 (86, 203)	0.035[*]	152 (117, 184)	179 (140, 217)	0.017[*]
Mild, n (%)	5 (11.4)	17 (25.4)	0.062[#]	9 (19.6)	23 (33.8)	0.249[#]
Moderate, n (%)	18 (40.9)	31 (46.3)		30 (65.2)	37 (54.4)	
Severe, n (%) 21 (47.7) 19 (28.4) 7 (15.2) 8 (11.8)	21 (47.7)	19 (28.4)		7 (15.2)	8 (11.8)	
Treatments						
Glucocorticoid therapy, n (%)	16 (36.4)	15 (22.4)	0.108	6 (13.0)	14 (20.6)	0.299
Immunoglobulin, n (%)	1 (2.3)	2 (3.0)	1.000	1 (2.2)	1 (1.5)	1.000
Sedative therapy, n (%)	25 (56.8)	25 (37.3)	0.043	25 (54.3)	21 (30.9)	0.012
Vasoactive agent therapy, n (%)	10 (22.7)	12 (17.9)	0.533	15 (32.6)	18 (26.5)	0.478
CRRT, n (%)	3 (6.8)	9 (13.4)	0.432	7 (15.2)	14 (20.6)	0.468
CVC, n (%)	19 (43.2)	26 (38.8)	0.646	36 (78.3)	44 (64.7)	0.121
IMV, n (%)	34 (77.3)	31 (46.3)	0.001	32 (69.6)	25 (36.8)	0.001
Length of IMV (days)	3 (2, 6)	3 (2, 10)	0.646	3 (2, 7)	3 (2, 8)	0.586
Length of IMV ≥ 3 days, n (%)	21 (61.8)	19 (61.3)	0.969	22 (68.8)	18 (72.0)	0.790
Mortality, n (%)	21 (47.7)	15 (22.4)	0.005	24 (52.2)	17 (25.0)	0.003

Data are presented as mean ± SD, median (IQR), or n (%). P values comparing DVT and non-DVT groups were from a two-sample t-test, Mann-Whitney U test, χ^2 test, or Fisher exact test. P < 0.05 was considered statistically significant
[*]χ^2 test comparing DVT and non-DVT groups
[#]χ^2 test comparing all subcategories
Abbreviations: APACHE Acute Physiology and Chronic Health Evaluation, ARDS acute respiratory distress syndrome, BMI body mass index, CRRT continuous renal replacement therapy, CVC central venous catheterization, DVT deep venous thrombosis, FiO$_2$ fraction of inspired oxygen, ICU intensive care unit, IMV invasive mechanical ventilation, IQR interquartile range, LMWH low molecular weight heparin, mild 200 mmHg<PaO$_2$/FiO$_2$ ≤ 300 mmHg, moderate 100 mmHg<PaO$_2$/FiO$_2$ ≤ 200 mmHg, PaO$_2$ partial pressure of arterial oxygen, SD standard deviation, severe, PaO$_2$/FiO$_2$ ≤ 100 mmHg, SOFA Sequential Organ Failure Assessment, VTE venous thromboembolism

after being diagnosed with ARDS than those without DVT in both groups (P = 0.005 and P = 0.003, respectively). There were no differences in APACHE II scores and SOFA scores between patients with and without DVT regardless of ARDS subgroup.

Independent predictors of DVT in patients with direct and indirect ARDS

Multivariable logistic regression models for DVT were applied in the overall study cohort and then in the direct and indirect ARDS groups, respectively (Table 5). In order to reduce data duplication, we did not include thrombus prediction scores and disease severity scores in the multiple regression models. Because all patients with sedation received IMV, there was a certain degree of overlap between these two variables, so we did not incorporate sedative therapy in the multivariate regression. In the combined and direct ARDS cohorts, age, serum creatinine level, and IMV were independently associated with DVT. In the indirect ARDS group, the independent contributors to DVT were age ($P = 0.015$) and IMV ($P = 0.024$). However, in contrast, the occurrence of DVT increased more significantly with increasing age in those with direct ARDS than in those with indirect ARDS (test for interaction, $P = 0.030$; Fig. 2). Distinct from direct ARDS, the serum creatinine level was not independently associated with increased DVT in the indirect ARDS group (test for interaction, $P = 0.006$; Fig. 3).

Comparison of diagnostic accuracy for screening for DVT of different ROCs in three ARDS cohorts

We propose three new ways of combining forecasting models for screening for DVT based on the significant risk factors. The sensitivity and specificity of the corresponding ROC curves of the proposed models were not inferior to those of the Padua prediction score and the Caprini score for screening for DVT (Fig. 4 A - C).

Survival curves for patients with and without DVT in three ARDS cohorts

Kaplan-Meier survival curves showed that patients with DVT had a significantly lower survival rate within 28 days after ARDS than patients without DVT, not only in the overall ARDS cohort but also in the direct and indirect ARDS groups ($P < 0.001$ [Fig. 5A]; $P = 0.004$ [Fig. 5B]; and $P = 0.007$ [Fig. 5C], respectively).

The 28-day cumulative incidence rate of DVT in ARDS and non-ARDS patients

To further explore the incidence rate of DVT in patients with ARDS in ICU, we selected non-ARDS patients ($n = 266$) in ICU during the same period consecutively (with the same exclusion criteria as for the ARDS group) as controls (Fig. 6). The 28-day cumulative incidence rate (95% CI) of DVT in patients with ARDS and non-ARDS were 40.2% (33.8, 46.6%) and 15.2% (10.5, 19.9%) respectively. Fine-Gray test showed that the 28-day cumulative incidence of DVT in ARDS group was significantly higher than that in non-ARDS group ($P < 0.001$). In addition, the 28-day mortality in ARDS group was significantly higher than that in non-ARDS group ($P < 0.001$).

Discussion

We eventually enrolled 225 patients with ARDS in this study, 111 of whom had direct ARDS and 114 had indirect ARDS. The prevalence of DVT on ultrasound scans in the overall group of patients with ARDS was as high as 40.0%, followed by an undifferentiated prevalence between the cohorts with direct and indirect ARDS (39.6% vs 40.4%, $P = 0.913$). Advanced age, serum creatinine level, and IMV were independently associated with DVT in the overall ARDS group as well as in the direct ARDS cohort. In the indirect ARDS cohort, however, increased DVT was only associated with advanced age and IMV. Patients with DVT had more adverse outcomes than those without DVT, not only in the overall ARDS cohort but also in the direct and indirect ARDS groups.

To the best of our knowledge, this research is the earlier systematic description of DVT in patients with ARDS and of distinct associations among clinical characteristics and DVT in patients with direct and indirect ARDS.

Table 5 Independent Predictors of Deep Vein Thrombosis in Patients with Direct and Indirect Acute Respiratory Distress Syndrome

Characteristics	Total ARDS (N = 225)		Direct ARDS (N = 111)		Indirect ARDS (N = 114)		P Value for Interaction With ARDS Type
	Adjusted OR (95% CI)	P value	Adjusted OR (95% CI)	P value	Adjusted OR (95% CI)	P value	
Age (per 10 years)	1.422 (1.147–1.763)	0.001	1.504 (1.025–2.207)	0.037	1.410 (1.070–1.856)	0.015	0.030
Serum creatinine (per 10 µmol/L)	0.939 (0.908–0.970)	< 0.001	0.857 (0.789–0.930)	< 0.001	0.971 (0.936–1.008)	0.120	0.006
Procalcitonin (ng/mL)	1.033 (0.997–1.070)	0.071	1.035 (0.975–1.099)	0.264	1.035 (0.989–1.084)	0.134	
D-dimer (µg/ml)	1.065 (0.985–1.151)	0.114	1.059 (0.852–1.317)	0.606	1.056 (0.971–1.149)	0.205	
PaO_2/FiO_2	0.996 (0.990–1.002)	0.223	0.996 (0.986–1.006)	0.453	0.995 (0.987–1.004)	0.295	
IMV	3.168 (1.579–6.356)	0.001	5.272 (1.536–18.100)	0.008	2.787 (1.144–6.792)	0.024	

Multivariable logistic regression was performed in the overall ARDS cohort and then in the direct ARDS and indirect ARDS groups separately. The interactions of ARDS type (direct or indirect) with age, serum creatinine level, level of procalcitonin, level of D-dimer, PaO_2/FiO_2, and IMV were included in the regression analysis

Abbreviations: ARDS acute respiratory distress syndrome, CI confidence interval, DVT deep venous thrombosis, FiO_2 fraction of inspired oxygen, IMV invasive mechanical ventilation, OR odds ratio, PaO_2 partial pressure of arterial oxygen

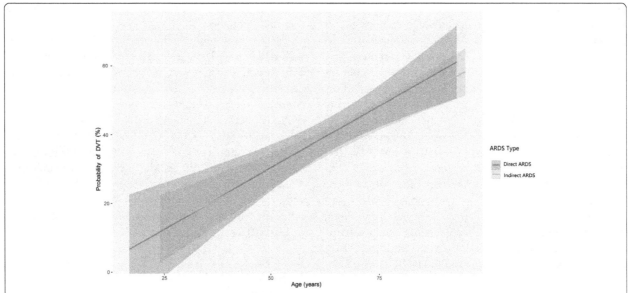

Fig. 2 Prevalence of DVT increased with age in patients with ARDS. The prevalence of DVT increased with age in patients with both direct (red line) and indirect ARDS (blue line). However, the occurrence of DVT increased more significantly with increasing age in the direct ARDS than in the indirect ARDS group (test for interaction; $P = 0.030$). Data are adjusted for level of serum creatinine, procalcitonin levels, D- dimer levels, PaO_2/FiO_2, and invasive mechanical ventilation. Abbreviations: ARDS, acute respiratory distress syndrome; DVT, deep vein thrombosis; FiO_2, fraction of inspired oxygen; PaO_2, partial pressure of arterial oxygen

Prevalence of DVT in patients with ARDS

In 2002, Greets et al. reported that the rates of objectively confirmed DVT in 4 prospective studies ranged from 13 to 31% [27]. In recent years, some research showed that, despite the use of guideline-recommended thromboprophylaxis, the incidence of DVT is still as high as 14 to 37.2% in critically ill patients [2, 3]. Zhang et al. reported that the cumulative incidence of VTE at 7, 14, 21, and 28 days was 4.45, 7.14, 7.53, and 9.55%, respectively, in patients admitted to ICUs in China, even

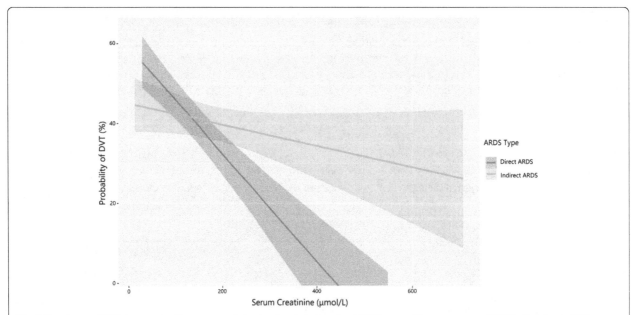

Fig. 3 Prevalence of DVT decreased with serum creatinine levels only in the direct ARDS group. The occurrence of DVT in the direct ARDS group (red line) decreased with increasing serum creatinine levels, whereas serum creatinine levels had no association with DVT in the indirect ARDS group (blue line; test for interaction, $P = 0.006$). Data are adjusted for age, procalcitonin levels, D-dimer levels, PaO_2/FiO_2, and invasive mechanical ventilation. Abbreviations: ARDS, acute respiratory distress syndrome; DVT, deep vein thrombosis; FiO_2, fraction of inspired oxygen; PaO_2, partial pressure of arterial oxygen

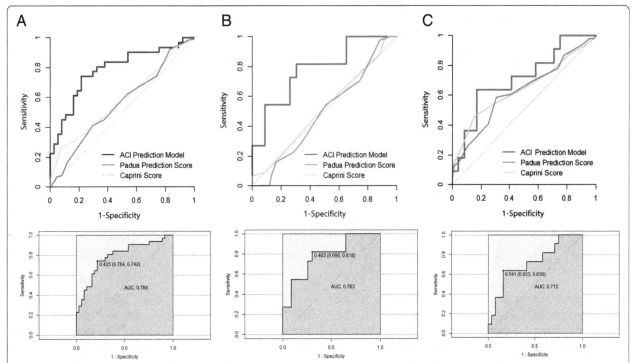

Fig. 4 A-C, Comparison of diagnostic accuracy for screening for DVT of different ROCs in three ARDS cohorts. Patients were split by generating random numbers to produce a training data set (n*0.7) and a validation data set (n*0.3) in the overall, direct, and indirect groups respectively. A, the ACI model which including age, serum creatinine level, and IMV shows satisfactory forecasting ability for DVT (AUC = 0.786; 95% CI: 0.673–0.898; sensitivity: 74.2%; specificity: 78.4%; $P < 0.001$) significantly higher than that of the Padua prediction score (AUC = 0.587; $P = 0.005$ for these two curves) and the Caprini score (AUC = 0.558; $P = 0.001$ for these two curves). B, the ACI model shows a satisfactory ability to predicting DVT (AUC = 0.783; 95% CI: 0.612–0.953; sensitivity: 81.8%; specificity: 69.6%; $P = 0.004$) significantly surpassed the Padua prediction score (AUC = 0.521; $P = 0.001$ for these two curves) and the Caprini score (AUC = 0.492; $P = 0.006$ for these two curves). C, the ACI model shows satisfactory ability for predicting DVT (AUC = 0.712; 95% CI: 0.519–0.905; sensitivity: 63.6%; specificity: 83.3%; $P = 0.024$) has no obvious difference compared with the Padua prediction score (AUC = 0.644; $P = 0.551$ for these two curves) and the Caprini score (AUC = 0.627; $P = 0.451$ for these two curves). Abbreviations: ACI = age + creatinine + IMV; ARDS, acute respiratory distress syndrome; AUC, area under the curve; CI, confidence interval; DVT, deep vein thrombosis; IMV, invasive mechanical ventilation; ROC, receiver operating characteristic

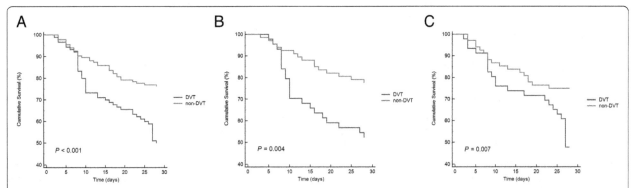

Fig. 5 A-C, Survival curves for patients with and without DVT in the different ARDS cohorts (log-rank test). A, The 28-day survival for patients with and without DVT in the overall ARDS cohort ($P < 0.001$); B, the 28-day survival for patients with and without DVT in the direct ARDS cohort ($P = 0.004$); C, the 28- day survival for patients with and without DVT in the indirect ARDS cohort ($P = 0.007$). Abbreviations: ARDS, acute respiratory distress syndrome; DVT, deep vein thrombosis

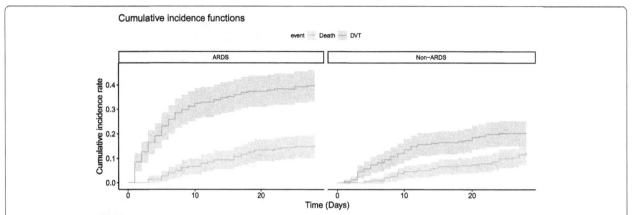

Fig. 6 The 28-day cumulative incidence curves of DVT in ICU patients with and without ARDS. Fine-Gray test showed that the 28-day cumulative incidence of DVT and the 28-day mortality in ARDS group were significantly higher than that in non-ARDS group (*P* < 0.001 for both). Abbreviations: ARDS, acute respiratory distress syndrome; DVT, deep vein thrombosis; ICU, intensive care unit

though the patients received guideline-recommended thromboprophylaxis [4]. Several factors probably account for the notably higher prevalence of DVT in our patients. First, most of the previously mentioned studies focused on critically ill patients who were in the ICU for different diseases. ARDS is a more serious type of critical illness that shows an overwhelming systemic inflammatory process accompanied by alveolar epithelial and vascular endothelial injury and an abnormal blood coagulation mechanism associated with significant death and may have a higher risk of DVT. We compared the 28-day cumulative incidence of DVT between ARDS group and non-ARDS group and found a significantly higher incidence of DVT in ARDS group than that in non-ARDS group. Multiple studies have also suggested that the incidence of DVT in patients with ARDS for coronavirus disease 2019 or influenza A (H_1N_1) was as high as 42.2 to 85.4% [28–31]. These conditions indicate that direct ARDS itself may be a risk factor for DVT. As the results shown, both direct and indirect ARDS had extremely high incidence rates of DVT. Second, some researchers defined VTE as a pulmonary embolism, proximal DVT, and/or symptomatic distal DVT, thereby excluding asymptomatic isolated distal DVT, which could probably be identified only by screening ultrasound [3]. Furthermore, the heterogeneous patient populations, such as those with different primary conditions, different numbers of days in the hospital, and different preventive measures, may represent a variety incidence.

In recent years, a study of COVID-19 showed a low proportion (14.7%, 23/156) of asymptomatic DVT in a cohort of patients admitted in non-ICUs [32]. The incidence is similar to that reported in other studies about asymptomatic DVT in internal medicine settings and orthopedic surgery settings [33, 34]. Compared with these studies above, the incidence of asymptomatic DVT

in ARDS was higher in our study. Also of note is the distal DVT rate (92.2%, 83/90) in patients with ARDS would be significantly higher than that reported in many other hospitalized patients (24.4%, 202/831) [35]. From this article, the conclusions drawn are high proximal DVT or PE recurrent rates (7.9%,16/202) and high mortality (52/202, 25.7%) after isolated distal DVT. So, we ought to pay more attention to the distal DVT in patients with ARDS in order to reduce the mortality.

Risk factors for DVT in patients with ARDS

Advanced age is a well-recognized risk factor for DVT in hospitalized patients, especially in critically ill patients, which has been included in a variety of thrombosis prevention scoring systems [22, 23]. As expected, in this study, the independent association of increased DVT with advanced age was found in both the direct and indirect ARDS cohorts. Interestingly, however, the contribution of advanced age to DVT differed in the different ARDS cohorts. The prevalence of DVT increased more significantly with advancing age in patients with direct ARDS than in those with indirect ARDS. The reason for this phenomenon may be partly, as previous studies have shown [14, 36] that, in our study, the patients in the indirect ARDS group also displayed more severe disease (higher APACHE II scores and higher SOFA scores) than those in the direct ARDS group, so the effect of advanced age on the overall condition of indirect ARDS was relatively small.

We found an independent association between serum creatinine levels and DVT in our patients. To our knowledge, however, this study earlier assessed the differences in DVT related to renal function in ARDS by direct or indirect etiology. We found that the independent association between the serum creatinine level and the incidence of DVT in ARDS is modified by the underlying

ARDS risk factors, with the protective effect on DVT of higher levels of serum creatinine being limited to patients with direct ARDS. However, we did not find a correlation between serum creatinine level and DVT in patients with indirect ARDS, which may be due to the more serious renal impairment and coagulation dysfunction in indirect ARDS, thus weakening the correlation between these two factors. Renal function was associated with dysregulation in coagulation in proportion to the severity of the renal impairment [37]. Some studies have demonstrated that chronic kidney disease and acute kidney injury (AKI) are independent risk factors for VTE [38, 39]. Al-Dorzi et al. pointed out that, for critically ill patients, neither AKI nor end-stage renal disease was an independent risk factor for VTE [40]. McMahon et al. reported that AKI increases the risk for hospitalization-related VTE in a large, heterogeneous population that includes medical and surgical patients. However, this relationship was not seen in patients with traumatic injuries [41]. Some studies have shown that LWMH may have different levels of bioaccumulation in the case of renal insufficiency [42, 43]. The study by Cook et al. indicated that the incidence of DVT for patients with renal insufficiency in ICU who received dalteparin 5000 IU once daily was 5.1% [44], which was far lower than that in the overall population of critically ill patients who received preventive treatment recommended by the guidelines [2–4]. So, we speculate that the same dose of LWMH may play a stronger role in the prevention of DVT in the case of renal insufficiency. Unfortunately, due to the retrospective nature of the study, the decrease of LWMH metabolism in patients with AKI and higher level of serum creatinine was based on the conjecture of clinical data analysis, and we did not detect the activity of anti-factor Xa.

ARDS is a clinical syndrome with high mortality manifested by severe acute hypoxemia, which usually requires MV, especially IMV [8]. With IMV, sedation and immobilization are often performed simultaneously, which would aggravate blood stasis and increase the risk of DVT. Some studies have shown that IMV is a high-risk factor for DVT [29, 45]. Knudso et al. pointed out that IMV administered for more than 3 days is an independent risk factor for VTE [46]. As the duration of IMV increased, the risk of DVT increased [3]. Our research showed that both IMV and sedation were risk factors for DVT. Because all sedated patients in our study were treated with IMV, we only included IMV in the multivariate regression analysis. The results showed that IMV was an independent risk factor for DVT in both direct and indirect ARDS cohorts. However, in this study, compared with patients in the non-DVT group, the duration of IMV in the DVT group did not increase significantly, possibly because our small number of cases resulted in no statistically significant difference.

In direct and indirect ARDS cohorts, neither the APACHE II score nor the SOFA score was associated with the occurrence of DVT, presumably because the serum creatinine level, which was negatively correlated with the occurrence of DVT, was included in these two scoring systems [24, 25], thus weakening the correlation between severity scores and DVT.

Different ROCs for screening for DVT in ARDS cohorts
Differences in predictors of DVT between direct and indirect ARDS partly support the growing body of literature suggesting that there are subphenotypes of ARDS that affect clinical outcomes [12–14, 16]. Our results suggest that subgroup analyses of ARDS are probably beneficial for stratifying and predicting the risk of DVT. We used age, IMV, and serum creatinine levels to predict DVT in the overall and the direct and indirect ARDS cohorts, respectively, and found that, in ARDS, the combined application of these indicators was not inferior to the current commonly used thrombus prediction scores, such as the Padua prediction score [23] and the Caprini score [22], for screening for DVT. Especially for direct ARDS, the combination of age, IMV, and serum creatinine level yielded a sensitivity of 81.8% and a specificity of 69.6% for scanning for DVT. A possible reason is that the Padua prediction score and the Caprini score apply to the general medical and surgical patients in the hospital. As a serious clinical pathophysiological syndrome with an overwhelming inflammatory response and coagulation abnormalities, ARDS has unique clinical characteristics and serious complications. The predictive value of the commonly used thrombus prediction method may be limited to screening for DVT in a patient with a critical illness such as ARDS.

Prognosis of DVT in patients with ARDS
Similar to the results of some previous studies [30, 47, 48], our results showed that DVT was associated with adverse outcomes in all the ARDS cohorts. Although there was no significant difference between length of stay in hospital and length of stay in ICU, Kaplan-Meier curves showed that the 28-day survival rate of patients with DVT was significantly lower than that of patients without DVT in all the ARDS cohorts. To validate the prognosis of DVT in patients with ARDS, we further plotted 28-day cumulative incidence curve of DVT, with death as the competitive risk, and found that the mortality increased with increasing incidence of DVT. The relationship between inflammation and thrombosis has been identified in different clinical scenarios where the inflammatory process and coagulation abnormalities are clearly interlinked [49, 50]. The high incidence of DVT in ARDS may be a manifestation of a severe

inflammatory response with significant coagulation and fibrinolytic dysfunction [50]. In addition, there is a 50% chance for patients with untreated proximal DVT to develop symptomatic PE within 3 months [51]. PE might aggravate the hypoxemia of ARDS patients and then result in lower actuarial survival rates. If there was any clinical suspicion of PE, a CTPA would be considered and obtained, if possible. Unfortunately, due to the critical condition of ARDS patients, CTPA examination was restricted. We only underwent CTPA examination on 3 patients with highly suspected PE and diagnosed with PE, which significantly underestimated the incidence of PE. The presence of PE associated with DVT may also be a cause of poor survival in patients with DVT.

Our study has some limitations. First, our sample size was small, which may underestimate the influence on DVT of factors such as obesity, being bedridden, and the insertion of a central venous catheter. Second, some patients had ultrasound scans only in the early stage of ARDS and did not have continuous dynamic monitoring, which may cause the incidence of DVT to be underestimated. Third, due to the critical condition of patients with ARDS, CTPA examinations were restricted. We performed CTPA examinations on only 3 patients with a high suspicion of PE and then confirmed the diagnosis of PE, which significantly underestimated the incidence of PE. Finally, this study is a retrospective study. We hope to conduct a prospective larger cohort to further clarify the incidence of DVT in patients with different subtypes of ARDS, to determine the corresponding risk factors, and to explore optimized individualized preventive measures in the case of ARDS to reduce DVT-related adverse prognoses.

Conclusions
The incidence of DVT is extremely high in patients with ARDS and may be associated with adverse outcomes. The risk factors for DVT are age, serum creatinine level, and IMV in ARDS. We suspect that DVT is probably an additional risk factor for the death of ARDS in hospitalized patients. The classification and analysis of ARDS may help to provide more accurate screening for DVT and risk stratification and lead to corresponding measures to improve the clinical outcome of patients with ARDS.

Abbreviations
AKI: Acute kidney injury; APACHE: Acute Physiology and Chronic Health Evaluation; ARDS: Acute respiratory distress syndrome; AUC: Area under the curve; CI: Confidence interval; CTPA: Computed tomography pulmonary angiography; DVT: Deep vein thrombosis; FiO$_2$: Fraction of inspired oxygen; ICU: Intensive care unit; IMV: Invasive mechanical ventilation; IQR: Interquartile range; MV: Mechanical ventilation; OR: Odds ratio; PaO$_2$: Partial pressure of arterial oxygen; PCT: Procalcitonin; PE: Pulmonary embolism; ROC: Receiver operating characteristic; SD: Standard deviation; SOFA: Sequential Organ Failure Assessment; VTE: Venous thromboembolism

Acknowledgements
We would like to thank the following doctors for taking part in the diagnosis and treatment of patients with ARDS: Jing Wang, Ling Wang, Jun Zhang and Song Mi from the Department of Pulmonary and Critical Care Medicine, Beijing Chao-Yang Hospital, Capital Medical University, Beijing, People's Republic China.

Authors' contributions
NC designed the study, collected clinical data, analyzed the data, and wrote the manuscript. CJ and HC collected clinical data. XF and LZ helped manage the research, performed the statistical analyses, and revised the paper. XF and LZ contributed equally to this article and share corresponding authorship. All authors read and approved the final manuscript.

Author details
[1]Department of Pulmonary and Critical Care Medicine, Beijing Chao-Yang Hospital, Capital Medical University, No. 8, Gongti South Road, Chaoyang District, Beijing 100020, People's Republic of China. [2]Beijing Institute of Respiratory Medicine, Beijing 100020, People's Republic of China. [3]Department of Intensive Care Unit, Shandong Provincial Qianfoshan Hospital, The First Affiliated Hospital of Shandong First Medical University, Ji'nan, People's Republic of China.

References
1. Di Nisio M, van Es N, Büller HR. Deep vein thrombosis and pulmonary embolism. Lancet. 2016;388(10063):3060–73. https://doi.org/10.1016/S0140-6736(16)30514-1.
2. Gibson CD, Colvin MO, Park MJ, Lai Q, Lin J, Negassa A, et al. Prevalence and predictors of deep vein thrombosis in critically ill medical patients who underwent diagnostic duplex ultrasonography. J Intensive Care Med. 2020; 35(10):1062–6. https://doi.org/10.1177/0885066618813300.
3. Kaplan D, Casper TC, Elliott CG, Men S, Pendleton RC, Kraiss LW, et al. VTE incidence and risk factors in patients with severe sepsis and septic shock. Chest. 2015;148(5):1224–30. https://doi.org/10.1378/chest.15-0287.
4. Zhang C, Zhang Z, Mi J, Wang X, Zou Y, Chen X, et al. The cumulative venous thromboembolism incidence and risk factors in intensive care patients receiving the guideline-recommended thromboprophylaxis. Medicine (Baltimore). 2019;98(23):e15833. https://doi.org/10.1097/MD.0000000000015833.
5. Chang JC. Acute respiratory distress syndrome as an organ phenotype of vascular microthrombotic disease: based on hemostatic theory and endothelial molecular pathogenesis. Clin Appl Thromb Hemost. 2019;25: 1076029619887437. https://doi.org/10.1177/1076029619887437.
6. Gando S, Kameue T, Matsuda N, Sawamura A, Hayakawa M, Kato H. Systemic inflammation and disseminated intravascular coagulation in early stage of ALI and ARDS: role of neutrophil and endothelial activation. Inflammation. 2004;28(4):237–44. https://doi.org/10.1023/B:IFLA.0000049049.81688.fe.
7. Fan E, Brodie D, Slutsky AS. Acute respiratory distress syndrome: advances in diagnosis and treatment. JAMA. 2018;319(7):698–710. https://doi.org/10.1001/jama.2017.21907.
8. Definition Task Force ARDS, Ranieri VM, Rubenfeld GD, et al. Acute respiratory distress syndrome: the Berlin definition. JAMA. 2012;307(23): 2526–33.
9. Bellani G, Laffey JG, Pham T, Fan E, Brochard L, Esteban A, et al. Epidemiology, patterns of care, and mortality for patients with acute respiratory distress syndrome in intensive care units in 50 countries. JAMA. 2016;315(8):788–800. https://doi.org/10.1001/jama.2016.0291.
10. Eworuke E, Major JM, Gilbert McClain LI. National incidence rates for acute respiratory distress syndrome (ARDS) and ARDS cause-specific factors in the United States (2006- 2014). J Crit Care. 2018;47:192–7. https://doi.org/10.1016/j.jcrc.2018.07.002.

11. Li S, Zhao D, Cui J, Wang L, Ma X, Li Y. Prevalence, potential risk factors and mortality rates of acute respiratory distress syndrome in Chinese patients with sepsis. J Int Med Res. 2020;48(2):300060519895659. https://doi.org/10.1177/0300060519895659.

12. Shaver CM, Bastarache JA. Clinical and biological heterogeneity in acute respiratory distress syndrome: direct versus indirect lung injury. Clin Chest Med. 2014;35(4):639–53. https://doi.org/10.1016/j.ccm.2014.08.004.

13. Anan K, Kawamura K, Suga M, Ichikado K. Clinical differences between pulmonary and extrapulmonary acute respiratory distress syndrome: a retrospective cohort study of prospectively collected data in Japan. J Thorac Dis. 2018;10(10):5796–803. https://doi.org/10.21037/jtd.2018.09.73.

14. Luo L, Shaver CM, Zhao Z, Koyama T, Calfee CS, Bastarache JA, et al. Clinical predictors of hospital mortality differ between direct and indirect ARDS. Chest. 2017;151(4):755–63. https://doi.org/10.1016/j.chest.2016.09.004.

15. Morisawa K, Fujitani S, Taira Y, et al. Difference in pulmonary permeability between indirect and direct acute respiratory distress syndrome assessed by the transpulmonary thermodilution technique: a prospective, observational, multi-institutional study. J Intensive Care. 2014;2(1):24. https://doi.org/10.1186/2052-0492-2-24.

16. Calfee CS, Janz DR, Bernard GR, May AK, Kangelaris KN, Matthay MA, et al. Distinct molecular phenotypes of direct vs indirect ARDS in single-center and multicenter studies. Chest. 2015;147(6):1539–48. https://doi.org/10.1378/chest.14-2454.

17. Perl M, Lomas-Neira J, Venet F, Chung CS, Ayala A. Pathogenesis of indirect (secondary) acute lung injury. Expert Rev Respir Med. 2011;5(1):115–26. https://doi.org/10.1586/ers.10.92.

18. Gong MN, Wei Z, Xu LL, Miller DP, Thompson BT, Christiani DC. Polymorphism in the surfactant protein-B gene, gender, and the risk of direct pulmonary injury and ARDS. Chest. 2004;125(1):203–11. https://doi.org/10.1378/chest.125.1.203.

19. Pelosi P, D'Onofrio D, Chiumello D, et al. Pulmonary and extrapulmonary acute respiratory distress syndrome are different. Eur Respir J Suppl. 2003;42:48s–56s.

20. Rudski LG, Lai WW, Afilalo J, et al. Guidelines for the echocardiographic assessment of the right heart in adults: a report from the American Society of Echocardiography endorsed by the European Association of Echocardiography, a registered branch of the European Society of Cardiology, and the Canadian Society of Echocardiography. J Am Soc Echocardiogr. 2010;23(7):685–713 quiz 786-8.

21. Singer M, Deutschman CS, Seymour CW, Shankar-Hari M, Annane D, Bauer M, et al. The third international consensus definitions for sepsis and septic shock (Sepsis-3). JAMA. 2016;315(8):801–10. https://doi.org/10.1001/jama.2016.0287.

22. Cronin M, Dengler N, Krauss ES, Segal A, Wei N, Daly M, et al. Completion of the updated Caprini risk assessment model (2013 version). Clin Appl Thromb Hemost. 2019;25:1076029619838052. https://doi.org/10.1177/1076029619838052.

23. Barbar S, Noventa F, Rossetto V, et al. A risk assessment model for the identification of hospitalized medical patients at risk for venous thromboembolism: the Padua prediction score. J Thromb Haemost. 2010;8(11):2450–7. https://doi.org/10.1111/j.1538-7836.2010.04044.x.

24. Knaus WA, Draper EA, Wagner DP, Zimmerman JE. APACHE II: A severity of disease classification system. Crit Care Med. 1985;13(10):818–29. https://doi.org/10.1097/00003246-198510000-00009.

25. Lambden S, Laterre PF, Levy MM, Francois B. The SOFA score—development, utility and challenges of accurate assessment in clinical trials. Crit Care. 2019;23(1):374. https://doi.org/10.1186/s13054-019-2663-7.

26. DeLong ER, DeLong DM, Clarke-Pearson DL. Comparing the areas under two or more correlated receiver operating characteristic curves: a nonparametric approach. Biometrics. 1988;44(3):837–45. https://doi.org/10.2307/2531595.

27. Geerts W, Cook D, Selby R, Etchells E. Venous thromboembolism and its prevention in critical care. J Crit Care. 2002;17(2):95–104. https://doi.org/10.1053/jcrc.2002.33941.

28. Chen S, Zhang D, Zheng T, Yu Y, Jiang J. DVT incidence and risk factors in critically ill patients with COVID-19. J Thromb Thrombolysis. 2021;51(1):33–9. https://doi.org/10.1007/s11239-020-02181-w

29. Ren B, Yan F, Deng Z, Zhang S, Xiao L, Wu M, et al. Extremely high incidence of lower extremity deep venous thrombosis in 48 patients with severe COVID-19 in Wuhan. Circulation. 2020;142(2):181–3. https://doi.org/10.1161/CIRCULATIONAHA.120.047407.

30. Zhang L, Feng X, Zhang D, Jiang C, Mei H, Wang J, et al. Deep vein thrombosis in hospitalized patients with COVID-19 in Wuhan, China: prevalence, risk factors, and outcome. Circulation. 2020;142(2):114–28. https://doi.org/10.1161/CIRCULATIONAHA.120.046702.

31. Obi AT, Tignanelli CJ, Jacobs BN, Arya S, Park PK, Wakefield TW, et al. Empirical systemic anticoagulation is associated with decreased venous thromboembolism in critically ill influenza a H1N1 acute respiratory distress syndrome patients. J Vasc Surg Venous Lymphat Disord. 2019;7(3):317–24. https://doi.org/10.1016/j.jvsv.2018.08.010.

32. Demelo-Rodríguez P, Cervilla-Muñoz E, Ordieres-Ortega L, Parra-Virto A, Toledano-Macías M, Toledo-Samaniego N, et al. Incidence of asymptomatic deep vein thrombosis in patients with COVID-19 pneumonia and elevated D-dimer levels. Thromb Res. 2020;192:23–6. https://doi.org/10.1016/j.thromres.2020.05.018.

33. Ciuti G, Grifoni E, Pavellini A, Righi D, Livi R, Perfetto F, et al. Incidence and characteristics of asymptomatic distal deep vein thrombosis unexpectedly found at admission in an internal medicine setting. Thromb Res. 2012;130(4):591–5. https://doi.org/10.1016/j.thromres.2012.05.018.

34. Kassaï B, Boissel JP, Cucherat M, Sonie S, Shah NR, Leizorovicz A. A systematic review of the accuracy of ultrasound in the diagnosis of deep venous thrombosis in asymptomatic patients. Thromb Haemost. 2004;91(4):655–66. https://doi.org/10.1160/TH03-11-0722.

35. Barco S, Corti M, Trinchero A, Picchi C, Ambaglio C, Konstantinides SV, et al. Survival and recurrent venous thromboembolism in patients with first proximal or isolated distal deep vein thrombosis and no pulmonary embolism. J Thromb Haemost. 2017;15(7):1436–42. https://doi.org/10.1111/jth.13713.

36. Sevransky JE, Martin GS, Mendez-Tellez P, Shanholtz C, Brower R, Pronovost PJ, et al. Pulmonary vs nonpulmonary sepsis and mortality in acute lung injury. Chest. 2008;134(3):534–8. https://doi.org/10.1378/chest.08-0309.

37. Dobrowolski C, Clark EG, Sood MM. Venous thromboembolism in chronic kidney disease: epidemiology, the role of proteinuria, CKD severity and therapeutics. J Thromb Thrombolysis. 2017;43(2):241–7. https://doi.org/10.1007/s11239-016-1437-1.

38. Kuo TH, Li HY, Lin SH. Acute kidney injury and risk of deep vein thrombosis and pulmonary embolism in Taiwan: a nationwide retrospective cohort study. Thromb Res. 2017;151:29–35. https://doi.org/10.1016/j.thromres.2017.01.004.

39. Christiansen CF, Schmidt M, Lamberg AL, Horváth-Puhó E, Baron JA, Jespersen B, et al. Kidney disease and risk of venous thromboembolism: a nationwide population-based case-control study. J Thromb Haemost. 2014;12(9):1449–54. https://doi.org/10.1111/jth.12652.

40. Al-Dorzi HM, Al-Heijan A, Tamim HM, Al-Ghamdi G, Arabi YM. Renal failure as a risk factor for venous thromboembolism in critically ill patients: a cohort study. Thromb Res. 2013;132(6):671–5. https://doi.org/10.1016/j.thromres.2013.09.036.

41. McMahon MMJ, Collen CJF, Chung CKK, et al. Acute kidney injury during hospitalization increases the risk of VTE. Chest. 2021;159(2):772–80. https://doi.org/10.1016/j.chest.2020.09.257.

42. Mahé I, Aghassarian M, Drouet L, Bal Dit-Sollier C, Lacut K, Heilmann JJ, et al. Tinzaparin and enoxaparin given at prophylactic dose for eight days in medical elderly patients with impaired renal function: a comparative pharmacokinetic study. Thromb Haemost. 2007;97(4):581–6. https://doi.org/10.1160/TH06-09-0513.

43. Schmid P, Brodmann D, Odermatt Y, Fischer AG, Wuillemin WA. Study of bioaccumulation of dalteparin at a therapeutic dose in patients with renal insufficiency. J Thromb Haemost. 2009;7(10):1629–32. https://doi.org/10.1111/j.1538-7836.2009.03556.x.

44. Cook D, Douketis J, Meade M, Guyatt G, Zytaruk N, Granton J, et al. Venous thromboembolism and bleeding in critically ill patients with severe renal insufficiency receiving dalteparin prophylaxis: prevalence, incidence and risk factors. Crit Care. 2008;12(2):R32. https://doi.org/10.1186/cc6810·

45. Rali P, O'Corragain O, Oresanya L, et al. Incidence of venous thromboembolism in coronavirus disease 2019: An experience from a single large academic center. J Vasc Surg Venous Lymphat Disord. 2020;S2213-333X(20):30524-2.

46. Knudson MM, Ikossi DG, Khaw L, Morabito D, Speetzen LS. Thromboembolism after trauma: an analysis of 1602 episodes from the American College of Surgeons National Trauma Data Bank. Ann Surg. 2004; 240(3):490–6; discussion 496-8. https://doi.org/10.1097/01.sla.0000137138.40116.6c.

47. Malato A, Dentali F, Siragusa S, Fabbiano F, Kagoma Y, Boddi M, et al. The impact of deep vein thrombosis in critically ill patients: a meta-analysis of major clinical outcomes. Blood Transfus. 2015;13(4):559–68. https://doi.org/10.2450/2015.0277-14.

48. Zerwes S, Hernandez Cancino F, Liebetrau D, Gosslau Y, Warm T, Märkl B, et al. Increased risk of deep vein thrombosis in intensive care unit patients with CoViD-19 infections?-preliminary data. [article in German]. Chirurg. 2020;91(7):588–94. https://doi.org/10.1007/s00104-020-01222-7.

49. van Deventer SJ, Büller HR, ten Cate JW, et al. Experimental endotoxemia in humans: analysis of cytokine release and coagulation, fibrinolytic, and complement pathways. Blood. 1990;76(12):2520–6. https://doi.org/10.1182/blood.V76.12.2520.2520.

50. Jezovnik MK, Fareed J, Poredos P. Patients with a history of idiopathic deep venous thrombosis have long-term increased levels of inflammatory markers and markers of endothelial damage. Clin Appl Thromb Hemost. 2017;23(2):124–31. https://doi.org/10.1177/1076029616670259.

51. Moheimani F, Jackson DE. Venous thromboembolism: classification, risk factors, diagnosis, and management. ISRN Hematol. 2011;2011:124610–7. https://doi.org/10.5402/2011/124610.

19

Superior vena cava thrombosis and dilated cardiomyopathy as initial presentations of Behcet's disease

Ahmed M. Elzanaty[1*], Mohammed T. Awad[1], Ashu Acharaya[1], Ebrahim Sabbagh[2], Eman Elsheikh[3] and Moshrik AbdAlamir[2]

Abstract

Background: Bechet's disease (BD) is a relatively rare disease that causes recurrent oral and genital ulcers in addition to a variety of systemic manifestations. Concomitant superior-vena-cava (SVC) thrombosis and cardiac involvement with dilated cardiomyopathy (DCM) as initial presentations for BD is considered rare.

Case presentation: A 32-year-old-man presenting with intractable headaches and dyspnea. He was later diagnosed with SVC thrombosis and DCM. A diagnosis of BD was made after detailed history-taking.

Conclusions: Cardiovascular manifisations can be the initial presentation of BD. We aim to highlight the importance of early clinical recognition of BD as a cause of DCM and SVC thrombosis.

Keywords: SVC thrombosis, Dilated cardiomyopathy, Behcet's disease

Introduction

BD is a rare disease, affecting 1 per 15,000 to 1 per 500,000 people in North America and European countries [1]. It is known to cause recurrent oral and genital ulcers alongside a wide variety of systemic presentation mostly related to vasculitis. Cardiac involvement, on the other hand, is rare in BD affecting from 7 to 31% of patients with the disease [2]. Cardiac involvement includes inflammation of all cardiac layers from the pericardium to myocardium, LV thrombus formation, endomyocardial fibrosis, and coronary arteritis [3–5].

Case report

A 32-year-old caucasian man with a past medical history of bronchial asthma presenting with generalized fatigue, orthopnea with intermittent fevers as well as recurrent

* Correspondence: Ahmedm.elzanaty@gmall.com
[1]Internal Medicine Departement, University of Toledo, 3000 Arlington Avenue, Toledo, OH 43614, USA
Full list of author information is available at the end of the article

sore throat for 9 months. Those symptoms triggered multiple emergency room visits and for which he received the diagnosis of recurrent viral upper respiratory tract infection (URTI). The patient started to develop intractable headaches with facial and chest wall swelling for 2 weeks prior to his admission to our hospital. Physical exam showed a positive Pemberton sign (facial plethora when raising the upper extremities). Lumbar puncture was performed which revealed a significantly elevated opening pressure of 36 mmH_2O. With the suspicion of superior vena cava syndrome in mind, the patient subsequently underwent CT angiogram that confirmed the presence of SVC thrombosis that extended to involve the brachiocephalic vein (Fig. 1). Extensive investigations including autoimmune, vasculitis, as well as thrombophilia workup were done and they were within normal. The patient's BNP, troponin I, and creatine kinase were also normal. The only lab abnormalities of significance were the raised ESR of 68 mm/, CRP of 7.3 mg/dl, anda reactive thrombocytosis with platelets of 506x10E9/L. The patient

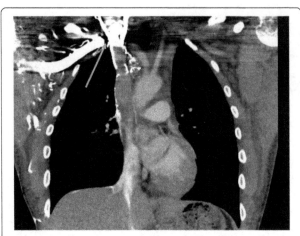

Fig. 1 CT chest on admission showed SVC thrombus that extended to involve the brachiocephalic vein

continued to have orthopnea despite initiation of heparin infusion and improvement of his SVC thrombosis symptoms for which a transthoracic echocardiogram was done which revealed global hypokinesia with ejection fraction (EF) of 20–25%.

Upon further detailed history taking, the patient reported having mouth ulcers that used to erupt whenever he had a sore throat (Fig. 2). He also reported unusual papules in his legs that matched the description of

pseudofolliculitis (Fig. 3). Furthermore, he reported a family history of BD in one of his distant family members. Pathergy test was not formally done, but there were skin reactions reported after blood draws. A diagnosis of BD was made after fulfilling the diagnostic criteria of the International Study Group for BD with recurrent oral ulcers alongside skin lesions of pseudofolliculitis and positive pathergy test. The patient was then started on methylprednisone.

The patient was also started on sacubitril/valsartan, carvedilol, aspirin, and atorvastatin given his new heart failure with reduced ejection fraction. He later underwent myocardium perfusion imaging that showed low normal EF with no reversible ischemia making the diagnosis of coronary artery disease with ischemic cardiomyopathy less likely. Coronary angiography wasn't pursued given low suspicion for coronary artery disease and ongoing SVC thrombosis. Aspirin was also discontinued given the same reason. Three days after the initiation of steroids, the patient continued to report significant improvement in his symptoms, he eventually underwent cardiac MRI that revealed an improvement of his EF to 52% with no evidence of myocardial scarring or fibrosis (Fig. 4). The patient was discharged on oral prednisone, lisinopril, metoprolol succinate, and warfarin. The patient was in good condition upon discharge with follow-up with rheumatology, vascular surgery, and cardiology for his BD, SVC thrombosis, and heart failure with recovered ejection fraction.

On outpatient follow up, the patient remained to do well. His steroids were gradually tapered and he was started on colchicine after which he continued to be symptom-free.

Case discussion

BD is a chronic relapsing autoimmune disorder of unknown etiology that is rare especially outside of the Silk-road area [6]. It is mostly diagnosed clinically, and that is why a thorough history and physical exam are needed to uncover it. A diagnosis is made when a patient is found to have recurrent oral ulcers alongside two of the following; recurrent genital aphthae, eye lesions like anterior or posterior uveitis, skin lesions like pseudofolliculitis, and a positive pathergy test [7].

BD's main pathophysiology is through vascular involvement [8], in the form of vasculitis, thromboembolic complication, as well as pseudoaneurysm [9]. Venous involvement is believed to be secondary to endothelial inflammation leading to eventual thrombosis [10]. Vascular involvement can be effectively managed with immunosuppression with anticoagulation being preserved if thrombotic events occurred [11]. In our case, the main symptom that prompted the patient to seek medical attention was the protracted headache, which

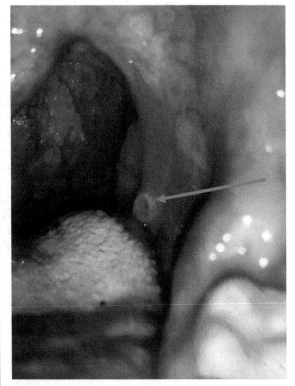

Fig. 2 Self-captured photo for prior oral ulcer

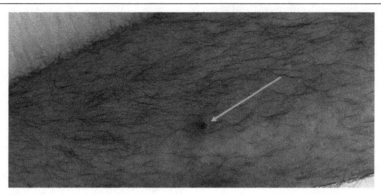

Fig. 3 Photo of psudo-folliculitis lesion

was later attributed to increased intracranial pressure secondary to SVC thrombosis. SVC involvement in BD is well known, Koc et al. in his review of vascular involvement in BD, report it as the 3rd most common venous site involvement [12]. The patient continued to have orthopnea and shortness of breath despite SVC thrombosis treatment for which a 2D echo was done that lead to the incidental discovery of DCM.

Cardiac involvement in BD is rare but reported in the medical literature [13, 14]. The cardiac presentation includes inflammation of one or all of cardiac layers, endomyocardial fibrosis, coronary arteritis with subsequent coronary artery disease, intracardiac thrombus, conduction system disturbances, and valvular disease [15]. Patients who have underlying cardiac complications have a poor prognosis with mortality reaching 20% [15]. However, to our knowledge the association of non-ischemic DCM with BD has been rarely reported with less than a handful of reported cases being found in our search

[16–18]. In our case, the patient was started early on steroids with a rapid and remarkable recovery of the symptoms as well the myocardium function over the course of 3 days, with symptoms as well as ejection fraction recovering from 25% on 2D echo to 52% on Cardiac MRI. Our case is different from prior case reports as it might point to the fact that early steroid use can rapidly convert heart failure with reduced ejection fraction to heart failure with recovered EF.

In our case, if an early emphasis was made on history taking as well as a detailed physical exam to uncover the recurrent oral ulcers alongside the skin lesions instead of initially fixating on the diagnosis of viralURTI would have saved the patient recurrent ER visits.

Conclusion

Recognizing the rare, but possibly grave, cardiac manifestation of BD including dilated non-ischemic cardiomyopathy

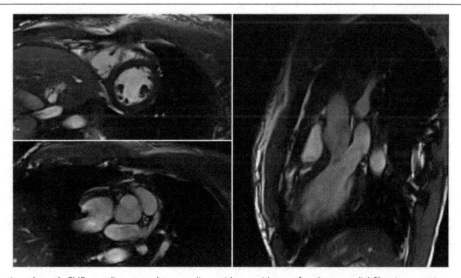

Fig. 4 Multiple Sections through CMR revealing normal myocardium with no evidence of endomyocardial fibrosis or scarring

is essential as it might aid in making the diagnosis and avoid the burden of over-testing.

Learning objectives

1. Recognize cardiovascular manifestation of BD including DCM and SVC thrombosis.
2. Emphasis the role of history taking in cases of unexplained cardiomyopathy to avoid the burden of over-testing.

Abbreviations
DCM: Dilated cardiomyopathy; BD: Behcet's disease; SVC: Superior vena cava

Acknowledgments
Not applicable.

Disclosures
No conflicts of interest or relationship with the industry to disclose by any of the authors.

Authors' contributions
All authors read and approved the final manuscript. All authors contributed equally to this work.

Author details
[1]Internal Medicine Departement, University of Toledo, 3000 Arlington Avenue, Toledo, OH 43614, USA. [2]Cardiology Departement, University of Toledo, Toledo, Ohio, USA. [3]Cardiology Departement, Tanta University Hospital, Tanta, Egypt.

References

1. Calamia KT, Wilson FC, Icen M, Crowson CS, Gabriel SE, Kremers HM. Epidemiology and clinical characteristics of Behcet's disease in the US: a population-based study. Arthritis Rheum. 2009;61(5):600–4.
2. Roguin A, Edoute Y, Milo S, Shtiwi S, Markiewicz W, Reisner SA. A fatal case of Behcet's disease associated with multiple cardiovascular lesions. Int J Cardiol. 1997;59(3):267–73.
3. Gurgun C, Ercan E, Ceyhan C, Yavuzgil O, Zoghi M, Aksu K, et al. Cardiovascular involvement in Behcet's disease. Jpn Heart J. 2002;43(4):389–98.
4. Wang H, Guo X, Tian Z, Liu Y, Wang Q, Li M, et al. Intracardiac thrombus in patients with Behcet's disease: clinical correlates, imaging features, and outcome: a retrospective, single-center experience. Clin Rheumatol. 2016; 35(10):2501–7.
5. Pu L, Li R, Xie J, Yang Y, Liu G, Wang Y, et al. Characteristic echocardiographic manifestations of Behcet's disease. Ultrasound Med Biol. 2018;44(4):825–30.
6. Yazici H, Fresko I, Yurdakul S. Behcet's syndrome: disease manifestations, management, and advances in treatment. Nat Clin Pract Rheumatol. 2007; 3(3):148–55.
7. International Study Group for Behcet's Disease. Criteria for diagnosis of Behcet's disease. Lancet (London, England). 1990;335(8697):1078–80.
8. Sarica-Kucukoglu R, Akdag-Kose A, Kayabal IM, Yazganoglu KD, Disci R, Erzengin D, et al. Vascular involvement in Behcet's disease: a retrospective analysis of 2319 cases. Int J Dermatol. 2006;45(8):919–21.
9. Mouine N, Bennani R, Amri R. A giant left ventricular pseudoaneurysm in Behcet's disease: a case report. Cardiol Young. 2014;24(2):382–3.
10. Barnes CG. Treatment of Behcet's syndrome. Rheumatology (Oxford). 2006; 45(3):245–7.
11. Tayer-Shifman OE, Seyahi E, Nowatzky J, Ben-Chetrit E. Major vessel thrombosis in Behçet's disease: the dilemma of anticoagulant therapy - the approach of rheumatologists from different countries. Clin Exp Rheumatol. 2012;30(5):735–40.
12. Koc Y, Gullu I, Akpek G, Akpolat T, Kansu E, Kiraz S, et al. Vascular involvement in Behcet's disease. J Rheumatol. 1992;19(3):402–10.
13. Cocco G, Gasparyan AY. Behcet's disease: an insight from a Cardiologist's point of view. Open Cardiovasc Med J. 2010;4:63–70.
14. Morelli S, Perrone C, Ferrante L, Sgreccia A, Priori R, Voci P, et al. Cardiac involvement in Behcet's disease. Cardiology. 1997;88(6):513–7.
15. Geri G, Wechsler B, Thi Huong du L, Isnard R, Piette JC, Amoura Z, et al. Spectrum of cardiac lesions in Behcet disease: a series of 52 patients and review of the literature. Medicine. 2012;91(1):25–34.
16. Scheuble A, Belliard O, Robinet S, Boccara F, Bardet J, Cohen A. Symptomatic left ventricular dysfunction and Behcet disease. Report of 2 cases. Arch Mal Coeur Vaiss. 2003;96(2):131–4.
17. Kaatz M, Gornig M, Bocker T, Zouboulis CC, Wollina U. Late manifestation of a fatal Behcet's disease with cardiac involvement and lethal outcome. Deutsche Medizinische Wochenschrift (1946). 1998;123(8):217–22.
18. Al Izzi M, El Bur M, Arif M. A diagnosis not to be missed: Behcet's disease as a cause of dilated cardiomyopathy in a young Arab male patient. Int J Rheum Dis. 2010;13(1):97–9.

20

Von Willebrand factor: Antigen and ADAMTS-13 level, but not soluble P-selectin, are risk factors for the first asymptomatic deep vein thrombosis in cancer patients undergoing chemotherapy

Budi Setiawan[1*], Cecilia Oktaria Permatadewi[2], Baringin de Samakto[2], Ashar Bugis[2], Ridho M. Naibaho[1,3], Eko Adhi Pangarsa[1], Damai Santosa[1] and Catharina Suharti[1]

Abstract

Background: There is a high incidence of deep vein thrombosis (DVT) among cancer patients undergoing chemotherapy. Chemotherapy-induced vascular endothelial cell activation (VECA) is characterized by increased plasma levels of von Willebrand factor (vWF) and soluble P-selectin (sP-selectin), leading to the activation of endothelial cells and signaling cascades. The biological role of a disintegrin-like and metalloproteinase with thrombospondin type 1 motif, member 13 (ADAMTS-13) is to control the activity of vWF and consequently the risk of thrombosis. The objective of this study was to investigate the roles of sP-selectin, vWF, and ADAMTS-13 as risk factors for the first episode of DVT in cancer patients undergoing chemotherapy.

Methods: This prospective cohort study was conducted at Dr. Kariadi Hospital, Indonesia, on 40 cancer patients. Prechemotherapy (baseline) and postchemotherapy sP-selectin, vWF antigen (vWF:Ag), and ADAMTS-13 plasma levels were determined with ELISAs before and 3 months after chemotherapy. The clinical characteristics of the patients, cancer type, cancer stage, chemotherapy regimen, ABO blood type, D-dimer level and Khorana risk score were also analyzed using logistic regression. Patients were observed for the possibility of developing DVT during chemotherapy.

Results: DVT was confirmed in 5 patients (12.5%) after a period of 3 months. In patients with DVT, sP-selectin and vWF were significantly higher while ADAMTS-13 was lower than in their counterparts. The levels of baseline vWF:Ag and ADAMTS-13, with cut-off points $\geq$ 2.35 IU/mL and $\leq$ 1.03 IU/mL, respectively, were found to independently predict the incidence of DVT. In the multivariate logistic regression analysis, the relative risk (RR) for DVT in patients with high vWF: Ag was 3.80 (95% CI 1.15–12.48, $p = 0.028$), and that for patients with low ADAMTS-13 was 2.67 (95% CI 1.22–23.82, $p = 0.005$). The vWF:Ag/ADAMTS-13 ratio and both vWF:Ag and ADAMTS-13 dynamics during treatment were also able to differentiate those with prospective DVT. However, sP-selectin and other covariates showed no statistical significance.

Conclusion: We found that prechemotherapy plasma levels of vWF:Ag $\geq$ 2.35 IU/mL and ADAMTS-13 $\leq$ 1.03 IU/mL are independent risk factors for DVT incidence among cancer patients.

Keywords: Deep vein thrombosis, sP-selectin, vWF, ADAMTS-13, Cancer, Chemotherapy

* Correspondence: boedhi_smg73@yahoo.com
[1]Division of Hematology and Medical Oncology, Department of Internal Medicine, Medical Faculty of Diponegoro University and Dr. Kariadi Hospital, Semarang, Indonesia
Full list of author information is available at the end of the article

Introduction

Deep vein thrombosis (DVT) and pulmonary embolism (PE), collectively referred to as venous thromboembolism (VTE), are major burdens in cancer that could lead to significant morbidity, prolonged hospitalization, increased treatment costs and a notable cause of death for patients [1]. Of all medical conditions, cancer is the strongest risk factor for thrombosis (up to 50-fold relative risk (RR) in the first 6 months after diagnosis) [2]. DVT embolization from the lower extremities is considered the main cause of PE. Asymptomatic patients and those with untreated DVT are reported to have a 50% risk of developing PE within 3 months after disease onset, with a substantial mortality risk [3]. Thrombosis is indeed the second leading cause of death in cancer patients receiving chemotherapy, following death caused by cancer progression itself [4]. The number of cancer patients has continuously increased worldwide, and the adequate treatment of cancer-associated thromboembolism is therefore particularly important [1, 5].

The propensity of thrombosis in cancer patients is multifactorial and includes various types of patient-, tumor-, and treatment-related risk factors and biomarkers [1, 6]. This study aimed to identify the acquired risk factors for DVT in cancer patients, particularly those who received chemotherapy. Heit et al. [7] performed a population-based study and found that cancer patients had a higher risk of developing VTE than those without cancer (RR 4.1), and the RR increased to 6.5 with chemotherapy. In general, the cytotoxic effects of chemotherapy may lead to endothelial damage. Biochemically, chemotherapy-induced vascular endothelial cell activation (VECA) is indicated by an increasing number of endothelial cells in the circulation and other plasma markers, von Willebrand factor (vWF) in the plasma, adhesion molecules, and selectins. It is also highly probable that the liberation of such biochemical markers into the circulation by injured endothelial cells may precede alterations in their functions [8].

Selectins are adhesion molecules that mediate calcium-dependent cell-to-cell interactions among leukocytes (L-selectin), platelets (P-selectin) and endothelial cells (P- and E-selectins) [9]. P-selectin is constitutively expressed in endothelial cells of the lung and the choroid plexus, megakaryocytes, and platelets and is stored within the Weibel-Palade bodies (WPBs) of endothelial cells or the alpha granules of platelets [10]. The binding of P-selectin to its specific counterreceptor, P-selectin specific ligand-1 (PSGL-1), on the surface of leukocytes and platelets increases tissue factor expression and initiates various procoagulant activities [11]. P-selectin can be identified as a circulating plasma protein, sP-selectin, which is shed from activated platelets and endothelial cells, and its function remains enigmatic [10, 12]. Some

researchers have found that sP-selectin is a better biomarker of VTE than D-dimer [13].

The platelet-adhesive blood coagulation protein vWF is synthesized mainly in vascular endothelial cells and megakaryocytes and stored in WPBs and the alpha granules of platelets in the form of "ultra large" vWF (UL-vWF). vWF is a multimeric protein that promotes platelet adhesion and aggregation under high shear stress conditions. This glycoprotein also acts as a carrier for coagulation factor VIII and plays a bifunctional role in primary and secondary hemostasis [14]. Several studies have also demonstrated increased plasma vWF levels in cancer patients [15]. A disintegrin and metalloproteinase with a thrombospondin type 1 motif, member 13 (ADAMTS-13) specifically cleaves vWF multimers and regulates their prothrombotic properties, producing a smaller and less active vWF subunit [16]. ADAMTS-13 is secreted by hepatic stellate cells [17] and endothelial cells [18]. Data on ADAMTS-13 are highly ambiguous. Lancelotti et al. [19] revealed that decreased ADAMTS-13 activity was related to VTE, while Mazetto et al. [20] reported the opposite. The interrelationship between sP-selectin to vWF antigen (vWF:Ag) and vWF:Ag to ADAMTS-13 and the calculated ratios are also of particular interest.

Based on the abovementioned reasons, this single-center prospective study was designed to investigate the roles of sP-selectin, vWF, and ADAMTS-13 as risk factors for DVT incidence in cancer patients undergoing chemotherapy. As previously hypothesized, increased levels of soluble P-selectin indicate platelet activation [12, 13, 21], while vWF and ADAMTS-13 could be regarded as markers of endothelial disruption [14, 18, 21]. This study aimed to provide a better understanding of the pathophysiology of chemotherapy-induced thrombosis and contribute to an early primary evaluation for cancer patients at risk of DVT.

Methods

Study setting

This prospective cohort study was performed at Dr. Kariadi Hospital, the main teaching hospital for the Medical Faculty of Diponegoro University, Semarang, Indonesia. This hospital is a tertiary referral hospital for all patients with cancer in Central Java province. The endpoint of this study was objectively confirmed DVT within 3 months after first-line chemotherapy was given, without verification of either venous or arterial thrombosis at the time of enrollment. All patients were evaluated by the Wells' score probability test and D-dimer level. Patients with a positive D-dimer level ($\geq$500 ng/mL) and/or a high probability Wells' score ($\geq$2) were referred to undergo a vascular duplex ultrasound. Short-cycle chemotherapy was administered as outpatient therapy, while a protocol consisting of more than 2 days of chemotherapy was administered as inpatient therapy. None of the patients received primary prophylaxis with anticoagulation because the patients who were included in this study had an Eastern Cooperative Oncology Group (ECOG) performance status ≥2 to maintain their active mobilization. This study was approved by the Internal Review Board of Dr. Kariadi Hospital. Written informed consent was obtained from all subjects. This study was conducted in accordance with the Declaration of Helsinki.

Patient selection and data collection

From November 2016 to February 2017, a total of 246 consecutive and unselected newly diagnosed cancer patients were screened. Forty consecutive patients with active cancers undergoing chemotherapy were enrolled (see Fig. 1 for patient enrollment). The inclusion criteria were as follows: newly diagnosed cancer with a histological confirmation, age over 18 years, ECOG performance status ≤2, consent to participate, and signed written informed consent. The exclusion criteria were as follows: overt bacterial or viral infection within the last 2 weeks, hepatic and renal dysfunction, venous or arterial thromboembolism within the last 3 months and the use of an anticoagulant, aspirin or statin and surgery or radiotherapy within the last 2 weeks. Inherited VTE risk

factors were not taken into consideration. The probability test for Wells' score (which will be described later) should indicated "DVT unlikely" for all participants.

Before this study was conducted, all patients had been informed about the study's details in an individual interview. Then, anamneses on patients' cancer history, tumor site, tumor histology and tumor stage were documented. Patients who met the inclusion criteria were selected as study subjects. Samples were examined twice (before and after chemotherapy) to measure the plasma levels of sP-selectin, vWF:Ag and ADAMTS-13. Age, sex, smoking history, ABO blood group, body mass index, DVT-related history, diabetes, hypertension, history of atherosclerosis, drug, type of cancer, and chemotherapy regimen were carefully recorded.

Treatment and follow-up

All patients received chemotherapy or chemoradiotherapy. Cisplatin/carboplatin-based chemotherapy included gemcitabine, paclitaxel, docetaxel or pemetrexed. Fluorouracil-based chemotherapy was used in colorectal cancer patients as a component of the FOLFOX/FORFIRI/de Gramont protocol with or without bevacizumab or cetuximab. Anthracycline-based chemotherapy was used in several patients, including those with acute myeloid leukemia (AML) who received a 3 + 7 protocol containing daunorubicin or doxorubicin in the R-CHOP

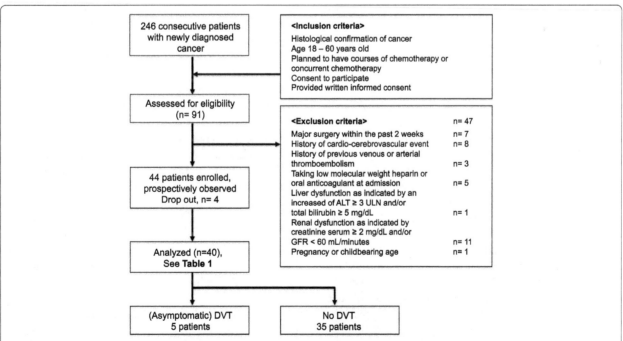

Fig. 1 Patient selection and enrollment of the cohort study. A total of 246 patients diagnosed with cancer between November 2016 and February 2017 were initially evaluated for study enrollment. Of those, only 44 fulfilled the inclusion and exclusion criteria. Four patients were excluded due to various reasons, leaving only 40 cancer patients undergoing chemotherapy. Five patients (12.5%) developed asymptomatic DVT at the end of the observation period. Abbreviations: ALT, alanine transaminase; DVT, deep vein thrombosis; GFR, glomerular filtration rate; ULN, upper limit of normal value

protocol. The patients were monitored for 3 months and evaluated during their follow-up visits at the Hematology and Medical Oncology Clinic by the attending staff. In the first, second and third months, evaluations of DVT occurrence were conducted clinically by examinations as well as the Wells' pretest probability model to assess DVT. If the Wells' score was ≥2, color duplex sonography was performed to establish the occurrence of DVT. Otherwise, color duplex sonography was conducted at the end of the third month.

Outcome measure: the deep vein thrombosis

The endpoint of this study was the occurrence of DVT, either asymptomatic, symptomatic or fatal VTE, confirmed by a duplex ultrasound. Color duplex sonography was performed at the Radiology Department of Dr. Kariadi Hospital, Semarang, Indonesia. Patients with clinically suspected DVT and a Wells' score ≥ 2 were assessed for DVT by using a Logiq 7 Pro US imaging system (Logiq 7 Pro; GE Healthcare, USA) with a 7–10 Hz linear probe. The diagnosis of DVT was based either on the presence of a noncompressible segment (compression ultrasound test – CUS) or flow impairment on color Doppler imaging. Patients were examined for both proximal (popliteal, femoral, and common femoral veins) and distal (peroneal and tibial veins) DVT. The first duplex ultrasound was performed within the first 7 days after inclusion and then during chemotherapy or if the Wells' score was ≥2 or at the final observation in the third month.

Prediction score

Two prediction scores were used in this study: the Khorana risk score and Wells' score. For each patient, we calculated the Khorana risk score to stratify the risk of VTE in cancer patients undergoing chemotherapy [22]. Patients were assigned to three risk categories for VTE: low risk = 0, intermediate risk = 1–2, and high risk ≥3. A Wells' score of 1 point each was given for active cancer, paralysis, paresis, recent plaster immobilization of the lower limb, recently bedridden for > 3 days, major surgery in the past 4 weeks, localized tenderness along the distribution of the deep venous system, entire leg swollen, calf swelling > 3 cm compared to the asymptomatic leg, pitting edema and collateral superficial veins. Two points were subtracted from this score for an alternative diagnosis as likely DVT or more likely than DVT. A score of 3 or higher suggests that DVT is likely, the patient should receive a diagnostic US, and the results should be documented [23].

Laboratory measurements

Venous blood specimens were collected by sterile and atraumatic antecubital venipuncture into citrate vacutainer tubes (SST 5 mL) containing 0.5 mL of liquid anticoagulant. Measurements of plasma sP-selectin levels were carried out using a recombinant human P-selectin/CD62P immunoassay (catalog number ADP3; R&D Systems, Inc., 614 McKinley Place NE, Minneapolis, MN 55413, USA) [24]. vWF antigen was measured using an ELISA (catalog number 885_BcSD20121001; Sekisui Diagnostic, LLC, 500 West Avenue, Stamford) [25]. Plasma ADAMTS-13 levels were measured with a Quantikine ELISA human ADAMTS-13 immunoassay (R&D Systems, Inc., 614 McKinley Place NE, Minneapolis, MN 55413, USA) [26].

Blood samples were collected at the following time points: (i) baseline, before initial chemotherapy, and (ii) 3 months after initial chemotherapy. Samples for ELISA were immediately centrifuged at 2500 g for 15 min, and plasma samples were aliquoted, coded and stored at −80 °C until the assays were performed. Samples were prepared according to the manufacturer's instructions, and plates were read on an ELx808 plate reader (Biotek, Vermont) at a wavelength of 450 nm. The results were converted to total protein using a bicinchoninic acid (BCA) assay (Pierce Rockford, Illinois) and are reported as ng/mg total protein. Measurements were performed in a blinded manner. All samples were assayed in duplicate, and those showing values above the standard curve were retested with appropriate dilutions.

Cut-off points and normal reference values

sP-selectin, vWF:Ag and ADAMTS-13 activity cut-off points were determined based on fold changes. The minimum detectable dose for sP-selectin was 0.5 ng/mL, and the range in citrate plasma was 20–44 ng/mL [24]. With regard to vWF:Ag, the reported mean level was 1.03 ± 0.3 IU/mL in men and 1.08 ± 0.4 IU/mL in women [27]. According to Green et al., the mean vWF:Ag/ADAMTS-13 ratio is 1.05 ± 0.30 IU/mL [28]. The ADAMTS antigen level in noncancer patients was 0.70–1.42 IU/mL (median 1.08 IU/mL) [29]. According to the manufacturer, serum ADAMTS-13 levels range from 0.51–1.64 IU/mL (Quantikine ELISA Human ADAMTS Immunoassay, R&D Systems, Inc.) [26]. The cut-off values for sP-selectin, vWF:Ag, and ADAMTS-13 were set at 105.5 ng/mL, 2.35 IU/mL, and 1.03 IU/mL, respectively, according to the 75th percentiles of the levels observed in this cohort.

Response to chemotherapy and follow-up

All patients who underwent chemotherapy or chemoradiotherapy were followed up for 3 months. After obtaining informed consent, patients were evaluated either during routine visits at the Hematology and Medical Oncology Outpatient Clinic or at the medical ward every pre- and postchemotherapy cycle. The performance status, chemotherapy eligibility and Wells' score were assessed at each visit. DVT occurring after enrollment was documented as a new event, first lifetime thrombosis. Median differences between the baseline and post-chemotherapy levels of each independent variable were calculated and are reported as positive or negative delta values.

Statistical analysis

Quantitative variables were examined for normality with a Shapiro-Wilk test. Continuous variables are summarized as medians (minimum-maximum), whereas categorical data are described as absolute frequencies and percentages. Clinical and laboratory parameters, including sP-selectin, vWF:Ag, and ADAMTS-13 levels and their delta values between DVT and non-DVT subjects were compared using a nonparametric Mann-Whitney test. Correlations between two continuous variables were evaluated with Spearman's rank correlation coefficient. To create positive and negative predictive values, we computed a logistic regression model with three independent variables together with other possible confounding factors. Dichotomous variables were created for all patients in our data set by comparing the probability of DVT associated with the selected cut-off point.

Stepwise multiple regression analysis was used to examine differences in sP-selectin, vWF:Ag, and ADAMTS-13 levels between baseline and postchemotherapy. The vWF:ADAMTS-13 ratio and other potential determinants, such as age, sex, smoking history, cardiovascular risk factors (such as overweight/obesity, hypertension and diabetes), Khorana risk score, D-dimer, chemotherapy regimen, and other biological factors (type of cancer and stage of disease) were also included. First, all potential predictors were entered simultaneously into a multivariate logistic regression model that was reduced using a backward selection method as the final step. Multivariate logistic regression was adjusted for all independent predictors, and only variables with correlations to the outcome (defined as $p < 0.25$ in the univariate model) were included. We generated the final multivariate model for DVT outcome using a backward stepwise approach, and $p < 0.05$ from the likelihood ratio test was used to exclude excess factors. The precision of the specified model to detect DVT incidents was quantified by the Hosmer-Lemeshow goodness-of-fit statistic, where a value greater than 0.05 indicates adequate calibration for the corresponding area under the receiver operating characteristic (ROC) curve [30]. The Statistical Package for Social Sciences (IBM v. 21; SPSS, Inc., USA) was used for all data analyses. All tests with p values < 0.05 were considered statistically significant.

Results

Patient characteristics and anatomical distribution of DVT

Table 1 shows the characteristics of the study population. Overall, 55% of patients were male and 45% were female. One patient died prior to chemotherapy during week 6. The median age of the patients was 49 (20–71) years, and the mean body mass index was 19.4 (15.2–22.6) kg/m^2. The main cancer entities were colorectal (45%) and cervical (15%) cancers. Distant metastasis was found in 42.5% of patients. During the observation period, all patients received chemotherapy. Seven patients received chemotherapy as a radiosensitizer, and the remainder received chemotherapy as either neoadjuvant, adjuvant or palliative chemotherapy. At enrollment, 27.5% of patients were treated as outpatients and 63.5% as inpatients; however, patient mobilization was maintained during the study period. None of the study participants used an erythropoietic-stimulating agent at study inclusion.

Patients were followed up regularly for a minimum of 4 occasions, and during this time, no patient developed clinical signs and symptoms of DVT, and Wells' score was < 2 in all patients. At the end of the observation period, duplex ultrasound was performed in all participants, and objective findings compatible with DVT were found in 5 patients (12.5%). Two patients had proximal thrombosis involving the femoral vein, whereas the other 3 patients were diagnosed with leg vein thrombosis. Thrombosis was seen more often in males than in females (3 vs. 2 patients). DVT was "asymptomatic" in all patients and subsequently treated with an anticoagulant according to local practice.

Plasma concentration of D-dimer, the Khorana risk score, cancer stage and ABO blood group in cancer patients with and without DVT

D-dimer levels at admission were higher in cancer patients who developed DVT than in those who did not ($p = 0.013$). D-dimer showed a positive correlation with sP-selectin ($r = 0.536$, $p < 0.001$) and vWF:Ag ($r = 0.398$, $p = 0.011$) but no significant correlation with ADAMTS-13 ($r = -0.226$, $p = 0.162$). According to the Khorana risk score, the majority (57.5%) of the study population had an intermediate score, while 42.5% had a high score, and 0% had a low score. The Khorana risk score was assessed in all patients and showed no difference in risk group distribution between patients with and without DVT.

With increasing cancer stage, both sP-selectin and vWF:Ag levels were increased, whereas ADAMTS-13 levels were decreased at the time of inclusion. No statistically significant difference was observed between sP-selectin, vWF:Ag, and ADAMTS-13 levels in study participants with cancer sorted by stage or the Khorana risk score ($p > 0.05$ for all, Mann-Whitney U test). However,

Table 1 Clinical characteristics of study participants

Characteristics	All patients (*n* = 40)	No DVT after enrollment (*n* = 35)	DVT after enrollment (*n* = 5)
Age at study entry (years), median (minimum – maximum)	49 (20–71)	49 (21–71)	42 (20–59)
Sex, n (%)			
Male	22 (55%)	20 (57.2%)	2 (40%)
Female	18 (45%)	15 (42.8%)	3 (60%)
Blood group, n (%)			
O blood group	8 (20%)	8 (22.8%)	0 (0%)
Non-O blood group (A, B, AB)	32 (80%)	27 (77.1%)	5 (100%)
Body mass index (kg/m^2)	19.4 (15.2–22.6)	19.4 (16.5–22.6)	19.7 (15.2–20.2)
Underweight	11 (27.5%)	9 (25.7%)	2 (40%)
Normoweight	29 (72.5%)	26 (74.3%)	3 (60%)
Overweight/obese	0 (0%)	0 (0%)	0 (0%)
Primary site of cancer, n (%)			
Colorectal	18 (45%)	17 (48.6%)	1 (20%)
Genitourinary	6 (15%)	3 (8.6%)	3 (60%)
Pancreas	3 (7.5%)	2 (5.7%)	1 (20%)
Lung	2 (5%)	2 (5.7%)	0 (0%)
Upper gastrointestinal tract	2 (5%)	2 (5.7%)	0 (0%)
Leukemia and lymphoma	2 (5%)	2 (5.7%)	0 (0%)
Others	7 (17.5%)	7 (20%)	0 (0%)
Stage at diagnosis, n (%)			
Localized	23 (57.5)	21 (60%)	2 (40%)
Advanced/metastasis	17 (42.5)	14 (40%)	3 (60%)
Chemotherapy regimen			
de Gramont/FOLFOX/FOLFIRI	10 (25%)	9 (25.7%)	1 (20%)
Paclitaxel + Cisplatin/Carboplatin	7 (17.5%)	6 (17.1%)	1 (20%)
FOLFOX + Bevacizumab	4 (10%)	4 (11.4%)	0 (0%)
FOLFIRI + Cetuximab	3 (7.5%)	3 (8.6%)	0 (0%)
de Gramont + Bevacizumab	1 (2.5%)	1 (2.8%)	0 (0%)
Doxorubicin-Ifosfamide	2 (5%)	2 (5.7%)	0 (0%)
Cisplatin-Fluorouracil	2 (5%)	2 (5.7%)	0 (0%)
Cisplatin+XRT	3 (7.5%)	3 (8.6%)	2 (40%)
Gemcitabine + Cisplatin/Carboplatin	3 (7.5%)	3 (8.6%)	0 (0%)
UK-ALL protocol	1 (2.5%)	1 (2.8%)	0 (0%)
Gemcitabine	1 (2.5%)	0 (0%)	1 (20%)
Paclitaxel	1 (2.5%)	1 (2.8%)	0 (0%)
R-CHOP	1 (2.5%)	1 (2.8%)	0 (0%)
3 + 7 protocol	1 (2.5%)	1 (2.8%)	0 (0%)
Radiotherapy	7 (17.5%)	5 (14.3%)	2 (40%)
Laboratory parameters			
Hemoglobin (g/dL)	11.1 (5.9–16.3)	10.9 (5.9–16.3)	11.2 (10.0–12.5)
Leukocytes ($\times 10^3$/µL)	9.2 (3.9–99.1)	8.8 (3.88–99.1)	11.9 (6.3–50.3)
Platelets ($\times 10^3$/µL)	340.0 (51.0–766.0)	330.2 (51.0–766.0)	449.5 (200–561)
D-dimer (ng/mL)	1.859.8 (230–11,450)	1370.12 (230–11,450)	3920 (460–7140)

Table 1 Clinical characteristics of study participants *(Continued)*

Characteristics	All patients (*n* = 40)	No DVT after enrollment (*n* = 35)	DVT after enrollment (*n* = 5)
Khorana risk score			
Low risk	0 (0%)	0 (0%)	0 (0%)
Intermediate risk	23 (57.5)	20 (57.2%)	3 (60%)
Very high risk	17 (42.5)	15 (42.8%)	2 (40%)

this method did not appear to discriminate patients when taking into account the proportion of patients with high risk scores. Detailed information is given in Table 2.

The ABO blood group has a significant influence on vWF:Ag levels, where the O blood group has lower levels than the non-O groups (median 0.73 U/mL vs. 1.4 U/mL, $p < 0.001$), as shown in Table 3. In contrast, the level of ADAMTS-13 was higher in the O blood group than in the non-O groups (median 0.99 U/mL vs. 0.84 U/mL, $p = 0.062$). With regard to the sP-selectin level, there was no significant difference between the ABO blood groups ($p = 0.310$).

Plasma concentrations of vWF:Ag and ADAMTS-13 in cancer patients with and without DVT

In this study, the baseline levels of vWF:Ag measured by ELISA were relatively high compared to those in normal healthy individuals [27] and markedly increased after chemotherapy. The median baseline and postchemotherapy vWF:Ag levels were 1.30 (0.37–3.75) and 1.50 (0.72–3.97) IU/mL, respectively (Table 4). The levels of vWF:Ag were higher in patients with prospective DVT than in those without DVT (3.03 vs. 1.19 IU/mL, $p = 0.001$). The median level of ADAMTS-13 was similar to the normal reference at both baseline and postchemotherapy. However, as shown in Fig. 2, the baseline level of ADAMTS-13 was lower in patients with DVT than in those without DVT.

We also observed that the median level of ADAMTS-13 slightly increased over time after chemotherapy (0.86 to 0.94, delta value + 0.03; $p = 0.026$; see Table 2). The dynamics of ADAMTS-13 can differentiate cancer patients who will develop DVT with a further reduction in

ADAMTS-13 during chemotherapy, creating a negative delta value (Fig. 2a). High vWF:Ag values were not necessarily associated with the occurrence of DVT, and interestingly, we found that those who developed DVT had a higher vWF/ADAMTS-13 ratio than their counterparts. DVT was observed in patients with high vWF levels and low ADAMTS-13 levels. Correlation analyses between ADAMTS-13 and vWF activities were conducted and revealed a significant inverse correlation ($r = -0.513$, $p = 0.001$), as shown in Fig. 2b.

Plasma vWF:Ag/ADAMTS-13 ratios in cancer patients with and without DVT

Differences in the overall direction and dynamics for both vWF:Ag and ADAMTS-13 during the course of chemotherapy at baseline and postchemotherapy (delta value) can also illustrate the "risk" of developing DVT by dividing patients according to the ratio of vWF:Ag/ADAMTS-13 at the end of the observation period. A negative correlation between vWF:Ag and ADAMTS-13 was observed (0.513, $p = 0.001$), corresponding to the wide gap ratio in certain patients during the course of chemotherapy. A high vWF:Ag/ADAMTS-13 ratio and either increased vWF:Ag or decreased ADAMTS-13 were closely related to DVT occurrence. Figure 3b shows that overall, the highest deviation of the reverse correlation between vWF:Ag and ADAMTS-13 (+ 3.49 vs. + 0.16, $p = 0.025$) will differentiate cancer patients who will develop DVT within the first 3 months following chemotherapy.

The vWF:Ag/ADAMTS-13 ratio was significantly higher in cancer patients with DVT than in those without (+ 4.12 vs. + 1.40, $p = 0.001$). The vWF:Ag/ADAMTS-13 ratio increased by 57.7% before

Table 2 sP-selectin, vWF:Ag and ADAMTS-13 levels according to cancer stage and the Khorana risk score category

Covariate	sP-selectin (ng/mL)	vWF:Ag (IU/mL)	ADAMTS-13 (IU/mL)
Local disease (*n* = 23)	69.3 (39.10–230.60)	1.36 (0.53–3.01)	0.97 (0.76–1.22)
Advanced/metastasis (*n* = 17)	88.3 (31.30–185.40)	1.68 (0.37–3.75)	0.85 (0.42–1.33)
$p^§$	0.479	0.066	0.671
Low/intermediate Khorana risk score (*n* = 22)	68.8 (37.30–145.10)	1.15 (0.37–2.97)	0.92 (0.42–1.33)
High/very high Khorana risk score (*n* = 18)	99.0 (31.30–230.60)	1.76 (0.80–3.75)	0.85 (0.45–1.21)
$p^§$	0.203	0.626	0.149

NOTE: §Mann-Whitney U Test

Table 3 Comparison of vWF:Ag and ADAMTS levels in patients according to ABO blood groups

Covariate	Group O (n = 8)	Group non-O (n = 32)	$p^{\S}$
vWF: Ag (IU/mL)	0.73 (0.37–0.95)	1.4 (0.65–3.75)	< 0.001
ADAMTS-13 (IU/mL)	0.99 (0.76–1.33)	0.84 (0.42–1.22)	0.062
sP-selectin (ng/mL)	68.3 (39.1–104.2)	85.4 (31.3–230.6)	0.310

Data are presented as the median (minimum-maximum range)
NOTE: §Mann-Whitney U Test

thrombosis. The difference in the vWF:Ag/ADAMTS-13 ratio from presentation to the final observation was therefore more prominent in the DVT group than in the non-DVT group (+ 3.39 vs. + 0.16, $p = 0.026$). The overall trend indicated by regression modeling was that an increased RR was associated with increased vWF:Ag and decreased ADAMTS-13.

Plasma concentration of sP-selectin in cancer patients with and without DVT

As implied in Table 4, the concentration of sP-selectin significantly increased after chemotherapy (median 81.95 ng/mL vs. 92.5 ng/mL, $p < 0.001$), with a median of a + 7.7 ng/mL increment from baseline. In other words, though they might overlap, both platelets and endothelial cells seem to be activated by the administration of chemotherapy, as reflected by the positive delta value. However, the significance was lost when considering the magnitude of the sP-selectin increment over the chemotherapy cycle ($p = 0.106$). We also performed the same statistical analyses for sP-selectin levels determined by ELISA with another endothelial marker: the vWF:Ag level. As expected, both pre- ($r = 0.439$, $p = 0.005$, see Fig. 2c) and postchemotherapy ($r = 0.46$, $p = 0.003$, data not shown) sP-selectin levels showed a positive correlation with vWF:Ag.

Univariate and multivariate analyses of the risk of DVT in cancer patients undergoing chemotherapy

In the univariate analysis, there were no significant associations with age at diagnosis ($p = 0.739$) or treatment with cisplatin/carboplatin agents ($p = 0.228$), fluorouracil ($p = 0.182$), anthracycline ($p = 0.440$), or steroids ($p = 377$). Five patients used an anti-vascular endothelial

growth factor agent (bevacizumab), showing a negative correlation with DVT ($p = 0.739$). The incidence of DVT was not associated with sex ($p = 0.477$), cancer type (0.341), cancer stage (0.904), ABO blood group ($p = 0.825$), D-dimer level ($p = 0.242$ for cut-off 2320 U/L and $p = 0.123$ for 4622 U/L) or high Khorana risk score ($p = 0.07$). However, the following variables were significantly associated with the incidence of DVT: sP-selectin ($p = 0.004$), vWF:Ag ($p = 0.013$), and ADAMTS-13 ($p = 0.029$).

Finally, in a stepwise manner, multiple logistic regression analysis was performed using DVT incidence as the dependent variable vs. the Khorana risk score, clinical profile (D-dimer, type of chemotherapy) and three possible biomarkers (sP-selectin, vWF:Ag, and ADAMTS) starting with a full model and then removing the nonsignificant variable one by one. The potential independent variables were dichotomously categorized using a predetermined cut-off value. The final model obtained by stepwise regression analysis revealed that only vWF:Ag levels ≥2.35 IU/mL (RR 3.80; 95% CI 1.15–12.48, $p = 0.028$) and ADAMTS-13 levels ≤1.03 IU/mL (RR 2.67; 95% CI 1.12–23.82, $p = 0.005$) were related to DVT incidence, as shown in Table 5. As these variables are independent, the individual variables are multiplicative for the risk, indicating that more than one variable suggests a markedly increased risk for DVT. The Hosmer-Lemeshow statistics test for the entire model suggested a good fit, with a value of 3.349 ($p = 0.138$), and the ROC area was 0.873 (95% CI 0.675–0.925, $p = 0.004$), which indicates good differentiation [31].

Discussion

DVT is a blood clot that forms within a deep vein in the body, typically in the lower extremities [1]. The occurrence of DVT, as well as thrombosis in any part of the human body, relates to Virchow's triad, which states three primary reasons: alterations in blood flow, hypercoagulability and endothelial injury [1, 32]. This study focused on the first cause of DVT in cancer patients undergoing chemotherapy. In brief, we included forty cancer patients, of whom 5 (12.5%) developed asymptomatic DVT as early as 3 months following chemotherapy. A previous study by Blom et al. [2] also found that

Table 4 sP-selectin, vWF:Ag, and ADAMTS levels, vWF/ADAMTS-13 ratios and respective delta values between baseline and postchemotherapy (n = 40)

Covariate	Baseline	Postchemotherapy	Difference in the median (delta value)	$p^{\S}$
sP-selectin (ng/mL)	81.95 (31.30–230.60)	92.5 (40.9–278.3)	+ 7.70 (1.0–88.1)	< 0.001
vWF:Ag (IU/mL)	1.30 (0.37–3.75)	1.50 (0.72–3.97)	+ 0.21 (0.02–1.22)	< 0.001
ADAMTS-13 antigen (IU/mL)	0.86 (0.42–1.33)	0.94 (0.31–1.64)	+ 0.03 (−0.39–0.36)	0.026
vWF:Ag/ ADAMTS-13 ratio	1.46 (0.39–8.33)	1.7 (0.56–12.80)	+ 0.17 (−1.24–4.47)	0.001

Data are presented as the median (minimum-maximum range)
NOTE: §Wilcoxon signed-rank test (between baseline and postchemotherapy)

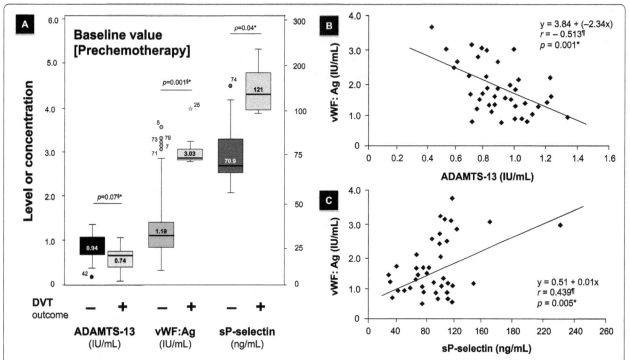

Fig. 2 a. Prechemotherapy (baseline) plasma levels of ADAMTS-13, vWF:Ag and sP-selectin in 40 cancer patients stratified based on the occurrence of DVT at the end of the observation period. Boxplot data are presented as the median value (minimum-maximum range), and the *p* value represents the difference between groups. **b.** Correlation coefficient, scatterplot and regression line between the vWF:Ag level and ADAMTS activity. **c.** Correlation coefficient, scatterplot and regression line between the vWF:Ag level and soluble P-selectin. NOTE: §Mann-Whitney U test; ¶Spearman's rank test; *Statistically significant at *p* < 0.05

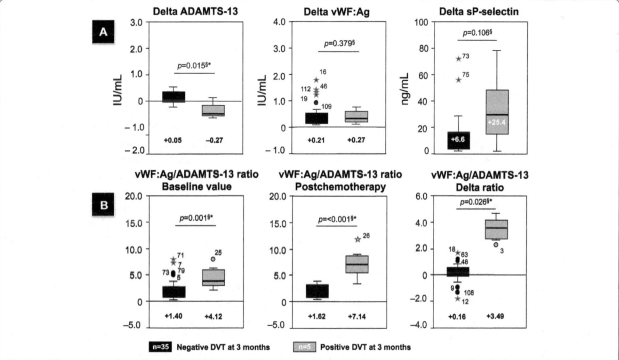

Fig. 3 a. Differences in each predictor (1. ADAMTS-13, 2. vWF:Ag, and 3. sP-selectin). Shifts in prechemotherapy (baseline) vs. postchemotherapy levels are reported as the delta values for prospective DVT. **b.** Respective vWF:ADAMTS-13 ratios (1. Prechemotherapy, 2. Postchemotherapy, and 3. Delta value for the ratio). NOTE: § Mann-Whitney U test; *Statistically significant at *p* < 0.05

Table 5 Univariate and multivariate analyses of the probability of predicting DVT incidence in cancer patients undergoing chemotherapy

Covariate	Univariate analysis		Multivariate analysis[a]	
	RR (95% CI)	P	RR (95% CI)	P
Age ≥ 55 years	1.50 (0.13–16.32)	0.739		
Male sex	2.00 (0.29–13.51)	0.477		
Type of cancer, low risk vs. high/very high risk	2.53 (0.37–17.24)	0.341		
Cancer stage, localized vs. advanced/metastasis	0.88 (0.13–6.00)	0.904		
Chemotherapy regimen				
Cisplatin/carboplatin-based	3.27 (0.47–22.46)	0.228	0.454 (0.208–26.68)	0.704
Fluorouracil-based	4.77 (0.48–46.90)	0.182	1.309 (0.606–17.14)	0.456
Bevacizumab	1.50 (0.13–16.32)	0.739		
Anthracycline	2.66 (0.22–32.17)	0.440		
Use of steroids	3.20 (0.24–42.18)	0.377		
Group O blood type	0.77 (0.77–7.71)	0.825		
D-dimer ≥2320 ng/mL (75th percentile)	2.55 (0.52–12.48)	0.242		
D-dimer ≥4622.4 ng/mL (90th percentile)	3.57 (0.707–18.04)	0.123	1.00 (0.99–2.01)	0.900
High Khorana risk score	8.07 (0.84–77.1)	0.07	0.537 (0.121–13.65)	0.537
Prechemotherapy sP-selectin ≥105.5 ng/mL	11.67 (2.22–61.27)	0.004	1.02 (0.98–11.05)	0.260
Prechemotherapy vWF:Ag ≥ 2.35 IU/mL	7.50 (1.53–36.71)	0.013	3.80 (1.15–12.48)	0.028
Prechemotherapy ADAMTS-13 ≤ 1.03 IU/mL	13.5 (1.31–38.65)	0.029	2.67 (1.22–23.82)	0.005

NOTE: [a]In the multivariate model, the area under the ROC curve = 0.873 (95% CI 0.675–0.925, $p = 0.004$). Hosmer-Lemeshow goodness-of-fit test: $X^2 = 3.349$, df = 8, $p = 0.138$. Null hypothesis = 0.5

the risk of developing thrombosis was highest in the first 3 months after cancer diagnosis (adjusted OR 53.4, 95% CI 8.6–334.3). Similarly, another study also observed these events over a median follow-up of 2.4 months in patients treated with chemotherapy [33].

Our present study confirmed that cancer is associated with increased levels of both sP-selectin and vWF:Ag, two molecules from the endothelial WPB. Endothelial cells, megakaryocytes and platelets can synthesize vWF, the largest multimeric glycoprotein involved in regulating hemostasis; thus, a high-level of vWF:Ag is a reliable marker of thrombosis. A recent study also found high vWF expression in tumor cells [34], contributing to a significant elevation of vWF levels in cancer patients. However, the baseline ADAMTS-13 level was lower than the normal reference level, and the response after chemotherapy varied.

Multivariate logistic regression revealed two independent risk factors related to DVT in cancer patients undergoing chemotherapy: vWF:Ag and ADAMTS-13. A vWF:Ag level above the 75th percentile was associated with a 3.8-fold increased risk of developing DVT, and an ADAMTS-13 level below the 25th percentile was associated with an approximately 2.7-fold increased risk of developing DVT in cancer patients after chemotherapy. Therefore, following cancer diagnosis, patients with a vWF:Ag level greater than 2.35 IU/mL and an ADAM

TS-13 level less than 1.03 IU/mL have a high probability of developing DVT during chemotherapy, suggesting that both vWF:Ag and ADAMTS-13 have a mechanistic effect. Similar studies were conducted by Pepin et al. [35] from France and Obermeier et al. [36] from Austria: these authors reported different perspectives on the role of ADAMTS-13 in relation to high vWF:Ag. Previous studies have shown that the activity and level of ADAM TS-13 are slightly lower in cancer patients than in healthy controls [37, 38]. Theoretically, a deficiency of ADAMTS-13 results in the presence of UL-vWF [39]. It is therefore believed that the circulating levels of ADAM TS-13 may influence the circulating levels of vWF and/ or its function and thereby the risk of thrombosis.

We explored the effect of high sP-selectin levels and then stratified patients into 2 groups based on the 75th percentile of sP-selectin levels (cut-off point 105.5 ng/mL). Surprisingly, sP-selectin was not an independent risk factor for DVT and failed to reach statistical significance in the multivariate analysis. Several studies have demonstrated elevated levels of sP-selectin in cancer patients with DVT [40–42], inconsistent with the results of the present study. Notably, our cut-off value was higher than that in other studies by Ay et al. (53.1 ng/mL) [41] and Ramaciotti et al. (90 ng/mL) [42], partly because of the higher sP-selectin levels at baseline in our study population.

This study showed that high sP-selectin levels cannot differentiate or identify cancer patients who will develop DVT early after undergoing chemotherapy.

The dynamics of plasma biomarkers should be accounted for in an absolute DVT risk assessment due to changes after chemotherapy. As shown in Fig. 3 and Table 4, temporal changes in sP-selectin, vWF:Ag, and ADAMTS-13 levels were observed following several courses of chemotherapy. There were no differences between baseline and postchemotherapy sP-selectin levels, as reflected by the nonsignificant delta value for DVT incidence (+ 6.6 vs. + 25. 4 ng/mL, $p = 0.106$, Mann-Whitney U test). However, when assessing its association with chemotherapy, there was a significant reduction in ADAMTS-13 from baseline in those who developed DVT (delta value – 0.27 with DVT vs. + 0.05, $p = 0.015$), while nearly all patients showed slightly increased vWF:Ag (delta value + 0.27 vs. + 0.21, $p = 0.379$) over time. Our findings revealed deficient levels of ADAMTS-13, which regulates the size and adhesive activity of plasma vWF. The corelationship between these two markers resulted in a wide gap in the vWF:Ag/ADAMTS-13 ratio.

Since the relation in the size of UL-vWF multimers via ADAMTS-13 is a relevant mechanism of thrombosis in cancer patients, reduced ADAMTS-13 levels as well as high plasma vWF:Ag levels, causing a high vWF:Ag/ADAMTS-13 ratio, may serve as independent predictive factors. However, there are no mechanistic or biochemical data that might explain this observed association between high vWF:Ag and low ADAMTS-13. We hypothesized several possible mechanisms for this phenomenon, including impaired protein synthesis in the liver or endothelial dysfunction associated with direct chemotherapy toxicity and consumption by increased vWF substrates [36, 43]. Various oncogenes have also been found to regulate the expression of extracellular proteinases, including matrix-degrading metalloproteinases, which can directly disrupt ADAMTS-13 activities [43]. Both the mechanisms of declination and to what extent ADAMTS-13 contributes require further study using different approaches.

In this study, we provide a piece of the puzzle regarding the cause-and-effect relationship of increased endothelial markers in cancer patients and DVT as a result of chemotherapy. In this respect, our study demonstrated a new perspective by determining that DVT in cancer patients is related to immunothrombosis. Thus, the coagulation process is not the sole mechanism that leads to thrombosis; rather, vascular inflammation on account of direct endothelial toxicity related to chemotherapy exposure may play a role. Biochemically, chemotherapy-induced VECA and vascular inflammation are indicated by increasing circulating endothelial cells and markers such as vWF:Ag

and sP-selectin. The rising endothelial activities as a result of inflammation induce various changes in endothelial cells, leukocytes and platelets, promoting procoagulant and prothrombotic surfaces in blood vessel walls that increase the risk of DVT.

The paradigm above provides new insights for studies concerning novel thromboprophylaxis strategies and suggests a role for anti-inflammatory agents, which could be used for DVT prevention with a lower risk of bleeding complications than conventional therapeutic approaches.

Despite these results, there were several limitations to the study that should be addressed. First, this was a single-center study with a relatively small sample size; thus, it was not large enough for a subgroup analysis for a deeper understanding. Therefore, the current findings must be confirmed in larger, multicenter and prospective studies. Second, this study incorporated only clinical probability testing at study enrollment to exclude the lack of CUS screening for DVT. Third, we did not accounted for PE incidence in the study outcome, even though 33% of PEs are not preceded by documented DVT, especially in patient with active cancer [44]. Fortunately, no study participants showed signs or symptoms suggesting PE during the observation period. Fourth, we acknowledge that there must be residual confounding by variables not measured in our study (e.g., smoking) that can influence DVT outcome or affect the levels of the covariates. Fifth, because we assessed the antigen level rather than activity, we could not assess the functional impact of the wide gap in the vWF:Ag: ADAMTS-13 ratio. Last, we were unable to investigate the relationship between DVT and other endothelial biomarkers, such as tissue factor activity, prothrombin fragments, the level of coagulation factor VIII, the dynamics of D-dimer, hereditary thrombosis risk factors or the effect of ADAMTS-13.

Conclusion

Our study demonstrated the following: 1) cancer is a prothrombotic stage as reflected by abnormal sP-selectin, vWF:Ag and ADAMTS-13 levels detected by ELISA; 2) following chemotherapy, patients who develop DVT show a particular pattern: high plasma levels of vWF:Ag and low plasma levels of ADAMTS-13, generating a wide gap in the vWF:Ag/ADAMTS-13 ratio; 3) by applying the 75th and 25th percentiles as cut-off points, we determined that a baseline level of vWF:Ag greater than 2.35 IU/mL and 4) an ADAMTS-13 level less than 1.03 IU/mL in cancer patients were independent risk factors for DVT after chemotherapy.

Further research is needed to understand the important role of the immune system and vascular inflammation in the pathogenesis of DVT in cancer patients undergoing chemotherapy and thus to provide insights into novel thromboprophylaxis strategies or suggest a role for anti-inflammatory agents, which could be used for DVT prevention with a lower risk of bleeding complications than conventional therapeutic approaches.

Abbreviations

AML: Acute myeloid leukemia; AST: Alanine transaminase; DVT: Deep vein thrombosis; ELISA: Enzyme-linked immunosorbent assay; GFR: Glomerular filtration rate; PE: Pulmonary embolism; PSGL-1: P-selectin glycoprotein ligand 1; VTE: Venous thromboembolism; VECA: Vascular endothelial cell activation; vWF: von Willebrand factor; sP-selectin: Soluble P-selectin; ULN: Upper limit of normal; UL-vWFM : Ultra large vWF molecule; VWF:Ag: von Willebrand factor antigen; ADAMTS-13: A disintegrin and metalloproteinase with a thrombospondin type 1 motif, member 13; ROC: Receiver Operating Characteristic; RR: Relative risk; WPB: Weibel-Palade bodies

Acknowledgments

Our sincere gratitude to Mika Lumbantobing, M.D., and Suyono, M.D. from the Department of Internal Medicine, Dr. Kariadi Hospital, Diponegoro University, Semarang, Indonesia for their contribution in cancer patient and to all colleagues at dr. Kariadi Hospital who supported us in patient recruitment. We also acknowledge support of the biomolecular laboratory at for providing assistance in ELISA analysis, Gunawan Santosa M.D., Ph.D. for his radiological expertise in performing dupplex ultrasound of the extremities, and Darminto, MD, MKes from the Clinical Epidemiology Unit of Diponegoro University for the statistical support. Lastly but not least, the authors would like to thank the participants and their family for contributing by enrolling in the study.

Authors' contributions

Budi Setiawan: Conceptualizing and design the study, reviewed data, wrote the first manuscript, analyzed the data and reviewed the final manuscript. Cecilia Oktaria Permatadewi: Included patients, collected the samples and data, and reviewed the manuscript. Baringin de Samakto: Included patients, collected the samples and data, and reviewed the manuscript. Ashar Bugis: Included patients, collected the samples and data, and reviewed the manuscript. Ridho M. Naibaho: Assissted with study oversight, collected the data, analyzed and carried out the statistical analysis, and drafted the revised version of the manuscript. Eko Adhi Pangarsa: Supervision the study, critically appraised the manuscript. Damai Santosa: Supervision the study, critically appraised the manuscript. Catharina Suharti: Conceptualization, supervision the study, critically appraised the manuscript. All authors participated in the interpretation and presentation of the results, then contributed, read and approved the final manuscript hereby submitted for publication.

Authors' information

Budi Setiawan and Eko Adhi Pangarsa are Hematologist and Medical Oncologist. They currently work as PhD candidate from the Faculty of Medicine, Diponegoro University/Dr. Kariadi Hospital, Semarang, Indonesia. Cecilia Oktaria Permatadewi, Baringin de Samakto, and Ashar Bugis are resident physician in Department of Internal Medicine, Faculty of Medicine Diponegoro University/Dr. Kariadi Hospital, Semarang, Indonesia. Ridho M. Naibaho is a clinical fellow in Hematology and Medical Oncology, Department of Internal Medicine, Faculty of Medicine, Diponegoro University/Dr. Kariadi Hospital, Semarang, Indonesia. Damai Santosa is chief of Division of Hematology and Medical Oncology, Department of Internal Medicine, Faculty of Medicine, Diponegoro University/Dr. Kariadi Hospital, Semarang, Indonesia. Catharina Suharti is professor of medicine in Division of Hematology and Medical Oncology, Department of Internal Medicine, Faculty of Medicine, Diponegoro University/Dr. Kariadi Hospital, Semarang, Indonesia.

Author details

[1]Division of Hematology and Medical Oncology, Department of Internal Medicine, Medical Faculty of Diponegoro University and Dr. Kariadi Hospital, Semarang, Indonesia. [2]Department of Internal Medicine, Medical Faculty of Diponegoro University and Dr. Kariadi Hospital, Semarang, Indonesia. [3]Fellow in Hematology and Medical Oncology, Department of Internal Medicine, Medical Faculty of Mulawarman University, Parikesit General Hospital, Kutai Kartanegara, Indonesia.

References

1.	Suharti C. Tromboemboli vena pada kanker [Article in Indonesian]. Med Hosp. 2013;1:143–9.
2.	Blom JW, Doggen CJ, Osanto S, Rosendaal FR. Malignancies, prothrombotic mutations, and the risk of venous thrombosis. JAMA. 2005;293:715–22.
3.	Kearon C. Natural history of venous thromboembolism. Semin Vasc Med. 2001;1:27–37.
4.	Khorana AA, Francis CW, Culakova E, Kuderer NM, Lyman GH. Thromboembolism is a leading cause of death in cancer patients receiving outpatient chemotherapy. J Thromb Haemost. 2007;5:632–4.
5.	Tambunan KL, Kurnianda J, Suharti C, et al. IDENTIA registry: incidence of deep vein thrombosis in medically ill subjects at high risk in Indonesia: a prospective study. Acta Med Indones. 2020;52:14–24.
6.	Khorana AA. Targeted prophylaxis in cancer: the evidence accumulates. Intern Emerg Med. 2013;8:187–9.
7.	Heit JA, Silverstein MD, Mohr DN, et al. Risk factors for deep vein thrombosis and pulmonary embolism: a population-based case-control study. Arch Intern Med. 2000;160:809–15.
8.	Kirwan CC, McCollum CN, McDowell G, Byrne GJ. Investigation of proposed mechanisms of chemotherapy-induced deep vein thrombosis: endothelial cell activation and procoagulant release due to apoptosis. Clin Appl Thromb. 2015;2:420–7.
9.	Varki A. Selectin ligands. Proc Natl Acad Sci U S A. 1994;91:7390–7.
10.	Kansas GS. Selectins and their ligands: current concepts and controversies. Blood. 1996;88:3259–87.
11.	Frenette PS, Denis CV, Weiss L, et al. P-selectin glycoprotein ligand 1 (PSGL-1) is expressed on platelets and can mediate platelet-endothelial interactions in vivo. J Exp Med. 2000;191:1413–22.
12.	Kappelmayer J, Nagy B Jr, Miszti-Blasius K, Hevessy Z, Setiadi H. The emerging value of P-selectin as a disease marker. Clin Chem Lab Med. 2004;42:475–86.
13.	Fernandes LFB, Fregnani JHTG, Strunz CMC, de Andrade Ramos Nogueira A, Longatto-Filho A. Role of P-selectin in thromboembolic events in patients with cancer. Mol Clin Oncol. 2018;8:188–96.
14.	Shahidi M. Thrombosis and von Willebrand factor. Adv Exp Med Biol. 2017; 906:285–306.
15.	Franchini M, Frattini F, Crestani S, Bonfanti C, Lippi G. Von Willebrand factor and cancer: a renewed interest. Thromb Res. 2013;131:290–2.
16.	Tsai HM. Physiologic cleavage of von Willebrand factor by a plasma protease is dependent on its conformation and requires calcium ion. Blood. 1996;87:4235–44.
17.	Uemura M, Tatsumi K, Matsumoto M, et al. Localization of ADAMTS13 to the stellate cells of human liver. Blood. 2005;106:922–4.
18.	Turner N, Nolasco L, Tao Z, Dong JF, Moake J. Human endothelial cells synthesize and release ADAMTS-13. J Thromb Haemost. 2006;4:1396–404.
19.	Lancelotti S, Basso M, Veca V, et al. Presence of portal vein thrmbosis in liver cirrhosis is strongly associated with low level of ADAMTS-13: a pilot study. Intern Emerg Med. 2016;11:959–67.
20.	Mazetto BM, Orsi FL, Barnabe A, et al. Increased ADAMTS13 activity in patients with venous thromboembolism. Thromb Res. 2012;130:889–93.
21.	Goncharov NV, Nadeev AN, Jenkins RO, Avdonin PV. Markers and biomarkers of endothelium: when something is rotten in the state. Oxidative Med Cell Longev. 2017. Article ID 9759735.
22.	Khorana AA, Kudener NM, Culakova E, Lyman GH, Francis CM. Development and validation of a predictive model for chemotherapy-associated thrombosis. Blood. 2008;111:4902–7.

23. Wells P, Anderson D, Rodger M, et al. Evaluation of D-dimer in the diagnosis of suspected deep-vein thrombosis. N Engl J Med. 2003;349:1227–35.

24. Human sP-selectin/CD62P immunoassay. Catalog number BBE6, SBBE6, PBBE6. Minneapolis: R&D Systems Inc.

25. Von Willebrand factor (vWF) ELISA kit. Stamford: Sekisui Diagnostic, LLC.

26. Quantikine ELISA human ADAMTS13 immunoassay. Catalog number DADT130. Minneapolis: R&D Systems Inc.

27. Blann AD. Normal levels of von Willebrand factor antigen in human body fluids. Biologicals. 1990;18:351–3.

28. Green D, Tian L, Greenland P, et al. Association of the von Willebrand factor–ADAMTS13 ratio with incident cardiovascular events in patients with peripheral arterial disease. Clin Appl Thromb Hemost. 2017;23:807–13.

29. Rieger M, Ferrari S, Hovinga JAK, et al. Relation between ADAMTS13 activity and ADAMTS13 antigen levels in healthy donors and patients with thrombotic microangiopathy (TMA). Thromb Haemost. 2006;95:212–20.

30. Hosmer DW, Lemeshow S. Applied logistic regression. New York: Wiley; 2000.

31. Brubaker PH. Do not be statistically cenophobic: time to ROC and roll! J Cardiopulm Rehab Prev. 2008;28:420–1.

32. Dickson BC. Venous thrombosis: on the history of Virchow's triad. Univ Tor Med J. 2004;81:166–71.

33. Khorana AA, Francis CW, Culakova E, Lymna GH. Risk factors for chemotherapy-associated venous thromboembolism in a prospective observational study. Cancer. 2005;104:2822–9.

34. Beuchat Z, Prevost N. Expression of von Willebrand factor by tumor cells – relevance to cancer-associated thrombosis and animal studies [abstract]. Melbourne: ISTH Congress; 2019.

35. Pepin M, Kleinjan A, Hajage D, Buller HR, Di Nisio M, et al. ADAMTS-13 and von Willebrand factor predict deep vein thrombosis in patients with cancer. J Thromb Haemost. 2016;14:306–15.

36. Obernier HL, Riedl J, Ay C, et al. The role of ADAMTS-13 and von Willebrand factor in cancer patients: results from the Vienna cancer and thrombosis study. Res Pract Thromb Haemost. 2019;3:503–14.

37. Bohm M, Gerlach R, Beecken WD, Scheer T, Stier-Bruck I, Scharrer I. ADAM TS-13 activity in patients with brain and prostate tumors is mildly reduced, but not correlated to stage of malignancy and metastasis. Thromb Res. 2003;111:33–7.

38. Manucci PM, Capoferri C, Canciani MT. Plasma levels of von Willebrand factor regulate ADAMTS-13, its major cleaving protease. Br J Haematol. 2004;126:213–8.

39. Dent JA, Galbuera M, Ruggeri ZM. Heterogeneity of plasma von Willebrand factor multimers resulting from proteolysis of the constituent subunit. J Clin Invest. 1991;88:774–82.

40. Papalambrosm E, Sigala F, Travlou A. P-selectin and antibodies against heparin-platelet factor 4 in patients with venous or arterial disease after a 7-day heparin treatment. J Am Coll Cardiol. 2004;199:69–77.

41. Ay C, Simanek R, Vormittag R, et al. High plasma levels of soluble P-selectin are predictive of venous thromboembolism in cancer patients: results from the Vienna Cancer and Thrombosis Study (CATS). Blood. 2008;112:2703–8.

42. Ramacciotti E, Blackburn S, Hawley AE, et al. Evaluation of soluble P-selectin as a marker for the diagnosis of deep vein thrombosis. Clin Appl Thromb Hemost. 2011;17:425–31.

43. Zheng XL. Structure-function and regulation of ADAMTS-13 protease. J Thromb Haemost. 2013;11(suppl 1):11–23.

44. Schwartz T, Hingorani A, Ascher E, et al. Pulmonary embolism without deep venous thrombosis. Ann Vasc Surg. 2012;26:973–6.

21

Frequency of deep vein thrombosis at admission for acute stroke and associated factors

Takahisa Mori[1*] ⓘ, Kazuhiro Yoshioka[1] and Yuhei Tanno[1,2]

Abstract

Background: Intermittent pneumatic compression (IPC) is commonly used to prevent deep vein thrombosis (DVT) during hospitalization in patients with acute stroke. However, if DVT exists at admission, IPC of the legs with DVT may cause migration of the thrombi, resulting in pulmonary emboli. Whole-leg ultrasonography (wl-US) is a practical tool to detect DVT; however, wl-US is not always performed at admission in all stroke patients. This retrospective cross-sectional study aimed to investigate DVT frequency and identify significant factors indicating the presence of DVT at admission for acute stroke.

Methods: We included patients admitted within 24 h of stroke onset between 2017 and 2019. Patients who did not undergo blood tests for D-dimer or wl-US within 72 h of arrival were excluded. We collected patient data on age; sex; anthropometric variables; presence of DVT on wl-US; and biomarkers such as D-dimer, high-sensitivity C-reactive protein (hs-CRP), and lipids.

Results: Of 1129 acute stroke patients, 917 met our inclusion criteria. DVT was detected in 161 patients (17.6 %). Patients with DVT were older; were more likely to be female; had lower body weight; had higher D-dimer and hs-CRP levels; had lower albumin, hemoglobin, and triglyceride levels; and had higher National Institutes of Health Stroke Scale and pre-stroke modified Rankin scale scores than patients without DVT ($n = 756$). In addition, multiple logistic regression analysis showed that sex (female) and D-dimer levels (≥ 1.52 µg/mL) were independent significant factors for the presence of DVT. Among 161 patients with DVT, 78 (48.4 %) had both these significant factors. Among 756 patients without DVT, 602 (79.6 %) had no or one significant factor. The odds ratio of the presence of DVT in patients with both significant factors was 6.29, using patients without any significant factors as the group for comparison.

Conclusions: The frequency of DVT is high in acute stroke patients at admission. Female sex and a high D-dimer level were independent significant factors for the presence of DVT. Therefore, in patients with these two significant factors at admission, IPC should be avoided or wl-US should be performed before IPC.

Keywords: Deep vein thrombosis, D-dimer, Frequency, Intermittent pneumatic compression, Stroke, Ultrasonography

* Correspondence: morit-koc@umin.net
[1]Department of Stroke Treatment, Shonan Kamakura General Hospital, Okamoto 1370-1, 247-8533 Kamakura City, Kanagawa, Japan
Full list of author information is available at the end of the article

Background

Venous thromboembolism (VT) is a common cause of death and morbidity in patients with acute stroke during hospitalization [1]. Anticoagulants reduce the frequency of pulmonary emboli due to VT; however, this benefit is offset by an increase in the frequency of extracranial hemorrhage [2]. In addition, anticoagulants cannot be administered to patients with hemorrhagic stroke. Therefore, intermittent pneumatic compression (IPC) is commonly used to reduce the risk of deep vein thrombosis (DVT) during hospitalization [3]. A DVT frequency of 8.0 or 8.7 % at admission was reported from Polish institutions [4, 5]; however, the DVT frequency at admission has been unknown in Japan. If the DVT frequency is high in Japan and IPC of the legs with DVT is started in patients with DVT at the time of admission, IPC may cause migration or fragmentation of thrombi and lead to pulmonary embolism. During hospitalization, D-dimer levels are often elevated in patients with DVT [6]. Whole-leg ultrasonography (wl-US) is a practical tool to detect DVT in outpatients or inpatients [7]. wl-US or D-dimer measurement should always be performed for detecting DVT at admission for stroke; however, wl-US is not routinely performed at admission in many facilities. Therefore, a practical index to estimate the presence of DVT at stroke admission is necessary. Our retrospective cross-sectional study aimed to investigate DVT frequency at admission and identify significant factors specific to the presence of DVT at admission for acute stroke.

Methods

To investigate DVT frequency at admission and identify related factors, we included patients admitted within 24 h of stroke onset between March 2017 and March 2019. We excluded patients whose plasma D-dimer level was not examined within 24 h of arrival or in whom whole-leg US was not performed within 72 h of arrival. We collected patient data on age, sex, anthropometric variables, and US findings of DVT. We evaluated biomarkers such as hemoglobin (Hb), serum albumin (Alb), high-sensitivity C-reactive protein (hs-CRP), glucose, HbA1c, total cholesterol, high-density lipoprotein cholesterol, triglycerides (TG), aspartate aminotransferase (AST), alanine aminotransferase (ALT), AST/ALT ratio, and plasma D-dimer. In addition, we evaluated the National Institutes of Health Stroke Scale (NIHSS) score [8] and pre-stroke modified Rankin scale (mRS) score at admission [9]. The low-density lipoprotein cholesterol concentration was calculated using the Friedewald formula: low-density lipoprotein cholesterol = total cholesterol – high-density lipoprotein cholesterol – TG/5. D-dimer levels were measured using latex turbidimetric immunoassay (LIAS AUTO D-Dimer NEO, Sysmex Co.,

Hyogo, Japan) [10]. DVT was diagnosed according to the findings of wl-US (Xario, Canon Medical Systems Co., Tochigi, Japan), performed by trained radiologists [11]. DVT was diagnosed based on the following US findings: presence of a non-compressible segment or flow impairment on color Doppler imaging [12]. Compression was performed at 2 cm intervals.

Statistical analysis

Non-normally distributed continuous variables are expressed as medians and interquartile ranges. We compared all possible pairs of variables with significant differences between patients with and without DVT. A dummy variable was used to represent categorical data, such as data on sex, and Spearman rank correlation coefficient (r_s) was calculated to measure the strength of the relationships. We defined $0 \leq |r_s| < 0.1$ as no correlation, $0.1 \leq |r_s| < 0.4$ as a weak correlation, $0.4 \leq |r_s| < 0.6$ as a moderate correlation, and $0.6 \leq |r_s|$ as a strong correlation. Multicollinearity was defined as the presence of a moderate or strong correlation between variables. When variables were moderately or strongly correlated with one another, we adopted the variable with a larger chi-squared value. After excluding variables with multicollinearity, we conducted a multiple logistic regression analysis to identify independent variables indicating the presence of DVT. We estimated the threshold values of independent variables indicating the presence of DVT using area under the curve values derived from the receiver operating characteristic curves of the logistic regression model. Statistical significance was set at a P-value < 0.05. We used JMP software (version 16.0; SAS Institute, Cary, NC, USA) for all statistical analyses.

Results

During the study period, 1129 acute stroke patients were admitted, and 917 met our inclusion criteria. Patient characteristics are summarized in Table 1. DVT was detected in 161 (17.6 %) of 917 patients at admission. Patients with DVT ($n = 161$) were older; were more likely to be female; had lower body weight; had higher plasma D-dimer and hs-CRP levels; had lower Hb, serum Alb, TG, and ALT levels; had a higher AST/ALT ratio; and had higher NIHSS and pre-stroke mRS scores than patients without DVT ($n = 756$) (Table 2). After excluding variables with significant differences between the two groups and variables with multicollinearity (Additional file 1), multiple logistic regression analysis showed that sex and D-dimer levels were independent variables for the presence of DVT (Table 3). Receiver operating characteristic curves demonstrated that female sex and a D-dimer level of ≥ 1.52 µg/mL were independent factors for the presence of DVT at the time of stroke admission (Table 4). Among 161 patients with DVT, 78 (48.4 %)

Table 1 Patient characteristics

Variables	Values
N	917
DVT, n (%)	161 (17.6 %)
Ischemic stroke, n (%)	734 (80.0 %)
Female sex, n (%)	449 (49.0 %)
Age, years	80 (71, 86)
BMI, kg/m²	22.0 (19.5, 24.4)
BW, kg	55 (47, 65)
Hb, g/dL	13.3 (12, 14.6)
Plt, /μL	20.8 (17.1, 25.5)
Alb, mg/dL	3.9 (3.6, 4.2)
AST, U/L	23 (19, 29)
ALT, U/L	16 (12, 23)
AST/ALT ratio	1.4 (1.1, 1.8)
Glucose, mg/dL	122 (105, 151)
HbA1c, % (NGSP)	5.8 (5.5, 6.4)
TC, mg/dL	196 (168, 225)
LDL, mg/dL	110 (85, 134)
HDL, mg/dL	56.2 (46.1, 68.4)
TG, mg/dL	93 (65, 136)
hs-CRP, mg/dL	0.14 (0.05, 0.53)
D-dimer, μg/mL	1.4 (0.7, 3.1)
NIHSS at admission	5 (2, 16)
Pre-stroke mRS	0 (0, 3)

All values except for categorical data are represented as median (interquartile range)

Abbreviations: ALT alanine aminotransferase, *AST* aspartate aminotransferase, *BW* body weight, *HDL* high-density lipoprotein cholesterol, *hs-CRP* high-sensitivity C-reactive protein, *DVT* deep vein thrombosis, *LDL* low-density lipoprotein cholesterol, *mRS* modified Rankin scale score, *NGSP* National Glycohemoglobin Standardization Program, *N* number, *NIHSS* National Institutes of Health Stroke Scale, *TC* total cholesterol, *TG* triglyceride

had both these significant factors. Among 756 patients without DVT, 602 (79.6 %) had no or one significant factor. The odds of the presence of DVT was 0.506 in patients with both significant factors, 0.182 in patients with one significant factor, and 0.081 in patients without any significant factors. On using patients without any significant factors as the group for comparison, the odds ratio of the presence of DVT was 6.29 in patients with both significant factors (Table 5).

Discussion

Our results demonstrated that DVT was present in 17.6 % of acute stroke patients at admission, and female sex and a high D-dimer level were significant factors indicating the presence of DVT at admission. The odds ratio of the presence of DVT in patients with both significant factors was 6.29. Therefore, in patients with

both these significant factors at admission, IPC should be avoided or wl-US should be performed before IPC.

wl-US has been shown to have high sensitivity (94.0 %) and specificity (97.3 %) for detecting DVT [7]. However, wl-US is not always performed for stroke patients in most facilities. In contrast, D-dimer levels can be measured easily in any institution. A cut-off value of 0.5 μg/mL for D-dimer levels showed a sensitivity of 82.9 % and specificity of 32.7 % for detecting DVT in patients during hospitalization [6]. Furthermore, our results demonstrated that D-dimer was a significant factor for the presence of DVT at stroke admission. Therefore, D-dimer levels should be examined routinely at stroke admission.

According to previous studies, DVT was found on day 3 after stroke onset in 8.0 % of acute stroke patients and within 7 days of stroke onset in 8.7 % of acute stroke patients in Polish institutions [4, 5]. In comparison, the DVT frequency was high in our study at 17.5 %; this may be because our patients were older than those in previous studies, and US was performed within 72 h of arrival in our patients, compared to the performance of US within 7 days of stroke onset in a previous study [4, 5]. Female sex, elevated CRP levels, and pre-stroke disability were risk factors for DVT within 7 days of stroke onset, and elevated CRP and pre-stroke disability were independent risk factors for the presence of DVT [5]. However, D-dimer was not examined in the previous study [5]. Elevated CRP levels and pre-stroke disability were also found to be significant factors for the presence of DVT in our patients (Table 2). However, they were not independent because of multicollinearity.

The incidence of DVT has been reported to be approximately 50 % within 2 weeks in the absence of heparin prophylaxis in patients with acute hemiplegic stroke [13]. Patients with proximal subclinical DVT had a 15 % risk of fatal pulmonary embolism [13, 14]. Untreated below-knee DVT is associated with a 20 % risk of proximal extension [13], and the pulmonary embolism rate is reportedly 6.1 % in trauma patients with below-knee DVT [15]. On admission to the stroke rehabilitation unit, the prevalence of DVT in patients with stroke ranges from 12 to 40 % [16]. Therefore, the onset of DVT during hospitalization in primary stroke centers must be prevented. When DVT is not detected at admission, IPC can be used safely. If DVT is detected at admission in patients with ischemic stroke, anticoagulants may be started soon. The disuse of IPC may not induce thrombi fragmentation in patients with DVT at admission. Early anticoagulant therapy may protect against thromboembolism caused by DVT present at admission, and early IPC or anticoagulant therapy may prevent DVT development after admission. Overall, the frequency of symptomatic or critical DVT may decrease

Table 2 Comparison of variables between the two groups

	Patients with DVT	Patients without DVT	Chi-square value	P-value
N	161	756		
Ischemic stroke, n (%)	132 (82.0 %)	602 (79.6 %)	0.5	0.4924
Female sex, n (%)	106 (65.8 %)	343 (45.4 %)	22.4	< 0.0001
Age, years	82 (77, 89)	79 (71, 86)	21.0	< 0.0001
BMI, kg/m²	21.5 (19.1, 23.7)	22.1 (19.6, 24.5)	3.6	0.0569
BW, kg	52 (44, 60)	56 (47, 65)	11.5	0.0007
Hb, g/dL	12.6 (11.5, 13.8)	13.4 (12.3, 13.9)	21.3	< 0.0001
Plt, /µL	20.5 (17.1, 25.5)	20.9 (17.2, 25.7)	0.2	0.6772
Alb, mg/dL	3.7 (3.4, 4.1)	4.0 (3.7, 4.2)	25.7	< 0.0001
AST, U/L	22 (19, 31)	23 (19, 28)	0.0	0.9744
ALT, U/L	15 (12, 21)	17 (12, 23)	6.3	0.0123
AST/ALT ratio	1.53 (1.22, 1.87)	1.38 (1.13, 1.73)	10.7	0.0011
Glucose, mg/dL	122 (106, 149)	123 (105, 153)	0.4	0.5314
HbA1c, % (NGSP)	5.8 (5.5, 6.3)	5.8 (5.5, 6.4)	0.2	0.6810
TC, mg/dL	194 (159, 226)	197 (170, 224)	0.3	0.5873
LDL, mg/dL	110 (82, 131)	111 (87, 135)	1.2	0.2794
HDL, mgl/dL	56.7 (44.3, 71.7)	55.8 (46.2, 68.2)	0.1	0.7125
TG, mg/dL	82 (61, 123)	95 (66, 141)	4.8	0.0279
hs-CRP, mg/dL	0.17 (0.07, 0.77)	0.13 (0.05, 0.47)	6.6	0.0103
D-dimer, µg/mL	2.7 (1.3, 6.0)	1.2 (0.6, 2.6)	60.2	< 0.0001
NIHSS at admission	8 (3,18)	5 (2,15)	12.3	0.0004
Pre-stroke mRS	2 (0, 3.5)	0 (0, 3)	16.1	< 0.0001

All values except for categorical data are represented as median (interquartile range)

Alb albumin, *ALT* alanine aminotransferase, *AST* aspartate aminotransferase, *BMI* body mass index, *BW* body weight, *Hb* hemoglobin, *HDL* high-density lipoprotein cholesterol, *hs-CRP* high-sensitivity C-reactive protein, *DVT* deep vein thrombosis, *LDL* low-density lipoprotein cholesterol, *mRS* modified Rankin scale score, *N* number, *NGSP* National Glycohemoglobin Standardization Program, *NIHSS* National Institutes of Health Stroke Scale, *P* probability, *Plt* platelet, *TC* total cholesterol, *TG* triglyceride

during hospitalization in primary stroke centers. Plasma D-dimer levels must be measured at the time of stroke, and patients with both significant factors, i.e., female sex and a D-dimer level ≥ 1.52 µg/mL, should immediately undergo wl-US, if possible.

Table 3 Multiple logistic regression for deep vein thrombosis presence at the admission of stroke using receiver operating characteristics curves

	Odds ratio	P-value	AUC	BIC
		< 0.0001	0.687	774
Sex	2.04 (1.40–3.00)	0.0002		
D-dimer	1.05 (1.02–1.08)	0.0003		
TG	1.00 (0.99–1.00)	0.0560		
hs-CRP	1.08 (0.99–1.17)	0.0680		
ALT	0.99 (0.98–1.00)	0.2479		
NIHSS	1.01 (0.99–1.03)	0.2698		

ALT alanine aminotransferase, *AUC* area under the curve, *BIC* Bayesian information criterion, *hs-CRP* high-sensitivity C-reactive protein, *NIHSS* National Institutes of Health Stroke Scale at admission, *P* probability, *TG* triglyceride

Limitations

Our study had several limitations. First, the sample size was small, and the study had a retrospective, cross-sectional design. Second, although US has a sensitivity of 94 % for detecting DVT, it cannot always detect DVT. Third, because most of the patients were Japanese, generalization of the study outcomes to non-Japanese populations may not be possible. There might be racial differences in the association between DVT-related factors and threshold values of factors associated with the

Table 4 Threshold values for DVT presence using receiver operating characteristics curves from logistic regression analysis

	Sens (%)	Spec (%)	Odds ratio	P-value	AUC	BIC
Sex (1 vs. < 1)	65.8	54.5	2.31 (1.62–3.31)	< 0.0001	0.602	843
D-dimer (≥ 1.52 vs. < 1.52) µg/mL	70.0	59.6	1.06 (1.03–1.09)	< 0.0001	0.695	836

AUC area under the curve, *BIC* Bayesian information criterion, *DVT* deep vein thrombosis, *P* probability, *Sens* sensitivity, *Spec* specificity, *TG* triglyceride

Table 5 Cross tabulation table between patients with significant factors, DVT, Odds, and Odds ratio

	DVT presence	DVT absence	Odds	Odds ratio
N	161	756		
Patients with the two significant factors	78	154	0.5065	6.29
Patients with one significant factor	62	341	0.1818	2.26
Patients without any significant factors	21	261	0.0805	

The two significant factors are female sex and D-dimer ≥ 1.52 μg/mL
DVT deep vein thrombosis, N number

presence of DVT. A prospective study including US and plasma D-dimer examination is required to determine the frequency of DVT at stroke admission and significant associated factors.

Conclusions

The frequency of DVT at admission in acute stroke patients was high at 17.6 % in our institution. Female sex and high D-dimer levels were significant factors for the presence of DVT. Therefore, in patients with these two significant factors at admission, IPC should be avoided or wl-US should be performed before IPC.

Abbreviations

Alb: Albumin; ALT: Alanine aminotransferase; AST: Aspartate aminotransferase; DVT: Deep vein thrombosis; hs-CRP: High-sensitivity C-reactive protein; IPC: Intermittent pneumatic compression; mRS: Modified Rankin scale; NIHSS: National Institutes of Health Stroke Scale; US: Ultrasonography; VT: Venous thromboembolism; wl-US: Whole-leg ultrasonography

Acknowledgements

We would like to thank Nozomi Chiba, BA., for her secretarial assistance and the ultrasonographers at our stroke center for specialized support.

Authors' contributions

Conceptualization: T.M. Methodology: T.M. Validation: T.M. Formal analysis: T.M. Investigation: T.M., K.Y., Y.T. Resources: T.M., K.Y., Y.T. Data curation: T.M., K.Y., Y.T. Writing–original draft preparation: T.M. Writing–review and editing: T.M. Visualization: T.M. All authors have read and agreed to the published version of the manuscript.

Author details

[1]Department of Stroke Treatment, Shonan Kamakura General Hospital, Okamoto 1370-1, 247-8533 Kamakura City, Kanagawa, Japan. [2]Department of Neurology, Nakatsugawa Municipal General Hospital, Komaba 1522-1, Gifu 508-8502 Nakatsugawa City, Japan.

References

1. House of Commons Health Committee. The prevention of venous thromboembolism in hospitalised patients. Second Report of Session 2004–05, HC 99. London: Stationery Office; 2005.
2. Sandercock PA, Counsell C, Kamal AK. Anticoagulants for acute ischaemic stroke. Cochrane Database Syst Rev. 2008:CD000024. https://doi.org/10.1002/14651858.CD000024.pub3.
3. CLOTS (Clots in Legs Or sTockings after Stroke) Trials Collaboration. Effectiveness of intermittent pneumatic compression in reduction of risk of deep vein thrombosis in patients who have had a stroke (CLOTS 3): a multicentre randomised controlled trial. Lancet. 2013;382:516–24.
4. Bembenek J, Karlinski M, Kobayashi A, Czlonkowska A. Early stroke-related deep venous thrombosis: risk factors and influence on outcome. J Thromb Thrombolysis. 2011;32:96–102.
5. Bembenek JP, Karlinski M, Kobayashi A, Czlonkowska A. Deep venous thrombosis in acute stroke patients. Clin Appl Thromb Hemost. 2012;18:258–64.
6. Canan A, Halicioglu SS, Gurel S. Mean platelet volume and D-dimer in patients with suspected deep venous thrombosis. J Thromb Thrombolysis. 2012;34:283–7.
7. Bhatt M, Braun C, Patel P, Patel P, Begum H, Wiercioch W, et al. Diagnosis of deep vein thrombosis of the lower extremity: a systematic review and meta-analysis of test accuracy. Blood Adv. 2020;4:1250–64.
8. Lyden P, Brott T, Tilley B, Welch KM, Mascha EJ, Levine S, et al. Improved reliability of the NIH Stroke Scale using video training. NINDS TPA Stroke Study Group. Stroke. 1994;25:2220–6.
9. van Swieten JC, Koudstaal PJ, Visser MC, Schouten HJ, van Gijn J. Interobserver agreement for the assessment of handicap in stroke patients. Stroke. 1988;19:604–7.
10. Suzuki H, Masaki Y, Okubo M, Yotsui S, Ogura M, Imanishi K, et al. A comparative study of Sysmex Latex Test BL-2 P-FDP and LIAS AUTO D-Dimer NEO with similar assay reagents of two other companies on the fully automated blood coagulation analyzer CS-5100. Sysmex J Int. 2014;24. https://www.sysmex.co.jp/en/products_solutions/library/journal/vol24_no1/vol24_1_10.pdf .
11. Konstantinides SV, Torbicki A, Agnelli G, Danchin N, Fitzmaurice D, Galie N, et al. 2014 ESC guidelines on the diagnosis and management of acute pulmonary embolism. Eur Heart J. 2014;35:3033–69, 3069a–3069k.
12. Needleman L, Cronan JJ, Lilly MP, Merli GJ, Adhikari S, Hertzberg BS, et al. Ultrasound for lower extremity deep venous thrombosis: multidisciplinary recommendations from the Society of Radiologists in Ultrasound Consensus Conference. Circulation. 2018;137:1505-15.
13. Kelly J, Rudd A, Lewis R, Hunt BJ. Venous thromboembolism after acute stroke. Stroke. 2001;32:262–7.
14. Khan MT, Ikram A, Saeed O, Afridi T, Sila CA, Smith MS, et al. Deep vein thrombosis in acute stroke - a systemic review of the literature. Cureus. 2017;9:e1982.
15. Olson EJ, Zander AL, Van Gent JM, Shackford SR, Badiee J, Sise CB, et al. Below-knee deep vein thrombosis: an opportunity to prevent pulmonary embolism? J Trauma Acute Care Surg. 2014;77:459–63.
16. Wilson RD, Murray PK. Cost-effectiveness of screening for deep vein thrombosis by ultrasound at admission to stroke rehabilitation. Arch Phys Med Rehabil. 2005;86:1941–8.

22

A thrombophilia family with protein S deficiency due to protein translation disorders caused by a Leu607Ser heterozygous mutation in *PROS1*

Yan-ping Zhang[1,2†], Bin Lin[1,2†], Yuan-yuan Ji[1,2†], Ya-nan Hu[1,2†], Xin-fu Lin[1,3†], Yi Tang[1,2], Jian-hui Zhang[1,2], Shao-jie Wu[1,2], Sen-lin Cai[1,2], Yan-feng Zhou[1,2], Ting Chen[1,2*], Zhu-ting Fang[1,2*] and Jie-wei Luo[1,4*] [iD]

Abstract

Background: Protein S deficiency (PSD) is an autosomal dominant hereditary disease. In 1984, familial PSD was reported to be prone to recurrent thrombosis. Follow-up studies have shown that heterozygous protein S (*PROS1*) mutations increase the risk of thrombosis. More than 300 *PROS1* mutations have been identified; among them, only a small number of mutations have been reported its possible mechanism to reduce plasma protein S (PS) levels. However, whether *PROS1* mutations affect protein structure and why it can induce PSD remains unknown.

Methods: The clinical phenotypes of the members of a family with thrombosis were collected. Their PS activity was measured using the coagulation method, whereas their protein C and antithrombin III activities were measured using methods such as the chromogenic substrate method. The proband and her parents were screened for the responsible mutation using second-generation whole exon sequencing, and the members of the family were verified for suspected mutations using Sanger sequencing. Mutant and wild type plasmids were constructed and transfected into HEK293T cells to detect the mRNA and protein expression of *PROS1*.

Results: In this family, the proband with venous thrombosis of both lower extremities, the proband's mother with pulmonary embolism and venous thrombosis of both lower extremities, and the proband's younger brother had significantly lower PS activity and carried a *PROS1* c. 1820 T > C:p.Leu607Ser heterozygous mutation (NM_000313.3). However, no such mutations were found in family members with normal PS activity. The PS expression in the cell lysate and supernatant of the Leu607Ser mutant cells decreased, while mRNA expression increased. Immunofluorescence localization showed that there was no significant difference in protein localization before and after mutation.

* Correspondence: cttc1990@126.com; 470389481@qq.com; docluo0421@aliyun.com
†Yan-ping Zhang, Bin Lin, Yuan-yuan Ji, Ya-nan Hu and Xin-fu Lin contributed equally to this work.
[1]Shengli Clinical Medical College of Fujian Medical University, Fuzhou 350001, China
Full list of author information is available at the end of the article

Conclusions: The analysis of family phenotype, gene association, and cell function tests suggest that the *PROS1* Leu607Ser heterozygous mutation may be a pathogenic mutation. Serine substitution causes structural instability of the entire protein. These data indicate that impaired PS translation and synthesis or possible secretion impairment is the main pathogenesis of this family with hereditary PSD and thrombophilia.

Keywords: Protein S, Deficiency, PROS1, Mutation, Vein thrombosis

Background

Protein S (PS) is a vitamin K-dependent plasma glycoprotein that is mainly synthesized by hepatocytes or macrophages [1]. Forty percent of PS is free and has anticoagulant activity, while 60% of PS is bound to C4b and has no activity [2]. On the one hand, PS exerts an anticoagulant effect mainly by serving as a cofactor of activated protein C (APC) to promote the inactivation of factor V (FV) a and FVIIIa [3]. On the other hand, PS also serves as a cofactor of tissue factor pathway inhibitor (TFPI), which inhibits the activity of tissue factors by promoting the binding interaction of TFPI and FXa [4]. Hereditary protein S deficiency (PSD) is an autosomal dominant hereditary disease, which may be caused by genetic and acquired factors [5]. It is classified into three subtypes: Type I (total PS, free PS levels, and PS activity are decreased), type II (total PS and free PS levels are normal, but PS activity is decreased), and type III (total PS level is normal, but free PS level and PS activity are decreased) [6]. There is no significant difference among these three types of clinical manifestations, which are only identified by laboratory testing; 95% of patients with PSD develop type I and type III PSD [7].

As of September 6, 2021, there are more than 360 mutations in PSD-related genes in the Human Gene Mutation Database (HGMD) (http://www.hgmd.org). There are 276 types of missense/nonsense, 48 types of splicing, 4 types of regulatory, 54 types of small deletions, 25 types of small insertions, 6 types of small indels, 28 types of gross deletions, 7 types of gross insertions, as well as complex repeats that have not yet been identified. The most common causes of PSD are missense or nonsense substitutions, followed by splice site mutations, small or large repeats, insertions, or deletions [8]. The main clinical manifestations of most patients with heterozygous mutations in the protein S gene *(PROS1)* are lower extremity deep venous thrombosis and pulmonary embolism [9]. *PROS1* mutations are associated with an increased risk of venous thrombosis [10], and some reports suggest that *PROS1* variants increase the risk of arterial embolism, such as cerebral infarction and myocardial infarction [11]. About half of patients with PSD develop symptoms before the age of 55, while some of them have no complications for the rest of their lives [12]. In the past, we detected a new mutation in *PROS1* in a family prone to thrombosis,

which had not been previously reported. In this study, we discuss the pathogenicity and pathogenesis of this mutation.

Materials and methods
Research subjects

The 16-year-old female proband (III5), of Han nationality, complained of "swelling and pain in the left lower limb for 3 days". She was in good health and had no bad lifestyle-related habits, such as, smoking, drinking etc. Among the family members, her mother (II8) had a history of bilateral deep venous thrombosis of the lower extremities and pulmonary embolism, and her parents were from non-consanguineous marriages. Physical examination showed that the left lower limb of the proband had edema, especially on the dorsal foot, shank, and thigh. There were no obvious varicose veins, hyperpigmentation, skin ulceration, palpable nodules, or deep vein tenderness with a positive Homan's sign. The circumference of both lower limbs was measured and was as follows: 15 cm above the left patella, 44 cm; 15 cm above the right patella, 39 cm; 15 cm below the left patella, 39 cm; and 15 cm below the right patella, 36 cm.

At the age of 39, II8 had complained of "distension and pain of the left lower limb for 2 days" in another hospital. She was in good health and had no special bad habits. Physical examination revealed swelling of the left lower limb. She was diagnosed with "deep venous thrombosis of the left lower limb" and was treated with anticoagulation and thrombolysis. After that, she improved and was discharged from the hospital and took anticoagulants regularly for a long time. A year ago, she visited the hospital again due to "sudden chest pain with loss of consciousness" and was diagnosed with "pulmonary embolism." .

Methods
Clinical phenotype detection

Clinical phenotypes and clinical biochemical indicators were collected from the proband and her related family members. Clinical biochemical indexes included PS activity, as measured using the coagulation method. Its principle is that protein C can hydrolyze coagulation factors VA and VIIIa in the coagulation waterfall reaction activated by RVV. The extension of coagulation time can reflect the activity of PS in the sample. The coagulation time of patients can calculate the content of free PS (FPS) from the standard curve. The sample must be centrifuged twice to remove platelets from the plasma sample (platelets in the plasma should be less than 10×10^9 / L) and frozen for inspection. The operation was performed according to the protein S kit instructions and completed by KingMed Diagnostics (Guangzhou, China). The activity of protein C (PC) and antithrombin III (AT), as measured using the chromogenic substrate method, blood routine, coagulation function, and biochemistry. FPS: Ag and TPS: Ag were used ELISA method (KingMed Diagnostics, Guangzhou, China) to measure.

Extraction of genomic DNA
Peripheral blood (8 mL) of the proband and peripheral blood (2 mL) of each family member were collected in ethylenediaminetetraacetic acid anticoagulant tubes, and genomic DNA of the proband and her family members was extracted using the QIAGEN DNA Blood Mini Kit (Cat# 51106, QIAGEN Co. Ltd., Shanghai, China).

Location and screening strategy of mutant genes
The TargetSeq® liquid probe hybridization and capture technique independently developed by Igen iGeneTech® (Beijing, China) was used to establish a genomic DNA library and capture the promoter and exon regions (16.06 Mbp) of 5,081 genes related to genetic diseases. Paired end 150 bp sequencing was performed using the Illumina X10 or NovaSeq 6000 platform. The captured target genes were *PROS1* and Serpin family C member 1 (*SERPINC1*). Based on the results of BAM alignment with the genome reference sequence, single-nucleotide variants and indels in the samtools, GATK, and ANNO-VAR sequencing results were used to remove the variation sites with intermediate frequency higher than 0.01 in ExAC, gnomAD, iGeneTechDB (local database with more than 10,000 samples), benign and likely benign mutations in ClinVar, and synonymous_variant mutations in the Human Genome Variation Society. Combined with the exon sequencing data of the parents, the sources of mutation were annotated and divided into three types: those from the father, from the mother, and suspected to be new mutations. The Hemostasis Thrombosis Expert Panel of the OMIM Phenotypic Series-PS188050 and CLINGENE were used to search for genes. Mutations from the father were excluded (the mutations from the mother and the suspected new mutations were retained), and two mutations in *SERPINC1* and *PROS1* were obtained. Sorting Intolerant from Tolerant (SIFT, http://sift.jcvi.org/), Polymorphism Phenotyping (PolyPhen-2, http://genetics.Bwh.harvard.edu/pPH2/) and Mutation Taster (http://mutationtaster.org/) were used to predict the pathogenicity and harmfulness of the mutations. The upper and downstream positions of the sequence of the target mutation site were designed using Premier 5.0, and the target area was amplified. The corresponding suspected pathogenic mutations were verified by Sanger sequencing using the ABI3500Dx platform. The amplified fragment length of c. 1820 T > C:p, the Leu607Ser sequence of the mutation point in *PROS1* (NM_000313.3), was 498 bp. The primers F: CTGGCTGGGATAGCCAAATGA and R: CTTGCT TATATTGAATCTTTGCTCTGC were used for amplification (melting temperature, 62.5 °C). The amplified fragment length of c.883G > A:p, the Val295Met sequence of *SERPINC1* (NM_000488.3), was 407 bp. The primers F: CTTGCAGCTGCTCCTTCAAACT and R: TGTCTTGT GTCAATAACTATCCTCCTA were used for amplification (melting temperature, 61 °C). Synbio Technologies Co., Ltd. (Suzhou, China) synthesized all primers.

Construction and identification of *PROS1* wild type (WT) and p.Leu607Ser mutant plasmids
The plasmid synthesis scheme pcDNA3.1–3 × Flag-C was used as the expression vector to synthesize *PROS1* with a KpnI/XhoI cleavage site. The WT plasmid 1 (pcDNA 3.1-PROS1WT-3 × Flag-C) and the mutant plasmid 2 (pcDNA3.1-PROS1mut-3 × Flag-C) were constructed, both with a KpnI/XhoI restriction enzyme site. The mutant plasmid 2 contained the 1820 T > C mutation in *PROS1*. Target genes were amplified and sequenced. The cloning of *PROS1* (WT) and *PROS1* (1820 T > C) and the synthesis of related polymerase chain reaction (PCR) primers were performed by Wuhan Gene Create Biological Engineering Co. Ltd.(Wuhan, China).

Cell transfection
HEK293T cells were digested and collected using trypsin, and the cells were placed into a 10 cm petri dish at a density of $1–2 \times 10^7$ cells/plate in an appropriate complete culture medium. After adhesion, the total area of the cells reached 80–90% confluence. According to the conditions of cell adhesion, cells were incubated at 37 °C in an incubator containing 5% CO_2 for 8–24 h, and transient transfection was started after the cells were completely adhered. According to the instructions for TurboFect (R0531, Thermo, Massachusetts, USA), TurboFect-DNA Mix was prepared and mixed with DNA plasmids (10 µg/*PROS1* WT, mutant, or control plasmid + 5 µg green fluorescent protein [GFP]) and 30 µL TurboFect in 1000 µL Opti-Medium. After incubation at room temperature for 15 min, TurboFect-DNA Mix was added to the petri dish. After 12 h, the complete medium was changed, and HEK293T cells were cultured for 48 h. Cells were observed to be in good condition by microscopy and the culture medium was collected for further evaluation.

Quantitative real-time (qRT)-PCR detection

HEK293T total RNA was extracted according to the TriPure Isolation Reagent kit (11,667,165,001, Roche, Shanghai, China), and the difference in the *PROS1* transcription levels was detected by reverse transcription and qRT-PCR. The first chain of cDNA was synthesized according to HiFiScript (CW2020M, CWBIO, Beijing, China). The reaction system contained 2.5 mM dNTP Mix, 4 µL; primer mix, 2 µL (primers in Table 1); RNA Template, 7 µL; 5× RT Buffer, 4 µL; 1× dithiothreitol, 0.1 M, 2 µL; 10 mM HiFiScript, 200 U/µL; and RNase-free water, 20 µL. After mixing the liquid using a vortexer, the tube was centrifuged for a short time. The product was incubated at 42 °C for 50 min and at 85 °C for 5 min. The cDNA obtained by reverse transcription was diluted 20-fold, and 40 RT-qPCR cycles were performed in a Roche LightCycler 480 (Roche, Beijing, China).

Western blot detection

HEK293T cells were cultured, lysed, total protein was extracted, and PROS1 expression was detected. Protein samples were separated using electrophoresis and then wet transferred to a polyvinylidene fluoride (PVDF) membrane, soaked in 5% skim milk prepared in Tris-buffered saline with 0.1% Tween® 20 (TBST), and sealed at room temperature for 1 h. Next, the membrane was washed once and anti-protein S antibody (97,387, Abcam, UK, 1: 500) or actin antibody (ab8227, Abcam, UK, 1: 5000) was added. The Flag antibody (F3165, Sigma, USA, 1:500), diluted with 5% bovine serum albumin (BSA), was added to the membrane overnight at 4 °C, and the membrane was washed thrice. Horseradish peroxidase-labeled secondary antibodies (goat anti-rabbit IgG, 1:2000 or goat anti-mouse IgG 1:2000, diluted with 5% BSA, ab6721 and ab6789, respectively, Abcam, UK) were added to the membrane and then incubated in a shaker at room temperature for 1 h. The PVDF membrane was washed with TBST five times and with ddH$_2$O once before exposure.

Enzyme linked immunosorbent assay (ELISA) of PROS1 in HEK293T cell lysates and cell supernatants

According to the instructions of the Human Protein S ELISA Kit (ab190808, Abcam, UK), the working standard liquid was prepared, and PROS1 expression in HEK293T cell lysates and cell supernatant was detected.

Table 1 Primers for qRT-PCR

hPROS1 qRT F	CCCGGAAACGGATTATTTTT
hPROS1 qRT R	CTCCTTGCCAACCTGGTTTA
hGAPDH F	AGAAGGCTGGGGCTCATTTG
hGAPDH R	AGGGGCCATCCACAGTCTTC
CopGFP qRT F	AGGACAGCGTGATCTTCACC
CopGFP qRT R	CTTGAAGTGCATGTGGCTGT

A microplate reader (Varioskan Lux, Thermo, Massachusetts, USA) was used to measure the optical density at 450 nm immediately after the substrate solution was added to stop the reaction. A standard curve was created and PROS1 levels in the sample were calculated.

Immunofluorescence localization experiment

After being fixed, permeabilized, and blocked, the transfected HEK293T cells were incubated at 4 °C overnight with the PROS1 primary antibody (diluted 1:200). The transfected HEK293T cells were rinsed with phosphate-buffered saline (PBS) thrice, the fluorescent secondary antibody (diluted 1:500) was added and incubated at room temperature in the dark for 2 h, rinsed with PBS thrice, and stained with 4′,6-diamidino-2-phenylindole. The transfected HEK293T cells were incubated at room temperature for 5 min and rinsed twice with 1× PBS for 3 min each time. A laser confocal microscope (Nikon A1, Shanghai, China) was used to capture images.

Statistics

Experimental data were statistically analyzed using GraphPad Prism 6.02. An unpaired *t*-test was used to compare the two groups. The mean value was expressed as the mean ± standard error of the mean (SEM), and $p < 0.05$ indicated that the difference was statistically significant.

Results
Clinical phenotypes

The 16-year-old proband (III5) was examined for blood coagulation function (Table 2). The indices related to blood coagulation had no significant changes. Color Doppler ultrasound of the lower limb vein showed thrombosis of the left external iliac vein and deep vein of the left lower limb. Digital subtraction angiography showed the distal left superficial femoral vein and the left inferior vena cava had thrombosis. PS activity, total protein S (TPS) and free protein S (FPS) was significantly decreased, while the PC and AT activities were normal; thus, it was considered asthrombosis caused by type I PSD. The mother of the proband (II8), 42 years old, had a history of recurrent venous thrombosis. For the first time, when lower limb swelling and pain occurred, Color Doppler ultrasound and Computed tomographic angiography (CTA) indicated thrombosis of the left lower extremities. The second time, when chest pain occurred, CTA showed pulmonary embolism. Color Doppler ultrasound showed that the deep vein of the left lower extremity and the right popliteal vein were partly recanalized after thrombosis. PS activity, TPS and FPS was significantly decreased and the activity of AT and PC was normal, so it was suspected that type I PSD caused thrombosis in II8 many times. The 13-year-old

Table 2 Coagulation function indexs of proband and family members in hereditary protein S deficiency family

Items	Propositus (III5)	Father (II7)	Mother (II8)	Brother (III6)	Member (II1)	Member (II6)	Member (II10)	reference value
PT (s)	13.3	11.2	11.8	12.3	9.8	11.9	12.1	9.9–12.9
APTT (s)	27.9	26.4	28.8	32	27.1	24.3	23.9	23.3–32.5
TT (s)	15.5	15.8	17.0	30.9	17.1	16.4	19.2	14–21
Fg (g/L)	2.57	2.32	2.7	1.9	2.41	2.79	2.34	1.8–3.5
D-dimer	25.8	0.24	13.2	15.5	0.23	0.01	0.01	0–0.55
TPS (mg/L)	67	208	85	71	–	–	–	160–260
FPS (mg/L)	19	66	22	23	–	–	–	48–67
PS(%)	< 16	84.4	< 16	16.7	102.7	97.4	112.3	Male:75–130 Female:52–118
PC(%)	66.9	90.1	100.2	60.2	113.4	124.2	98.1	70–140
AT-III(%)	92	107.6	97.4	85.9	121.2	109.1	97.1	75–125

Note: *PT* prothrombin time; *INR* international normalized ratio; *APTT* activated partial thromboplastin time; *TT* thrombin time; *Fg* fibrinogen; *FDP* fibrin degradation products; *TPS* total protein S; *FPS* free protein S; *PS* protein S; *PC* protein C; *AT* antithrombin III

younger brother of the proband (III6) had no history of thrombosis. His PS activity, TPS and FPS was significantly decreased and the PC and AT activities were normal; thus, he was diagnosed with typeIPSD. The father of II8 (I1) at the age of 63 died of "pulmonary embolism". The older sister of II8 (II3), 45 years old, died of "pulmonary embolism". Another older sister (II4) died of "pulmonary embolism",when she was 49 years old. The father of III5 (II7), 43 years old, was in good health. To date, no thrombosis has been found in other family members (II1, II10, II6, III1, III2, III3, III4, III7, III8). Blood coagulation function of all members are displayed in the Table 2. A pedigree map of the genetic family was drawn (Fig. 1).

Screening for a thrombophilia gene mutation

The members of the family were analyzed by whole exon sequencing, and two mutation sites were identified in proband III5. One was a heterozygous mutation of exon 14 in *PROS1* (NM_000313.3): c.1820 T > C(p.Leu607Ser);

the transformation from TTG to TCG was not recorded in the ClinVar and HGMD databases. Thus, this is a newly discovered mutation, and its pathogenicity is unclear. The other was a heterozygous mutation of exon 3 in *SERPINC1* (NM_000488.3): c.883G > A (p.Val295Met) (rs201381904). This mutation has not been recorded in the ClinVar and HGMD databases, and its pathogenicity is not clear, but the AT plasma levels in the members of this family were normal, which ruled out the diagnosis of hereditary AT deficiency. According to SIFT [13] and PolyPhen-2 [14] scores, the *PROS1* mutation SIFT score is 0, PolyPhen-2 score is 1, and Mutation Tester [15] predicts that protein function is moderately affected. The *SERPINC1* mutation SIFT score was 0.036, and the PolyPhen-2 score was 0.996. The lower the SIFT score, the greater the harm and the closer the PolyPhen-2 score to 1, the stronger the pathogenicity. The *PROS1* L607S heterozygous mutation and *SERPINC1* V295M heterozygous mutation were identified in II8, and a *PROS1* L607S heterozygous mutation was also identified

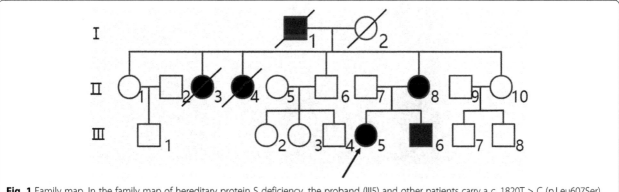

Fig. 1 Family map. In the family map of hereditary protein S deficiency, the proband (III5) and other patients carry a c. 1820T > C (p.Leu607Ser) *PROS1* heterozygous mutation

in III6. Except for the heterozygous mutation V295M carried by II1, there were no L607S and V295M mutations in other family members.

Cloning of PROS1 WT and p.Leu607Ser gene mutations

The *PROS1* WT and *PROS1*/p.Leu607Ser cloning and eukaryotic expression vectors were successfully constructed. Fragments of WT *PROS1* and mutant *PROS1*/p.Leu607Ser digested by KpnI/XhoI were approximately 1138 bp, which was consistent with plasmid design. The constructed vectors were verified by sequencing and transfected successfully into HEK293T cells.

Localization of WT PROS1 and its mutants in cells

The localization of WT and mutant PROS1 was detected by immunofluorescence (Fig. 2), which showed that PROS1 was distributed in the cytoplasm of the cells. There was no significant difference in intracellular fluorescence localization before and after introduction of the *PROS1* 1820 T > C mutation. However, the expression intensity of PROS1 protein after mutation decreased significantly, considering the reduction of PROS1 protein synthesis due to mutation.

Expression of WT *PROS1* and its mutants in HEK293T cells

The relative mRNA expression of the WT (*PROS1*-WT) and p.Leu607Ser mutant (*PROS1*-MUT) *PROS1* in HEK293T cells was detected using qRT-PCR. The difference between the *PROS1* mRNA expression groups was compared to that of actin (Fig. 3b) as an internal reference when there was no significant difference in transfection efficiency among groups (Fig. 3a). *PROS1* mRNA expression was significantly upregulated with the *PROS1* 1820 T > C mutation ($p < 0.05$). GFP was used as an external reference (Fig. 3c) to compare the difference between the *PROS1* mRNA expression between groups. Again *PROS1* mRNA expression was significantly upregulated with the *PROS1* 1820 T > C mutation ($p < 0.01$). PS expression (Fig. 3d) in the cell supernatant and lysate was detected by western blotting. PROS1 expression was significantly downregulated with the mutation. At the same time, PROS1 expression in the supernatant of the cell culture medium and cell lysate was detected using ELISA (Fig. 3e, f). PROS1 expression levels in the culture medium supernatant and cell lysate of the p.Leu607Ser mutant group was significantly lower than that of the WT group, which was consistent with the results of western blotting.

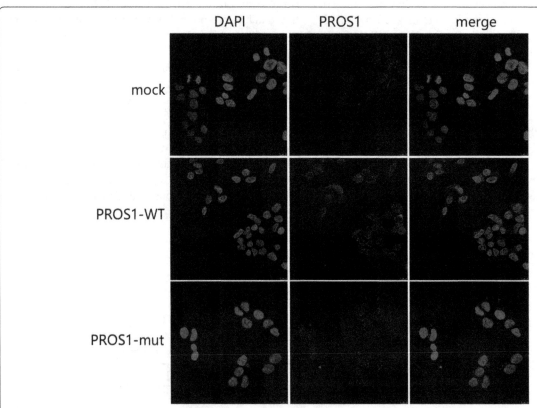

Fig. 2 Localization of protein S (PROS1). Localization of PROS1 mock, wild type (*PROS1*-WT), and the p.Leu607Ser mutation (*PROS1*-M) in HEK293T cells, as detected by immunofluorescence. There is no difference before and after introduction of the *PROS1* 1820T > C mutation. PROS1 expression was obviously downregulated after mutation

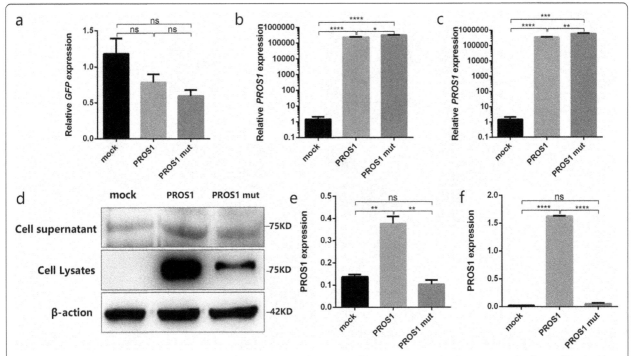

Fig. 3 Relative protein S (PROS1) mRNA and protein expression. (**a**) Relative green fluorescent protein (GFP) expression of cells transfected with mock, wild type (*PROS1*-WT), and the p.Leu607Ser mutation (*PROS1*-M) shows that there is no significant difference in transfection efficiency between the three groups. (**b**) Relative *PROS1* mRNA expression of mock, *PROS1*-WT, and *PROS1*-M in HEK293T cells with glyceraldehyde-3-phosphate dehydrogenase (GAPDH) as an internal reference. (**c**) Relative *PROS1* mRNA expression of mock, *PROS1*-WT, and *PROS1*-M in HEK293T cells using GFP as an external reference. (**d**) PROS1 expression of mock, *PROS1*-WT, and *PROS1*-M in the supernatant and lysate of HEK293T cells, as detected by western blot. (**e**) According to the enzyme-linked immunosorbent assay (ELISA) standard curve, the expression of PROS1 mock, *PROS1*-WT, and *PROS1*-M in the supernatant of HEK293T cells is calculated. (**f**) According to the ELISA standard curve, the expression of PROS1 mock, *PROS1*-WT, and *PROS1*-M in HEK293T cell lysate is calculated. *$p<0.05$,** $p<0.01$,*** $p<0.005$, $n = 3$

Protein of bioinformatics prediction

The mutant (https://swissmodel.expasy.org/interactive/7J8pZH/models/) and WT PROS1 (https://swissmodel.expasy.org/interactive/HxBw4h/models/) homologous proteins were constructed using the Swiss Model (Fig. 4a). The characteristics of the advanced structure were observedl. The number of amino acid residues in the Ca^{2+} region of the mutant protein was one less than that of the WT protein. In humans and other mammals, a comparison between Leu607 of PS and the adjacent flanking structures of PS show that this site is highly conserved (Fig. 4b). Prediction of protein phosphorylation pathway on Leu607Ser using GPS 5.0 software (http://gps.biocuckoo.org/index.php). The results show that L607S is more likely to pass through polo-like kinase (PLK) pathway (Fig. 5).

Discussion

In this study, we found a new mutation site *PROS1* c. 1820 T > C (p.Leu607Ser) for the first time. In previous studies a missense *PROS1* mutation (Gly222Arg) has been identified in a patient with pulmonary embolism, which causes PS activity to decrease to 5.0% [16]. The

PS activity of several codon mutations near L607, such as Ser627fs, Ser627 ins101fsX34 (acc HGMD nomenclature), p.Ala536Val, p.Asn583His, p.Thr617Ile, and p.Cys666Ser (acc HGVS nomenclature) are all less than 40%, and the lowest is 12%, suggesting that mutation of the corresponding domain causes serious functional defects [17]. *PROS1* is located near the centromere of chromosome 3 (3q11.1); it contains 15 exons and encodes PS [18]. From the N-terminal to the C-terminal, there is a γ-carboxyl glutamate domain, a region sensitive to cleavage by thrombin, four domains homologous to epidermal growth factor, and a region homologous to sex hormone binding globulin (SHBG). SHBG contains two tandem laminin G regions (LG1 and LG2) [19]. Mutations in *PROS1* are a risk factor for thrombosis in Asian populations and repeated spontaneous DVT and pulmonary embolism without obvious reasons are the most common symptoms [20]. Whether individuals with *PROS1* mutations have thrombosis greatly depends on the interaction between genes and the interaction between genes and the environment. However, compared to individuals without gene mutations, the risk of thrombosis with gene mutations is 2–11 times higher [21].

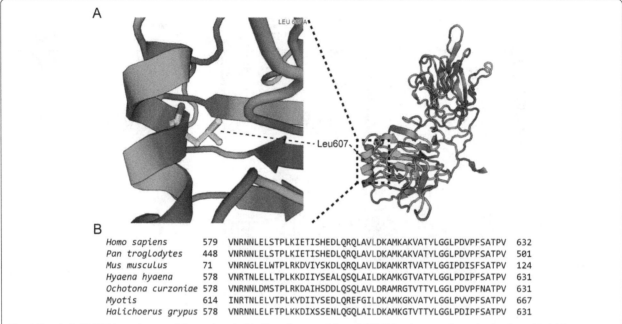

Fig. 4 Protein S (PROS1) homology modeling and analysis. **a** Homology modeling of PROS1 has been performed using Swiss-Model. Leu607 is labeled in the alpha helix. **b** Conserved analysis of amino acid sequences near Leu607 (marked with red) (https://swissmodel.expasy.org/repository/uniprot/P07225?template=1h30.1.A&range=266-673)

Although not every patient with PSD has a clinical phenotype, it will obviously increase the risk of thrombosis, especially in patients with heterozygous mutations and PS activity less than 30% [22]. The occurrence of clinical phenotypes is related to age, sex, and mutation type [23]. There are more male patients with hereditary PSD than female patients with hereditary PSD, but the peak age in females is younger, which is due to the influence of hormones and risk factors, such as trauma, surgery, and oral contraceptives [24]. If *PROS1* occurs as a homozygous mutation, the prognosis is poor and the child may die of fulminant purple spot caused by severe PSD in the neonatal period [25]. Similar to the results of an animal experiment, explosive bleeding in

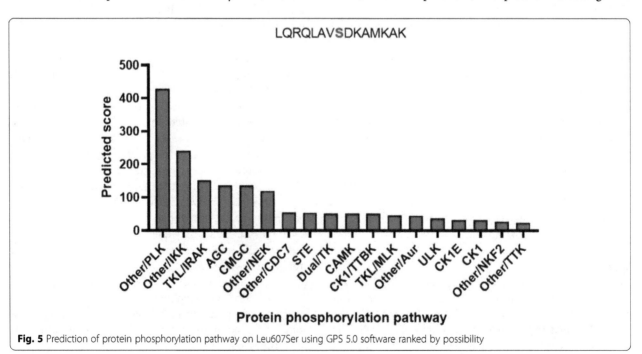

Fig. 5 Prediction of protein phosphorylation pathway on Leu607Ser using GPS 5.0 software ranked by possibility

$PROS1^{-/-}$ homozygous mice is observed in mice with *PROS1* knockout at the embryonic stage. $PROS1^{-/+}$ heterozygous mice survive to adulthood, but different degrees of vascular injury and dysplasia are observed [26]. At the same time, the level of PROS1 and the activity of auxiliary APC are detected, which are significantly lower than those of WT mice [26].

PROS1 L607S may be because the mutated residues affect the level of translation and post-translation modification, resulting in disordered protein processing and secretion, which is the main molecular disease mechanism of most missense and other mutations in genetic diseases [27]. Conformation of SHBG and may be important in the PS anticoagulant effect; about half of the *PROS1* mutations in the LamG domain involve the acquisition and loss of residues with unique physical and chemical properties, such as cysteine, proline, and glycine, which directly affect PS function [28]. Because most of the mutant residues are hydrophobic, changes in these residues may affect protein folding and secretion [29]. The PS level and activity of D38Y and P626L mutants is significantly decreased in transfected COS-7 cells [30]. In this study, the hydrophobic amino acid Leu at position 607 was replaced by the polar neutral amino acid Ser, which is easily phosphorylated by protein kinase. Phosphorylation is the most important post-translational modification and has the greatest effect on the local and overall structural changes in proteins; most phosphorylation occurs on serine residues [31]. The phosphate group formed after phosphorylation of the mutated Ser607 may form hydrogen bonds or salt bridges with the adjacent Lys609, making the local structure compact, which may change the overall conformation of the protein and the interaction between proteins to regulate function [32]. In the mutant protein structure, Ser607 phosphorylation may also affect the binding force of calcium binding region. Ca^{2+} regulates the binding of the C-terminal SHBG region of bound PS to C4 binding protein (C4BP) [33]. Both LG1 and LG2 are involved in PS binding to C4BP, showing anticoagulant activity independent of APC [34]. If PS residues Lys423, Lys427, and Lys429 are replaced by other polar amino acids, the binding force between PS and C4BP is reduced by 5–10-fold. Insertion of alanine at position 611 leads to the loss of binding to C4BP [35], which leads to a decrease in anticoagulant function. The anticoagulant activity of free PS through the tissue factor pathway inhibitor (TFPI) is also through the combination of SHBG and TFPI, which further promotes the interaction between TPFI and FX a, thus inhibiting the activity of tissue factor [2]. LG1 and LG2 are necessary for the binding of SHBG and TFPI, but LG1 plays a major role [36]. A R474C mutant in LG1 reduces PS secretion by eight-fold and shortens the half-life of radioactive markers in transfected cells [37]. Because R474C mutation may lead to PS secretion disorder and intracellular degradation [37]. Then, the mechanism of endoplasmic reticulum-associated protein degradation is initiated, which leads to the decomposition of related proteins in cells [38].

In recent years, the relatively new drug is Novel oral anticoagulants (NOAC). NOACs is a highly selective anticoagulant, including factor Xa inhibitor rivaroxaban and direct thrombin inhibitor dabigatran. NOACs drugs have been shown to be more effective and safer than warfarin in randomized controlled trials, which can significantly reduce the incidence of stroke and thrombotic events [39]. Its therapeutic effect in patients with severe inherited thrombophilia is unclear, although there was one case of good benefit after using dabigatran [40]. A recent report indicated patients with severe inherited thrombophilia had a good effect after receiving NOACs, but it was less effective in patients with PSD [41].

However, this research also has some limitations that only using bioinformatics analysis software to predict the possible effect of mutation sites on the structure of PROS1 protein, lacking experimental evidence, so we can further study the influence of 607Ser on protein. The specific mechanism remains undefined, and the mutation site affects which step in the secretion process, which needs to be further investigated.

Conclusions

In this study, a heterozygous mutation of *PROS1* c.1820 T > C:p.Leu607Ser, was identified as a pathogenic mutation that caused disorderly PS translation, synthesis, and secretion or intracellular degradation, and finally led to a decrease in PS levels and activity, resulting in type I PSD. Heterozygous mutation of *PROS1* c.1820 T > C: p.Leu607Ser was familial.

Abbreviations

PS: protein S; PROS1: protein S gene; PSD: protein S deficiency; SERPINC1: Serpin family C member 1; TFPI: tissue factor pathway inhibitor; APC: activated protein C; qRT-PCR: quantitative real-time-polymerase chain reaction; DVT: deep vein thrombosis; PC: protein C; AT: antithrombin III; WT: wild type; PVDF: polyvinylidene fluoride; BSA: bovine serum albumin; ELISA: Enzyme linked immunosorbent assay; PBS: phosphate-buffered saline; PT: prothrombin time; INR: international normalized ratio; FDP: fibrinogen degradation product; TT: thrombin time; CDFI: Color Doppler flow imaging; CTA: Computed tomographic angiography; SHBG: sex hormone binding globulin; LG: laminin G regions; C4BP: C4 binding protein; NOAC: Novel oral anticoagulants

Authors' contributions

Collection, data analysis, and drafting of the article: YPZ, BL, YYJ and YNH. Collection: YT, JHZ and SJW. Design, supervision, and editing of the manuscript: JWL and ZTF. Provision of the table and figures: YNH. Study supervision: SLC and YFZ. All authors have read and approved the final manuscript.

Author details
¹Shengli Clinical Medical College of Fujian Medical University, Fuzhou 350001, China. ²Department of Interventional Radiology, Fujian Provincial Hospital, Fuzhou 350001, China. ³Department of Pediatrics, Fujian Provincial hospital, Fuzhou 350001, China. ⁴Department of Traditional Chinese Medicine, Fujian Provincial Hospital, Fuzhou 350001, China.

References
1. Dahlback B. Vitamin K-dependent protein S: beyond the protein C pathway. Semin Thromb Hemost. 2018;44:176–84.
2. Gierula M, Ahnstrom J. Anticoagulant protein S-new insights on interactions and functions. J Thromb Haemost. 2020;18:2801–11.
3. Dahlback B. The tale of protein S and C4b-binding protein, story of affection. Thromb Haemost. 2007;98:90–6.
4. Hackeng TM, Sere KM, Tans G, Rosing J. Protein S stimulates inhibition of the tissue factor pathway by tissue factor pathway inhibitor. Proc Natl Acad Sci U S A. 2006;103:3106–11.
5. Wypasek E, Undas A. Protein C and protein S deficiency - practical diagnostic issues. Adv Clin Exp Med. 2013;22:459–67.
6. Wypasek E, Karpinski M, Alhenc-Gelas M, Undas A. Venous thromboembolism associated with protein S deficiency due to Arg451* mutation in PROS1 gene: a case report and a literature review. J Genet. 2017;96:1047–51.
7. Espinosa-Parrilla Y, Morell M, Souto J, Tirado I, Estivill X, Sala N. Protein S gene analysis reveals the presence of a cosegregating mutation in most pedigrees with type I but not type III PS deficiency. Hum Mutat. 1999;14:30–9.
8. Mrożek M, Wypasek E, Alhenc-Gelas M, Potaczek D, Undas A. Novel Splice Site Mutation in the PROS1 Gene in a Polish Patient with Venous Thromboembolism: c.602-2delA, Splice Acceptor Site of Exon 7. Medicina (Kaunas). 2020;56:485.
9. Lipe B, Ornstein DL. Deficiencies of natural anticoagulants, protein C, protein S, and antithrombin. Circulation. 2011;124:e365–8.
10. Chan N, Cheng C, Chan K, Wong C, Lau K, Kwong J, et al. Distinctive regional-specific PROS1 mutation spectrum in southern China. J Thromb Thrombolysis. 2018;46:120–4.
11. Wypasek E, Potaczek DP, Plonka J, Alhenc-Gelas M, Undas A. Protein S deficiency and Heerlen polymorphism in a polish patient with acute myocardial infarction and previous venous thromboembolism. Thromb Res. 2013;132:776–7.
12. Brouwer J, Lijfering W, Ten Kate M, Kluin-Nelemans H, Veeger N, van der Meer J. High long-term absolute risk of recurrent venous thromboembolism in patients with hereditary deficiencies of protein S, protein C or antithrombin. Thromb Haemost. 2009;101:93–9.
13. Kumar P, Henikoff S, Ng PC. Predicting the effects of coding non-synonymous variants on protein function using the SIFT algorithm. Nat Protoc. 2009;4:1073–81.
14. Adzhubei IA, Schmidt S, Peshkin L, Ramensky VE, Gerasimova A, Bork P, et al. A method and server for predicting damaging missense mutations. Nat Methods. 2010;7:248–9.
15. Schwarz J, Cooper D, Schuelke M, Seelow D. MutationTaster2: mutation prediction for the deep-sequencing age. Nat Methods. 2014;11:361–2.
16. Xu J, Peng G, Ouyang Y. A novel mutation Gly222Arg in PROS1 causing protein S deficiency in a patient with pulmonary embolism. J Clin Lab Anal. 2020;34:e23111.
17. Caspers M, Pavlova A, Driesen J, Harbrecht U, Klamroth R, Kadar J, et al. Deficiencies of antithrombin, protein C and protein S - practical experience in genetic analysis of a large patient cohort. Thromb Haemost. 2012;108:247–57.
18. Schmidel DK, Tatro AV, Phelps LG, Tomczak JA, Long GL. Organization of the human protein S genes. Biochemistry. 1990;29:7845–52.
19. Suleiman L, Negrier C, Boukerche H. Protein S: a multifunctional anticoagulant vitamin K-dependent protein at the crossroads of coagulation, inflammation, angiogenesis, and cancer. Crit Rev Oncol Hematol. 2013;88:637–54.
20. Kim HJ, Seo JY, Lee KO, Bang SH, Lee ST, Ki CS, et al. Distinct frequencies and mutation spectrums of genetic thrombophilia in Korea in comparison with other Asian countries both in patients with thromboembolism and in the general population. Haematologica. 2014;99:561–9.
21. Soare A, Popa C. Deficiencies of proteins C, S and Antithrombin and activated protein C resistance–their involvement in the occurrence of arterial Thromboses. J Med Life. 2010;3:412–5.
22. Alhenc-Gelas M, Plu-Bureau G, Horellou MH, Rauch A. Suchon P, group Ggt: PROS1 genotype phenotype relationships in a large cohort of adults with suspicion of inherited quantitative protein S deficiency. Thromb Haemost. 2016;115:570–9.
23. Ding Q, Shen W, Ye X, Wu Y, Wang X, Wang H. Clinical and genetic features of protein C deficiency in 23 unrelated Chinese patients. Blood Cells Mol Dis. 2013;50:53–8.
24. ten Kate M, van der Meer J. Protein S deficiency: a clinical perspective. Haemophilia. 2008;14:1222–8.
25. Estellés A, Garcia-Plaza I, Dasí A, Aznar J, Duart M, Sanz G, et al. Severe inherited "homozygous" protein C deficiency in a newborn infant. Thromb Haemost. 1984;52:53–6.
26. Burstyn-Cohen T, Heeb M, Lemke G. Lack of protein S in mice causes embryonic lethal coagulopathy and vascular dysgenesis. J Clin Invest. 2009;119:2942–53.
27. Andersen B, Bisgaard M, Lind B, Philips M, Villoutreix B, Thorsen S. Characterization and structural impact of five novel PROS1 mutations in eleven protein S-deficient families. Thromb Haemost. 2001;86:1392–9.
28. Garcia de Frutos P, Fuentes-Prior P, Hurtado B, Sala N. Molecular basis of protein S deficiency. Thromb Haemost. 2007;98:543–56.
29. Sasaki T, Knyazev P, Cheburkin Y, Göhring W, Tisi D, Ullrich A, et al. Crystal structure of a C-terminal fragment of growth arrest-specific protein Gas6. Receptor tyrosine kinase activation by laminin G-like domains. J Biol Chem. 2002;277:44164–70.
30. Ikejiri M, Tsuji A, Wada H, Sakamoto Y, Nishioka J, Ota S, et al. Analysis three abnormal protein S genes in a patient with pulmonary embolism. Thromb Res. 2010;125:529–32.
31. Nishi H, Shaytan A, Panchenko AR. Physicochemical mechanisms of protein regulation by phosphorylation. Front Genet. 2014;5:270.
32. Humphrey SJ, James DE, Mann M. Protein phosphorylation: a major switch mechanism for metabolic regulation. Trends Endocrinol Metab. 2015;26:676–87.
33. Sjöberg A, Trouw L, McGrath F, Hack C, Blom A. Regulation of complement activation by C-reactive protein: targeting of the inhibitory activity of C4b-binding protein. J Immunol. 2006;176:7612–20.
34. D'Angelo A, D'Angelo S. Protein S deficiency. Haematologica. 2008;93:498–501.
35. Villoutreix B, Dahlbäck B, Borgel D, Gandrille S, Muller Y. Three-dimensional model of the SHBG-like region of anticoagulant protein S: new structure-function insights. Proteins. 2001;43:203–16.
36. Reglińska-Matveyev N, Andersson H, Rezende S, Dahlbäck B, Crawley J, Lane D, et al. TFPI cofactor function of protein S: essential role of the protein S SHBG-like domain. Blood. 2014;123:3979–87.
37. Yamazaki T, Katsumi A, Kagami K, Okamoto Y, Sugiura I, Hamaguchi M, et al. Molecular basis of a hereditary type I protein S deficiency caused by a substitution of Cys for Arg474. Blood. 1996;87:4643–50.
38. Reitsma P, Ploos van Amstel H, Bertina R. Three novel mutations in five unrelated subjects with hereditary protein S deficiency type I. J Clin Invest. 1994;93:486–92.
39. Sander R. Dabigatran versus warfarin in patients with atrial fibrillation. Nurs Older People. 2017;29:11.
40. Lee WC, Huang MP. Lead thrombus under standard-dose edoxaban in a patient with normal to high creatinine clearance and protein S deficiency. Thromb J. 2021;19:50.
41. Undas A, Goralczyk T. Non-vitamin K antagonist oral anticoagulants in patients with severe inherited thrombophilia: a series of 33 patients. Blood Coagul Fibrinolysis. 2017;28:438–42.

23

Malignant tumor is the greatest risk factor for pulmonary embolism in hospitalized patients

Kaoru Fujieda[1,2]* (iD), Akiko Nozue[1], Akie Watanabe[1,2], Keiko Shi[1,2], Hiroya Itagaki[2], Yoshihiko Hosokawa[2], Keiko Nishida[2], Nobutaka Tasaka[2], Toyomi Satoh[2] and Ken Nishide[1]

Abstract

Background: This study aimed to investigate the background of patients who presented with pulmonary embolism (PE) on contrast-enhanced chest computed tomography (CT) and to explore the risk factors for PE.

Methods: This study included a review of the medical records of all 50,621 patients who were admitted to one community hospital between January 1, 2013 and December 31, 2017. Data on sex, age, risk factors related to blood flow stagnation (obesity, long-term bed rest, cardiopulmonary disease, cast fixation, long-term sitting), risk factors related to vascular endothelial disorder (surgery, trauma/fracture, central venous catheterization, catheter tests/treatments, vasculitis, antiphospholipid antibody syndrome, history of venous thromboembolism (VTE)), and risk factors related to hypercoagulability (malignant tumor, use of oral contraceptives/low-dose estrogen progestin/steroids, infection, inflammatory enteric disease, polycythemia, protein C or protein S deficiency, dehydration) were evaluated.

Results: Of all inpatients, 179(0.35%) out of 50,621 were diagnosed with PE after contrast-enhanced chest CT examination, in which 74 patients were symptomatic and 105 patients had no symptom. Among asymptomatic 105 patients, 71 patients got CT scans for other reasons including cancer screening and searching infection focus, and 34 patients got CT scans for searching PE due to either apparent or suspicious DVT. The rate of discovering PE was significantly greater in women (0.46%, 90/19,409) than men (0.29%, 89/31,212) ($P = 0.008$). Of the 179 patients with PE, 164 (92%) had some type of risk factor. For both men and women, the most frequent risk factor was a malignant tumor, followed by obesity, long-term bed rest and infection for men and long-term bed rest, obesity and infection for women. The most common malignant tumor was lung cancer. Although taking antipsychotic agent is not advocated as a risk factor, there is a possibility of involvement.

Conclusions: The risk factors for PE were identified in this single-center, retrospective study.

Keywords: Venous thromboembolism, Pulmonary embolism, Gynecological cancer

---

* Correspondence: fujieda-smr@umin.ac.jp
[1]Tsukuba Medical Center Hospital, Tsukuba, Ibaraki, Japan
[2]Department of Obstetrics and Gynecology, Faculty of Medicine, University of Tsukuba, 1-1-1 Tennoudai, Tsukuba, Ibaraki 305-8575, Japan

Background

The mortality of patients who develop acute pulmonary embolism (PE) is high, at 4.1–14.5% [1–3], indicating the seriousness of the condition. The mechanism of onset is as follows: first, the free-floating blood clots formed in the deep vein or right atrium rapidly occlude the pulmonary artery, and over 90% of the cases are caused by deep vein thrombosis (DVT) formed in the lower limbs or pelvis [4, 5]. Factors that cause venous thromboembolism (VTE), as proposed by Virchow in 1856 are (1) blood flow stagnation, (2) vascular endothelial disorder, and (3) hypercoagulability [6]. Numerous underlying conditions affect the onset of PE, and PE occurs in patients admitted to various departments. However, most reports of PE in Japan include cases from only a single department. This study aimed to investigate the background of patients who presented with PE on contrast-enhanced chest computed tomography (CT) and to explore the risk factors for PE.

Methods

Patients

This study included all 50,621 patients who were admitted to the Tsukuba Medical Center Hospital between January 1, 2013 and December 31, 2017. Because we used the records of hospitalized patients, same patients who admitted to hospital another period were counted separately.

Diagnosis of PE

PE was diagnosed after contrast-enhanced chest CT examination. There was no algorithm for diagnosing PE in our hospital. The condition of CT scanning was not unified, but there was possibility of PE or DVT, we used specific condition CT to find a VTE. After injection of a contrast medium, we scanned chest 15–20 s later and lower limbs 3 min later.

Examination medical records

A retrospective examination of medical records was conducted to extract data on sex, age, risk factors related to blood flow stagnation (obesity, long-term bed rest, cardiopulmonary disease, cast fixation, long-term sitting), risk factors related to vascular endothelial disorder (surgery, trauma/fracture, central venous catheterization, catheter tests/treatments, vasculitis, antiphospholipid antibody syndrome, history of VTE), and risk factors related to hypercoagulability (malignant tumor, use of oral contraceptives/low-dose estrogen progestin/steroids, infection, inflammatory enteric disease, polycythemia, protein C or protein S deficiency, dehydration). For patients with multiple risk factors, each factor was counted separately for the analysis. For patients with a malignant tumor, the frequency of PE was calculated by cancer type. The χ^2 test was used for analysis, and $P < 0.05$ was considered significant.

Summary of facilities

Our hospital is a 453-bed community hospital primarily equipped to handle emergency medicine. Emergency admission to the cardiology and neurology departments is relatively common, and perinatal conditions are not handled. This study was approved by the institutional review board at Tsukuba Medical Center Hospital.

Results

Patients' profile: symptomatic and asymptomatic, association with DVT

Of all inpatients, 179(0.35%) out of 50,621 were diagnosed with PE after contrast-enhanced chest CT examination, in which 74 patients were symptomatic and 105 patients had no symptom. Among asymptomatic 105 patients, 71 patients got CT scans for other reasons including cancer screening and searching infection focus, and 34 patients got CT scans for searching PE due to either apparent or suspicious of DVT. 74 patients had symptoms such as dyspnea, chest pain, fever, fainting, cough, wheezing, hemoptysis and palpitations [7]. 74 symptomatic patients and 34 asymptomatic patients (31 had lower limb edema and 3 had proximal DVT) were made CT scanning for a suspicious of PE. 5 symptomatic patient's vital signs were deadly, took only chest CT scan immediately. In asymptomatic patients, 4 patients with lower limb edema and 3 patients with elevated D-dimmer value were made lower limb ultrasonography prior to CT scan and had proximal DVT. Left 27 patients with lower limb edema searched for DVT by CT scan, 25 patients had DVT. 71 patients got a CT scan for other reasons and diagnosed PE coincidentally. 48 out of 71 patients searched for DVT and 31 had DVT. (Figs. 1,2).

PE was more proximal pulmonary artery than subregion branch in all patients. However, there was possibility of overlooking peripheral PE because it was not routine work to search the PE in asymptomatic patient.

Gender and age

The rate of discovering PE was significantly greater in women (0.46%, 90/19,409) than men (0.29%, 89/31,212) ($P = 0.008$). Table 1 show the number of patients with PE by sex and age group.

In men, the number of patients increased gradually from the 30s age group and reached a peak around the 60–70s age group. In contrast, in women, the number increased from the 40s age group, with a relatively steep peak at the 70–80s age group. In men, the rate of discovering PE was not different between those under age 60 years (0.32%, 37/11,609) and those 60 years and older (0.27%, 52/19,603) ($P = 0.3$). In contrast, in women, the

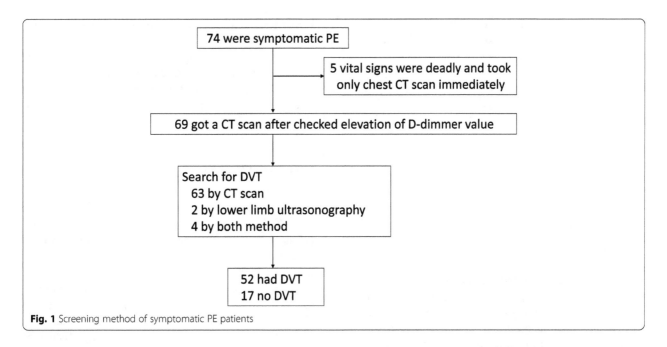

Fig. 1 Screening method of symptomatic PE patients

rate was significantly greater in those 60 years and older (0.63%, 69/11,009) than in those under 60 years of age (0.25%, 21/8400) (*P* = 0.0001).

Risk factors for DVT/PE
Of the 179 patients with PE, 164 (92%) had some type of risk factor (Table 2).

There was difference in the frequency of CT scanning between cancer and other diseases. 1 patient with colon cancer or lung cancer got a CT scan every 3 months, 1 patient with lung cancer got a CT scan every 6 months after the treatment. 8 cancer patients (6 patients with lung cancer, 1 patient with colon cancer, 1 patient with breast cancer) who were under the treatment got a CT scan every time judging the therapeutic effect. Other cancer patients got a CT scan one time only to investigate the causes of symptoms. Other than cancer patients, 17 patients got a second time CT scan, because 6 patients had hypoxia, 6 patients suspected DVT, 5 patients followed up trauma or infection. Other patients got a CT scan one time only.

We used Wells score and defined that long-term bed rest was more than 72 h [8] and sitting for a long time was more than 5 h [9]. 22 out of 41 patients, long-term

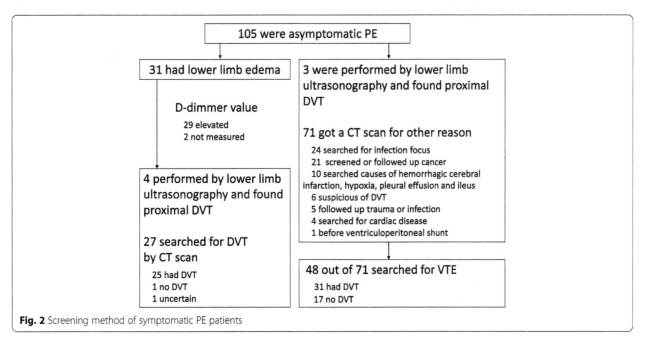

Fig. 2 Screening method of symptomatic PE patients

Table 1 Distribution of the number of patients by age and sex

Age(y)	Male(%)	Female(%)
10–19	1 (1)	0 (0)
20–29	1 (1)	1 (1)
30–39	8 (9)	2 (2)
40–49	13 (15)	7 (8)
50–59	14 (16)	11 (12)
60–69	18 (20)	15 (17)
70–79	17 (19)	28 (31)
80–89	13 (15)	22 (24)
90–99	4 (4)	4 (4)

bed rest was in-hospital outbreak. They were forced long-term bed rest due to consciousness or trauma.

Regarding to surgery, trauma/fracture and central venous catheterization, refer to Wells score, we determined that the time was less than 3 months before admission. The median time to onset, 10 (0–60) days at operation, 10 (0–72) days at trauma, fracture and cast fixed, and 8 days at central venous catheter. 1 patient after operation of osteoarthritis of the knee had 60 days, 2 patients after fractured had 17 days or 60 days before administration, other patients were admitted immediately after injured or already in the hospital to get surgery.

Only one patient who had past medical history of VTE took anticoagulant therapy, warfarin, other patients were self-interruption or not prescribed.

Patients for unknown reason were measured thrombus predisposition (Protein C or S, anti-cardiolipin antibody and lupus anti-core grant), and 2 patients were diagnosed protein C or S deficiency, 1 patient was diagnosed antiphospholipid antibody syndrome.

The risk factor for the development of PE could not be identified in 15 patients.

Although taking antipsychotic agent is not advocated as a risk factor, 9 patients with schizophrenia were taking antipsychotic agent.

Gender difference

Although there were no significant differences between men and women in the percentage of patients with each PE risk factor, long-term bed rest was more common in women, at 17%, compared with men, at 13%, and trauma/fracture/cast fixation was more common in men, at 8%, than in women, at 6%. A total of 33(89%) obese patients had another risk factor. For both men and women, the most frequent risk factor was a malignant tumor, followed by long-term bed rest and infection.

Contribution of cancer-bearing

47 patients with PE and a malignant tumor. 35 patients had advanced cancer. 27 patients were diagnosed cancer after PE diagnosis. Seventeen patients were under the treatment (15 patients had chemotherapy, 1 patient had hormone therapy, 1 patient had surgery). Ten out of 17

Table 2 The risk factors of patients with PE separated by gender

	Risk factor	Male(%)	Female(%)	P-value
Blood flow stagnation	Obesity	20 (15)	17 (13)	0.63
	Long-term bed rest	18 (13)	23 (17)	0.37
	Sitting for a long time	3 (2)	4 (3)	0.69
	Cardiopulmonary disease	4 (3)	7 (5)	0.34
	Trauma, Fracture, Cast fixed	11 (8)	8 (6)	0.50
	Central venous catheter	0 (0)	1 (1)	0.31
	Surgery	9 (7)	9 (7)	0.97
Vascular endothelial disorder	Antiphospholipid antibody syndrome and collagen disease	6 (4)	2 (1)	0.16
	Past medical history of VTE	2 (1)	1 (1)	0.57
	Cancer	24 (18)	23 (17)	0.92
Hypercoagulability	OCs, LEP, Steroids	2 (1)	5 (4)	0.24
	Infection	18 (13)	17 (13)	0.89
	Inflammatory enteric disease	1 (1)	2 (1)	0.55
	Polycythemia	1 (1)	1 (1)	0.99
	Protein C or Protein S deficiency	2 (1)	0 (0)	0.16
	Dehydration	4 (3)	6 (5)	0.50
	No risk factor	9 (7)	6 (5)	0.44

patients who were under the treatment got a CT scan to judge therapeutic effect, 7 patients were PD, 2 patients were PR, 1 patient was SD. 3 patients got a CT scan regularly to follow up after treatment and 1 patient had seen recurrence of cancer. 45 patients (95%) had active cancer.

Patients with lung cancer were the most common, accounting for 34% of the 47 patients. The rate of discovering PE by cancer type was greatest in ovarian cancer, at 3.3%, followed by endometrial cancer, at 2.4% (Table 3).

The rate of discovering PE in ovarian cancer was not significantly different from that of endometrial cancer, gallbladder cancer, and lung cancer, but it was significantly greater compared with that of colon cancer, stomach cancer, breast cancer, prostate cancer, kidney cancer, and cervical cancer ($P = 0.0001$ to 0.01).

Discussion

Although there are conflicting reports that the incidence of PE is higher in men [10, 11] or is not different between men and women [12], the incidence is 1.5-fold higher in Japanese women than men, peaking in the 60–70s age group [13]. The present results also showed that the discovery rate was greater in women and peaked around the 60–70s, corroborating previous reports from Japan. PE is thought to more likely occur in older individuals than in younger individuals because the morbidity of underlying conditions, such as cerebrovascular disease/neurological disease, long-term bed rest from a lumbar compression fracture, malignant tumor, and bacterial infections including aspiration pneumonia/pyelonephritis, that are likely to cause VTE increases with increasing age. In particular, in postmenopausal women, events such as cardiovascular diseases and fractures increase rapidly, and this is considered to be the reason why PE is frequently observed in older women.

In PE patients with a malignant tumor, lung cancer was the most common tumor. This is because patients with lung cancer are the most common cancer

inpatients at our hospital, and because smoking, a risk factor for lung cancer [14], is also a risk factor for VTE [15]. Thus, this was an expected outcome. Analysis of the PE discovery rate by cancer type showed that patients with ovarian cancer had the highest rate. Before treatment, PE was discovered in 8.8–13.3% of ovarian cancer [16, 17], 3.0–4.7% of endometrial cancer [16, 18], 1.1–1.4% of cervical cancer [16, 19], and 2.9% of advanced pancreatic cancer [20] cases. Moreover, whereas PE was not discovered in bladder cancer or stomach cancer cases, DVT was found in 13.9 and 4.4% of the patients, respectively [21]. VTE is common in ovarian cancer due to vascular dehydration caused by ascites [16] and venous compression by a large tumor [22]. In clear cell carcinoma, Factor VII is activated via the extrinsic blood coagulation pathway, leading to the production of tissue factors that augment coagulation [23, 24], and this is thought to be one of the causes for high VTE rates.

Although taking antipsychotic agent was not advocated as a risk factor, there was a possibility of involvement. Antipsychotics are known to induce pulmonary vasospasm and contraction, as well as platelet aggregation via the serotonin-like action of 5HT2/D2 antagonists [25]. Taking antipsychotics for more than 24 months increases the risk for VTE by 32%, and by 73% with atypical antipsychotics [26]. In Japan, the Ministry of Health, Labour and Welfare in 2010 recommended the addition of PE and DVT as serious side effects to the package inserts of antipsychotics such as haloperidol, blonanserin, clozapine, and risperidone. The use of antipsychotics should perhaps be noted as a risk factor for VTE.

Conclusions

In our hospital, the rate of discovering PE was high in women who were at least 60 years old. In 92% of the cases, some type of risk factor for onset was identified. The most frequently observed risk factor was a malignant tumor. Lung cancer was the most common by the number of patients, and ovarian cancer was the highest

Table 3 Numbers and incidence of patients with PE by each cancer type

Cancer type	Number of hospitalized patients	Number of patients with PE(%)
Ovarian cancer	152	5 (3.3)
Endometrial cancer	122	3 (2.4)
Gallbladder cancer	89	2 (2.2)
Lung cancer	1258	16 (1.3)
Colon cancer	1177	9 (0.8)
Gastric cancer	693	3 (0.4)
Breast cancer	1109	5 (0.5)
Prostate cancer	881	3 (0.3)
Kidney cancer	816	1 (0.1)
Cervical cancer	287	0 (0)

by frequency of discovery. Other risk factors were infection, long-term bed rest and obesity. 89% of obese patients had another risk factor. Antipsychotic drugs may have been associated with PE in some patients.

There are some limitations of this study. Firstly, the sample size is small. 179 patients were selected, but the number of patients would not be sufficient to collect relevant date. Secondly, patients had some risk factors, so we couldn't declare the most influence risk factors. Finally, there was limitation of department in our hospital, therefore there was the possibility of overlooking the risk factor or undiagnosed diseases. Furthermore, we were unable to fully analyze the date of patients who had not PE, because some medical records were disposed, so we couldn't do multivariate analysis.

Though there are limitations with this single-center retrospective study, it demonstrated the risk factors for PE in patients who presented with PE.

Abbreviations

PE: Pulmonary embolism; CT: Computed tomography; VTE: Venous thromboembolism; DVT: Deep vein thrombosis; BMI: Body mass index; OCs: Oral contraceptives; LEP: Low dose Estrogen Progestin; RECIST: Response evaluation criteria in solid tumors; NED: No evidence of disease; Rec: Recurrence; PD: Progressive disease; SD: Stable disease; PR: Partial response

Authors' contributions

AN, KF and NK were involved in study design and date interpretation. AN, KF, NK and TS were involved in the date analysis. All authors read and approved the final manuscript.

References

1. Akgüllü Ç, Ömürlü İK, Eryılmaz U, Avcil M, Dağtekin E, Akdeniz M, et al. Predictors of early death in patients with acute pulmonary embolism. Am J Emerg Med. 2015;33(2):214–21. https://doi.org/10.1016/j.ajem.2014.11.022.
2. Becattini C, Agnelli G, Mareike L, Masotti L, Pruszczyk P, Casazza F, et al. Acute pulmonary embolism: mortality prediction by the 2014 European Society of Cardiology risk stratification model. Eur Respir J. 2016;48(3):780–6. https://doi.org/10.1183/13993003.00024-2016.
3. Bach AG, Taute BM, Baasai N, Wienke A, Meyer HJ, Schramm D, et al. 30-day mortality in acute pulmonary embolism: prognostic value of clinical scores and anamnestic features. PLoS One. 2016;11(2):e0148728. https://doi.org/10.1371/journal.pone.0148728.
4. Moser KM. Venous thromboembolism. Am Rev Respir Dis. 1990;141(1):235–49. https://doi.org/10.1164/ajrccm/141.1.235.
5. Ro A, Kageyama N, Tanifuji T, Fukunaga T. Pulmonary thromboembolism: overview and update from medicolegal aspects. Leg Med (Tokyo). 2008; 10(2):57–71. https://doi.org/10.1016/j.legalmed.2007.09.003.
6. Virchow R. Gesammalte Abhandlungen Zur Wissenschaftlichen Medizin. Frankfurt: Medinger Sohn & CO; 1856. p. 219–732.
7. Maisso M, Renato P, Brouno F, Carlo M, Giorgio DR, Lucia T, et al. Accuracy of clinical assessment in the diagnosis of pulmonary embolism. Am J Respir Crit Care Med. 1999;159(3):864–71.
8. Wells PS, Owen C, Doucette S, Fergusson D, Tran H. Dose this patient have deep vein thrombosis? JAMA. 2006;295(2):199–207. https://doi.org/10.1001/jama.295.2.199.
9. Shirakawa T, Iso H, Yamagishi K, Yatsuya H, Tanabe N, Ikehara A, et al. Watching television and risk of mortality from pulmonary embolism among Japanese men and women: the JACC study (Japan collaborative cohort). Circulation. 2016;134(4):355–7. https://doi.org/10.1161/CIRCULATIONAHA.116.023671.
10. Naess IA, Christiansen SC, Romundstad P, Cannegieter SC, Rosendaal FR, Hammerstrøm J. Incidence and mortality of venous thrombosis: a population-based study. J Thromb Haemost. 2007;5(4):692–9. https://doi.org/10.1111/j.1538-7836.2007.02450.x.
11. Heit JA. The epidemiology of venous thromboembolism in the community. Arteriosclerosis Thromb Vasc Biol. 2008;28(3):370–2. https://doi.org/10.1161/ATVBAHA.108.162545.
12. Nordström M, Lindblad B, Bergqvist D, Kjellström T. A prospective study of the incidence of deep-vein thrombosis within a defined urban population. J Intern Med. 1992;232(2):155–60. https://doi.org/10.1111/j.1365-2796.1992.tb00565.x.
13. Nakamura M, Fujioka H, Yamada N, Sakuma M, Okada O, Nakanishi N, et al. Clinical characteristics of acute pulmonary thromboembolism in Japan: results of a multicenter registry in the Japanese Society of Pulmonary Embolism Research. Clin Cardiol. 2001;24(2):132–8. https://doi.org/10.1002/clc.4960240207.
14. Sobue T, Yamamoto S, Hara M, Sasazuki S, Sasaki S, Tsugane S. Cigarette smoking and subsequent risk of lung cancer by histologic type in middle-aged Japanese men and women: the JPHC study. Int J Cancer. 2002;99(2):245–51. https://doi.org/10.1002/ijc.10308.
15. Cheng YJ, Liu ZH, Yao FJ, Zeng WT, Zheng DD, Dong YG, et al. Current and former smoking and risk for venous thromboembolism: a systematic review and meta-analysis. PLoS Med. 2013;10(9):e1001515. https://doi.org/10.1371/journal.pmed.1001515.
16. Kodama J, Seki N, Fukushima C, Kusumoto T, Nakamura K, Hongo A, et al. Elevated preoperative plasma D-dimer levels and the incidence of venous thromboembolism in Japanese females with gynecological cancer. Oncol Lett. 2013;5(1):299–304. https://doi.org/10.3892/ol.2012.970.
17. Satoh T, Oki A, Uno K, Sakurai M, Ochi H, Okada S, et al. High incidence of silent venous thromboembolism before treatment in ovarian cancer. Br J Cancer. 2007;97(8):1053–7. https://doi.org/10.1038/sj.bjc.6603989.
18. Satoh T, Oki A, Uno K, Sakurai M, Ochi H, Okada S, et al. Silent venous thromboembolism before treatment in endometrial cancer and the risk factors. Br J Cancer. 2008;99(7):1034–9. https://doi.org/10.1038/sj.bjc.6604658.
19. Satoh T, Matsumoto K, Tanaka YO, Akiyama A, Nakao S, Sakurai M, et al. Incidence of venous thromboembolism before treatment in cervical cancer and the impact of management on venous thromboembolism after commencement of treatment. Thromb Res. 2013;131(4):127–32. https://doi.org/10.1016/j.thromres.2013.01.027.
20. Kondo S, Sakai M, Hosoi H, Sakamoto Y, Morizane C, Ueno H, et al. Incidence and risk factors for venous thromboembolism in patients with pretreated advanced pancreatic carcinoma. Oncotarget. 2018;9(24):16883–90. https://doi.org/10.18632/oncotarget.24721.
21. Schomburg JL, Krishna S, Cotter KJ, Soubra A, Rao A, Konely BR. Preoperative incidence of deep venous thrombosis in patients with bladder cancer undergoing radical cystectomy. Urology. 2018;116:120–4. https://doi.org/10.1016/j.urology.2018.01.052.
22. Liao TY, Hsu HC, Wen MS, Juan YH, Hung YH, Liaw CC. Iliofemoral venous thrombosis mainly related to iliofemoral venous obstruction by external tumor compression in cancer patients. Case Rep Oncol. 2016;9(3):760–71. https://doi.org/10.1159/000452943.
23. Uno K, Homma S, Satoh T, Nakanishi K, Abe D, Matsumoto K, et al. Tissue factor expression as a possible determinant of thromboembolism in ovarian cancer. Br J Cancer. 2007;96(2):290· 5. https://doi.org/10.1038/sj.bjc.6603552

24. Chanakira A, Westmark PR, Ong IM, Sheehan JP. Tissue factor-factor VIIa complex triggers protease activated receptor 2-dependent growth factor release and migration in ovarian cancer. Gynecol Oncol. 2007;145(1):167–75.
25. Boullin DJ, Woods HF, Grimes RP, Grahame-Smith DG. Increased platelet aggregation responses to 5-hydroxytryptamine in patients taking chlorpromazine. Br J Clin Pharmacol. 1975;2(1):29–35. https://doi.org/10.1111/j.1365-2125.1975.tb00468.x.
26. Parker C, Coupland C, Hippisley-Cox J. Antipsychotic drugs and risk of venous thromboembolism: nested case-control study. BMJ. 2010;341(sep21 1):c4245. https://doi.org/10.1136/bmj.c4245.

24

Time trends for pulmonary embolism incidence in Greece

Dimitrios G. Raptis[1], Konstantinos I. Gourgoulianis[1], Zoe Daniil[1] and Foteini Malli[1,2*] (ID)

Abstract

Background: Pulmonary embolism (PE) is a disease with a significant impact on public health. However, international epidemiological data are unclear and show considerable heterogeneity. The present study aims to investigate the incidence of PE at the Greek population and the associated demographic characteristics of patients with PE.

Methods: Data on hospital admissions for PE between 1999 and 2012 were provided by the Hellenic Statistical Authority of Greece. Data on age, gender and days of hospitalization from 1999 to 2007 were provided as well. The total population in each region was derived from the 1991, 2001, 2011 Census of the national statistical service of Greece.

Results: The mean annual incidence of PE during the study period was 18.5 per 100.000 population. The annual incidence of PE showed an upward trend ranging from 14 (1999) to 30 (2012) per 100.000 population. In the years before and after the economic crisis faced by Greece we observed statistically significant differences of PE incidence for the two different periods (1999–2008 versus 2009–2012, 14.49 versus 23.06 respectively, $p = 0.002$). The available data revealed a female predominance (16.48 cases for females per 100.000 population versus 13.69 cases for males per 100.000 population, $p = 0.031$). Incidence rate increased with age with a higher incidence in the "80–89" age group.

Conclusions: The incidence of PE appeared to increase in Greece, while it remains below the expected trend in an international context that may be attributed to Computed Tomography Pulmonary Angiography availability and/or PE awareness among clinicians.

Keywords: Pulmonary embolism, Incidence, Mortality, Epidemiology

Background

Pulmonary embolism (PE) can be difficult to diagnose and manage. The occurrence of PE is influenced by several factors including aging, cancer and/or hormone replacement therapy [1, 2]. Annual incidence rates of Venous Thromboembolism (VTE) vary significantly and ranges from 62 to 143 per 100,000 persons [3]. Data from United States of America (USA) VTE studies reported that the VTE incidence increased by 82% from 73 to 133 per 100.000 population in the period 1985–2009, that is mainly attributed to an increase in PE [4] and use of Computed Tomography Pulmonary Angiography

(CTPA) in the USA [5]. The differentiation may be based on characteristics of the population studied, including age and nationality, on availability of reliable data sources, data from the patients' medical records only, and on insufficient assessment of primary and recurrent episodes [6].

Data collection on PE hospitalizations is important at national level to evaluate patient outcome and disease incidence. Nevertheless, a small number of studies have examined trends in the incidence of PE during the last two decades. In the USA studies have shown increase in incidence and a significant fall in mortality [5, 7]. Similarly, in the United Kingdom and Australia, rates of admission for PE have increased in recent years [8, 9]. On the other hand, in China, the incidence of PE has remained stable over the past decade, while the mortality

* Correspondence: mallifoteini@yahoo.gr
[1]Respiratory Medicine Department, School of Medicine, University of Thessaly, Larissa, Greece
[2]Anatomy and Phsyiology Lab, Nursing Department, University of Thessaly, Larissa, Greece

rate has decreased [10]. The observed variation between countries may be partly attributed to differences in risk factors for PE or inconsistencies in PE diagnosis between countries.

The data taken together support that PE incidence is increased in recent years, however objective data on the burden of PE are not fully known. To our knowledge there are no available data on PE incidence for the Greek population. In Greece, early reports have shown negative consequences of financial crisis on public health, and notably on respiratory health. The impact of the Greek downturn on respiratory health was obvious although most studies applied data covering only the first years of the crisis and reported its' short-term outcomes [11].

The aim of the present study was to conduct a nationwide analysis of hospital discharge data of PE, collected from 1999 to 2012. These data were used to elucidate changes in the incidence of patients hospitalized for PE in Greece over a 14-year study period.

Methods

Information on hospital admissions for PE between 1999 and 2012 were provided by the Hellenic Statistical Authority of Greece. The Hellenic Statistical Authority (ELSTAT) is an independent organization enjoying operational, administrative and financial independence that coordinates the functions of the other agencies in the Hellenic Statistical System. Its' operation is subject to the control of the Hellenic Parliament but not to the control of governmental bodies or other administrative authority. ELSTAT coordinates all the agencies that have the responsibility or obligation to collect the country's official statistics and forwards these statistics to Eurostat. The services and agencies of the public sector, the Legal Entities under Private Law, the associations of individuals and natural persons are obliged to grant ELSTAT access to all the administrative sources, public registers and files they keep, in printed, electronic or other form, and provide, in an accurate and timely manner, ELSTAT with primary statistical data and information, which is required for the performance of its duties. The data provided to ELSTAT from government entities and administrative sources are subjected to controls by ELSTAT with a view to assessing their accuracy and reliability before being used in the production of statistics by Hellenic Statistical Authority. The mission of the Hellenic Statistical Authority is to safeguard and continuously improve the quality of the country's statistics by following in all areas the highest European and international standards of statistical practice, as well as by unswervingly observing the rules and responsibilities it is committed to [12]. Data on age, gender and days of hospitalization from 1999 to 2007 were provided as well.

The dataset of 1999 to 2007 contained data on deaths where PE was reported as a cause of death in the death certificate. The annual incidence of PE was estimated as the number of hospital discharges with PE diagnosis in 1 yr (including fatal cases of PE) to the total population and expressed as the number of events per 100.000 population. The discharges were recorded using the ICD 9 and ICD 10 system, depending on the system in force at the time of each discharge. Specifically, the calculation of PE incidence resulted from the quotient of new cases (discharges) during a comparable year in a region to the total population in the same year in that region expressed per 100.000 population. Briefly ICD 10 codes used for Pulmonary embolism cases were I26 (I26.0 and I26.9) and ICD 9 codes were 415.1. The total population in each region was derived from the 1991, 2001, 2011 Census of the national statistical service of Greece [12].

The incidence of PE (per 100.000 population) was calculated for each year from 1999 to 2012 in each of the 10 regional areas of Greece and in the total population of Greece. In addition, these 14 years were divided into two groups with a milestone in 2008 which presents the start of the economic crisis. In detail, two groups were created, a group of 1999–2008 and one of 2009–2012 in the average incidence wad calculated. For the processing of age, we used ten-year intervals from the age of 10 up to the age of 100 and over, and the outcome was 10 age-categories.

Data on all patients identifiers were not provided to the authors in order to assure patient confidentiality. The study protocol was approved by the ethics committee of our institution.

Statistical analysis

Demographic characteristics are reported as mean ± standard deviation unless otherwise indicated. All datasets were tested for normality using the Shapiro-Wilk normality test. Incidence rates comparison was performed using a parametric t-test.

All the statistical analysis was performed at the statistical significance level of 5% corresponding to p value of 0.05. Data were analyzed using SPSS software, version 22 (Statistical Package for Social Sciences Inc., 2003, Chicago, USA).

Results

The average annual incidence of PE in Greece for the 14 years of our study was 18.5 per 100.000 (95% CI: 15.61–21.39). We observed an upward trend in PE incidence during the period 1999 to 2012. During this period a total of 27.347 cases of PE in Greece were reported to the National Statistical Service of Greece, with incidence per 100.000 population ranging from 13 to 30 per year (Fig. 1). PE showed a higher incidence in 2012 when compared to previous years, with an average annual reported incidence of 30 outbreaks per 100.000 population (number of cases: 3096). Table 1 presents PE incidence in Greece per geographical area in the years before and after the economic crisis faced by Greece (at 2008). We observed statistically significant differences of PE incidence for the two different periods of time (1999–2008 versus 2009–2012, 14.49 versus 23.06, respectively, $p = 0.002$). When comparing the 10 regional areas with the intervals 1999–2008 and 2009–2012, we noticed that there are areas with a large increase in incidence, while only one remained approximately at the same level (Additional file 1: Table S1 and Figure S1A and S1B). Specifically, we observed that Thessaly and the Ionian Islands have the largest increase in the incidence, Epirus has a small increase, while Macedonia has a very small decrease ($p < 0.001$).

Incidence rate increases with age. Figure 2 presents the age distribution of PE from 1999 to 2007 where available data concerning age where provided. The number of cases reported during this period was 14.827 and showed an increasing trend from the age group "10–19" to "70–79", however, there is a downward trend after the age of 79. In more details, the disease showed a higher proportion in the "70–79" age group with approximately 30% ($n = 4446$) of cases, followed by "60–69" and "80–89" age groups with 17.50% ($n = 2595$) and 16.84% ($n = 2497$) of total cases respectively. As for the age groups "50–59", "40–49", "30–39" and "20–29" the proportion was 11.60% ($n = 1720$), 9.11% ($n = 1352$), 8.10% ($n = 1201$) and 4.10% ($n = 608$) of cases respectively. As expected, the age group with the fewest cases of PE was "10–19" with a percentage of 0.26% ($n = 40$).

The distribution of PE cases from 1999 to 2007 by sex is presented in Fig. 3. From the total number of patients examined during this period, 44.9% ($n = 6668$) of cases

Table 1 Incidence of PE per geographic area 2 time periods, 1999–2008 (before the economic crisis) and 2009–2012 (following the economic crisis). The values correspond to cases per 100.000 population. #p = 0.002

		1999–2008	2009–2012
Incidence rate	Attica	16	27
	Central Greece	9.38	16.07
	Peloponnese	12.51	17.22
	Ionian Islands	11	25
	Epirus	20.83	25.04
	Thessaly	11	32
	Macedonia	22.01	20.74
	Thrace	14	27
	Aegean Islands	11.2	16.52
	Crete	17	24
	Total Greece	14.49	23.06#

were males and 55.1% ($n = 8191$) were females. We observed a female predominance that was not present in all years studied (Additional file 1: Figure S2). Table 2presents annual incidence of PE from 1999 to 2007 sorted by age and sex. The mean incidence increases with age for both genders with a peak at the age group of 80–89 for females and > 90 for males. Corresponding graphs are presented as Additional file 1: (Figure S3A and Figure S3B).

The total incidence of PE for the years 1999 to 2007 for females was estimated at 16.48 cases per 100.000 population and for males at 13.69 cases per 100.000 population ($p = 0.031$, Table 2 and Fig. 3). We observed a female predominance in PE age-adjusted incidence for the age-groups of 70–79 and 80–89 and a male predominance for

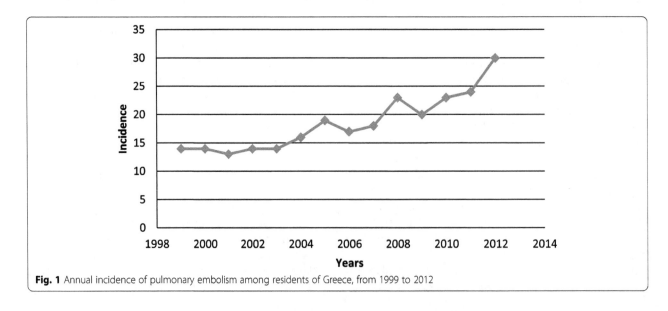

Fig. 1 Annual incidence of pulmonary embolism among residents of Greece, from 1999 to 2012

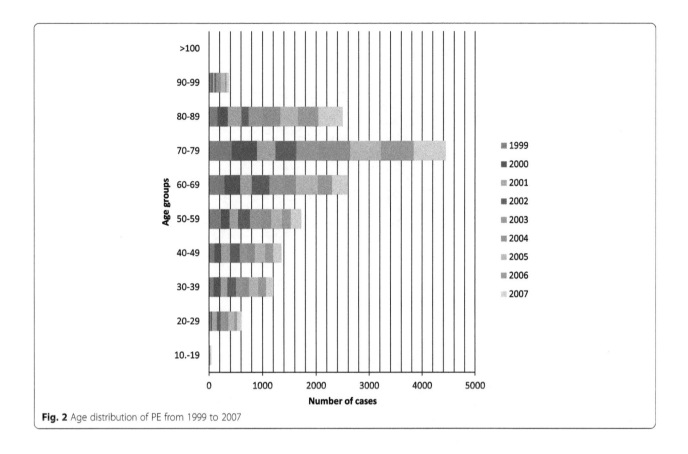

Fig. 2 Age distribution of PE from 1999 to 2007

the age groups 10–19, 20–29, 30–39, 40–49, 50–59, 60–69 and > 90 (Table 2).

Figure 4 shows the variation in the days of hospitalization per person in the years 1999 to 2007. Average nursing days in the study period are 11.44 ± 1.74. We observed that nursing days are approximately constant throughout the years.

Data on mortality were provided for the years 1999 to 2007 and are shown in detail in Additional file 1: Table S1. Mortality rate for the studied period was 2.01 ± 0.38

(95% CI: 1.72–2.31) per 100.000 population. We observed an increase in mortality rates from 1999 to 2007 although not statistically significant (Fig. 5).

Discussion

To our knowledge, this is the first study addressing PE incidence in the Greek population. According to our results, PE incidence is 30 cases per 100.000 population for 2012 that seems to be lower than previously

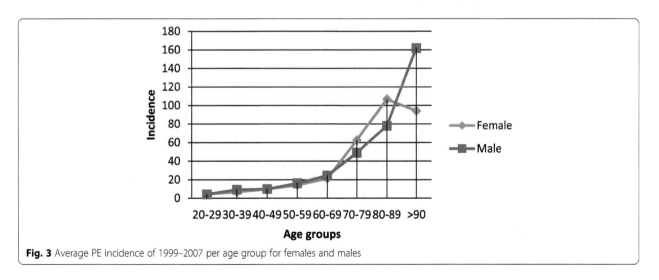

Fig. 3 Average PE incidence of 1999–2007 per age group for females and males

Table 2 Annual age-adjusted incidence of PE cases during the years 1999 to 2007 for females and males as distributed by age. Mean incidence corresponds to mean annual incidence per age group throughout the years studied

Age	Female												Male											
	Population*	1999	2000	2001	2002	2003	2004	2005	2006	2007	Mean incidence	95% CI	Population*	1999	2000	2001	2002	2003	2004	2005	2006	2007	Mean incidence	95% CI
10–19	626,778	0	0	0	0	2,55	0	0	0	1,28	0,4256	-0,2679-11,190	686,037	1,17	0	0	0	0	0	0	0	1,17	0,2600	-0,1366-0,6566
20–29	809,332	0,99	0,99	6,92	3,95	4,94	5,93	5,93	3,95	3,95	41,722	25,709-57,736	872,420	3,67	0,92	4,58	3,67	3,67	2,75	7,34	6,42	5,5	42,800	27,848-57,752
30–39	819,475	5,86	7,81	6,83	8,79	3,9	4,88	7,81	8,79	5,86	67,256	54,004-80,507	833,355	4,8	7,68	8,64	10,68	10,56	9,6	13,44	8,64	10,56	94,000	75,575-11,2425
40–49	752,130	7,45	9,57	10,64	14,89	5,32	11,7	11,7	8,51	10,64	10,0467	79,189-12,1745	743,368	6,46	6,46	11,84	9,69	11,84	8,61	14	11,84	9,69	10,0478	80,633-12,0323
50–59	638,375	15,04	16,29	10,03	17,54	12,53	12,53	16,29	16,29	12,53	14,3411	12,4091-16,2732	608,950	21,02	9,2	15,76	18,39	19,71	18,39	15,76	10,51	18,39	16,3478	13,2313-19,4643
60–69	673,592	13,21	24,94	19	27,32	17,96	16,63	32,07	20,19	20,19	21,2789	16,7997-25,7580	589,611	34,09	21,71	14,93	24,42	27,14	16,28	32,56	23,07	27,14	24,5933	19,5838-29,6028
70–79	482,051	61,474	59,74	49,79	54,77	46,88	76,55	69,7	84,85	59,95	62,6256	53,0973-72,1538	391,770	32,67	47,22	26,55	32,67	46,97	57,18	63,3	53,09	81,68	49,0367	35,7209-62,3524
80–89	168,725	75,86	56,9	118,54	56,9	85,35	137,5	104,31	170,69	156,47	106,9467	74,7534-139,1400	124,548	25,69	77,08	44,96	32,12	90,73	77,08	122,04	77,08	154,16	77,8822	45,9139-109,8505
>90	27,340	87,78	87,78	58,52	87,78	0	146,31	175,57	117,04	87,78	94,2844	55,6883-132,2806	9337	257,04	0	171,36	85,68	257,04	171,36	342,72	0	171,36	161,8400	71,9928-251,6872
Total	4,997,798	13,49	14,93	15,22	16,23	12,66	18,28	19,56	20,6	17,41	16,4867	14,4143-18,5591	4,859,396	11,85	10,81	10,35	11,55	14,95	13,16	18,48	13,31	18,77	13,6922	11,2893-16,0951

*According to the 2001 census
**Total Greek population with age group "0–9": 10932136

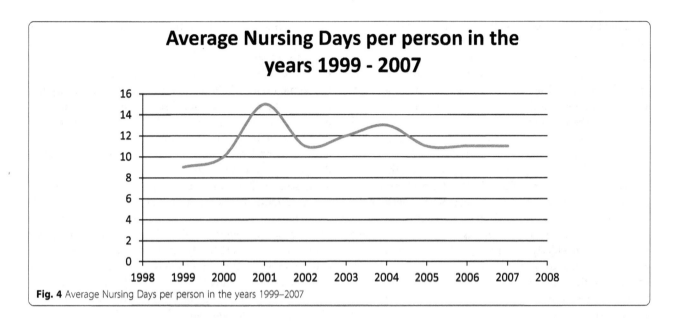

Fig. 4 Average Nursing Days per person in the years 1999–2007

published reports from other countries [3, 4]. Additionally, we demonstrated that there is an upward trend in PE incidence from 1999 to 2012, probably reflecting advances in available diagnostic tests among others. The available data revealed a female predominance that was mainly attributed to the age group of > 70 years. As expected, PE incidence rised with older age with a peak at years 80–89.

The annual incidence in PE for 2012 was estimated to 30 per 100.000 population. The reported incidence in PE is lower than previously reported by others. Dentali et al. [13] observed an incidence of 55.4 for females and 40.6 for males per 100.000 population in Northwestern Italy. Date from the USA report an incidence of VTE of 133

cases per 100.000 population [4]. The significant variation may be attributed to multiple factors including age distribution of the population studied, ethnicity, CTPA availability and/or PE awareness among clinicians [6]. The design of our study did not address this data and further studies are required to elicit the significant variation of PE incidence among studies.

We observed annual increases in PE incidence in the 14 years studied. We demonstrated a PE incidence of 30 cases per 100.000 population in 2012 and 14 cases per 100.000 population in 1999. The increase in PE incidence was evident in both genders. Our results are in agreement with previously published data [5, 8, 13–16] suggesting an upward trend in PE event rates throughout the years. The

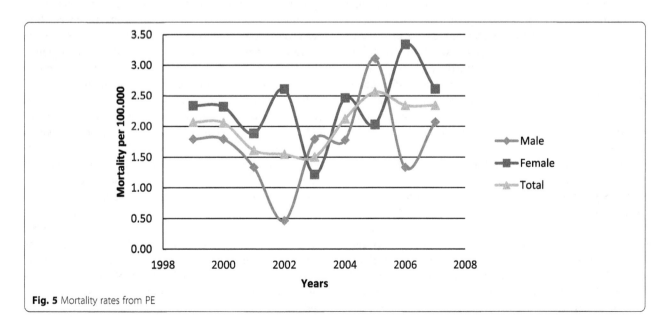

Fig. 5 Mortality rates from PE

observed trends may be partially explained by the continuous improvement in diagnostic strategies for the identification of the disease. The wide availability of CTPA along with the greater adoption of diagnostic algorithms may explain the rise in PE incidence. A greater awareness of PE among clinicians and the higher rate of incidental diagnosis of PE (when Computed Tomography was performed for other reasons, i.e. cancer staging) may to some extent account for the increased rates of PE [9].

Our results provide further support to the age-dependent increase in VTE risk. We have observed increased PE incidence in older subjects with a peak at the age groups > 80 years for both genders. Our findings are consistent with previously published data. Incidence rates of PE in elderly patients are three times as high when compared to younger patients [17]. The factors underlying the increase in VTE risk with age are multiple and include alterations in coagulation system proteins, platelet activity and inflammatory state among others [18].

Our data revealed a female predominance in PE incidence that was mainly attributed to the age groups of 70–79 and 80–89 years with no significant differences in age-adjusted incidence in the younger age groups for both genders. Traditionally the age-adjusted incidence of PE is considered higher among males with a male to female ratio of 1.2:1. Studied have previously shown a female predominance in PE incidence [13] although age-adjusted incidence of VTE among males and females presents no differences suggesting that sex does not significantly impact on VTE incident cases [13, 19]. We observed significant differences in total PE incidence among females and males. One possible explanation could be differences in life expectancy amongst sexes. The life expectancy of females is greater than males for the study period (ranging from 81.1 in 1999 to 83.4 years in 2012 for females and 75.90 in 1999 to 78 years in 2012 for males) [20]. Additionally, differences in thrombotic and fibrinolytic activity between the two sexes may implicate the sex-related discrepancies of PE incidence in older age [21]. The factors, contributing to the sex dependent increase in PE incidence in our population merits further research in future studies.

We have demonstrated a rather low rate of PE related deaths although the mortality rate seems to increase from 1999 to 2007. The mortality rate reported in our study is lower than the one reported in United Kingdom [8] and USA [7] and approximately the same with the one reported in Australia [9]. Additionally mortality rates increase over time in certain countries and decrease in others [22]. The reasons for the increase in PE related deaths throughout the year are uncertain and cannot be addressed with the data available in our study.

It is well known that the financial crisis in Greece has significantly reduced health expenses from 13.2% in 2006 to 11.5% in 2012 [23, 24]. Studies have demonstrated a deterioration of self-rated health during the economic crisis [25, 26], while the financial austerity has been associated with an increase in people reporting unmet medical needs [27]. Greece has ranked 4th out of 30 countries in terms of deaths from the A(H1N1) influenza virus and the Western Nile virus outbreak during the period 2009–2012 [28]. However, austerity has been associated with important positive steps including the standardization of the health benefits package for all citizens and new monitoring tools for hospital management and the development of e-health governance tools. We demonstrated a statistically significant increase in PE incidence between two time frames, 1999–2008 and 2009–2012 that corresponds to the economic crisis. We attribute the increase in PE diagnosis to the improvements of diagnostic tests and possibly to the increased awareness for the disease as well as the rise in the use of public services as opposed to private ones [29, 30]. Unfortunately, our study was not designed to address this question and no definite conclusions can be drawn regarding the explanation of our findings.

Our study has several strengths and limitations. This is the first report of PE incidence in Greece and covers data for a long period of time (14 years). However we acknowledge that data on age, sex, days of hospitalization and mortality are limited to the years 1999–2007 since the Hellenic Statistical Authority had no available data thereafter. Unfortunately, the reasons that underlie this are not available to us. One possible explanation could be that the economic downturn faced by Greece could influence the department(s) resourcing and that may have influenced the data reporting. To our knowledge there was no reduction in the personnel responsible for coding, although this merits further exploration. Additionally, our study is of retrospective nature while we did not have available data on demographics of the cases (besides age and gender) or VTE related risk factors like cancer or hormone-replacement therapy. Our study was based on the discharge diagnoses (including fatal cases) of PE from all the Greek provinces during the years 1999 and 2012. The Hellenic Statistical Authority provided data on gender and age distribution of PE diagnosis on each geographical department. Unfortunately, data on the risk factors associated with the reported cases (including comorbidities, hospitalization status, use of thromboprophylaxis, etc) were not available to us. We have included only PE cases that were recorded by hospital discharges irrespective of length of hopsitalization (including early discharfe or < 24 h hopsital stay). PE cases managed as outpatients were not included in the analysis. However, we have reason to believe that the proportion of patients managed as outpatients would be rather small. Analysis form the RIETE registry suggests that only a small proportion of PE patients are managed as outpatients for our study period (ranging from 0.03 to 1.7% for 2001 to 2013, respectively) suggesting a minimal estimation bias [31].

Conclusions

In conclusion, the results of our study confirm a not negligible incidence of PE in the Greek population. During the 14 years of observation the incidence of PE appeared to increase, while it remains below the expected trend in an international context. The frequency of CTPA testing has increased in emergency departments, and we suggest that further studies could analyze national data to determine how increased rates of diagnosis for PE compare with the utilization of outpatient management options for low-risk PE.

Abbreviations

CTPA: Computed Tomography Pulmonary Angiography; PE: Pulmonary Embolism; SPSS: Statistical Package for Social Sciences; USA: United States of America; VTE: Venous Thromboembolism

Acknowledgements

Not applicable.

Authors' contributions

KIG was involved in the study conception and design. FM was involved in the literature search and in the data interpretation. DR performed the literature search, the data collection, the statistical analysis and prepared and write the manuscript. KIG, ZD and FM were involved in revising the manuscript for important intellectual content. All authors read and approved the final manuscript.

References

1. Goldhaber SZ. Pulmonary embolism. Lancet. 2004;363:1295–305. https://doi.org/10.1016/S0140-6736(04)16004-2.
2. Kyrle PA, Eichinger S, et al. Lancet. 2005;365:1163–74. https://doi.org/10.1016/S0140-6736(05)71880-8.
3. Spencer FA, Emery C, Joffe SW, et al. Incidence rates, clinical profile, and outcomes of patients with venous thromboembolism. The Worcester VTE study. J Thromb Thrombolysis. 2009;28:401–9. https://doi.org/10.1007/s11239-009-0378-3.
4. Huang W, Goldberg RJ, Anderson FA, Kiefe CI, Spencer FA. Secular trends in occurrence of acute venous thromboembolism: the Worcester VTE study (1985-2009). Am J Med. 2014;127:829–39. https://doi.org/10.1016/j.amjmed.2014.03.041.
5. Wiener RS, Schwartz LM, Woloshin S. Time trends in pulmonary embolism in the United States: evidence of overdiagnosis. Arch Intern Med. 2011;171:831–7. https://doi.org/10.1001/archinternmed.2011.178.
6. Cushman M. Epidemiology and risk factors for venous thrombosis. SeminHematol. 2007;44:62–9. https://doi.org/10.1053/j.seminhematol.2007.02.004.
7. Horlander KT, Mannino DM, Leeper KV. Pulmonary embolism mortality in the United States, 1979-1998: an analysis using multiple-cause mortality data. Arch Intern Med. 2003;163:1711–7. https://doi.org/10.1001/archinte.163.14.1711

8. Aylin P, Bottle A, Kirkwood G, Bell D. Trends in hospital admissions for pulmonary embolism in England: 1996/7 to 2005/6. ClinMed. 2008;8:388–92. https://doi.org/10.7861/clinmedicine.8-4-388.
9. Shiraev TP, Omari A, Rushworth RL. Trends in pulmonary embolism morbidity and mortality in Australia. Thromb Res. 2013;132:19–25. https://doi.org/10.1016/j.thromres.2013.04.032.
10. Yang Y, Liang L, Zhai Z, et al. Pulmonary embolism incidence and fatality trends in Chinese hospitals from 1997 to 2008: a multicenter registration study. PLoS One. 2011;6:e26861. https://doi.org/10.1371/journal.pone.0026861.
11. Kotsiou OS, Zouridis S, Kosmopoulos M, Gourgoulianis KI. Impact of the financial crisis on COPD burden: Greece as a case study. Eur Respir Rev. 2018;27:170106. https://doi.org/10.1183/16000617.0106-2017.
12. Hellenic Statistical Authority of Greece. [www.statistics.gr]. Access 16/12/2019.
13. Dentali F, Ageno W, Pomero F, Fenoglio L, Squizzato A, Bonzini M. Time trends and case fatality rate of in-hospital treated pulmonary embolism during 11 years of observation in northwestern Italy. Thromb Haemost2016; 116: 399–405; doi:https://doi.org/10.1160/TH15-02-0172.
14. Park B, Messina L, Dargon P, Huang W, Ciocca R, Anderson FA. Recent trends in clinical outcomes and resource utilization for pulmonary embolism in the United States: findings from the nationwide inpatient sample. Chest. 2009;136:983–90. https://doi.org/10.1378/chest.08-2258.
15. de Miguel-Díez J, Jiménez-García R, Jiménez D, et al. Trends in hospital admissions for pulmonary embolism in Spain from 2002 to 2011. Eur Respir J. 2014;44:942–50. https://doi.org/10.1183/09031936.00194213.
16. Mellemkjaer L, Sorensen HT, Dreyer L, Olsen J, Olsen JH. Admission for and mortality from primary venous thromboembolismin women of fertile age in Denmark, 1977–95. BMJ. 1999;319:820–1. https://doi.org/10.1136/bmj.319.7213.820.
17. Cushman M, Tsai AW, White RH, et al. Deep vein thrombosis and pulmonary embolism in two cohorts: the longitudinal investigation of thromboembolism etiology. Am J Med. 2004;117:19–25. https://doi.org/10.1016/j.amjmed.2004.01.018.
18. Wilkerson WR, Sane DC. Aging and thrombosis. InSeminars in thrombosis and hemostasis. 2002;28:555–68. https://doi.org/10.1055/s-2002-36700.
19. Tagalakis V, Patenaude V, Kahn SR, Suissa S. Incidence of and mortality from venous thromboembolism in a real-world population: the Q-VTE study cohort. Am J Med. 2013;126:832–e13. https://doi.org/10.1016/j.amjmed.2013.02.024.
20. Countryeconomy.com [https://countryeconomy.com/demography/life-expectancy/Greece], Access 16/12/2019.
21. Stegnar M, Pentek M. Fibrinolytic response to venous occlusion in healthy subjects: relationship to age, gender, body weight, blood lipids and insulin. Thromb Res. 1993;69:81–92. https://doi.org/10.1016/0049-3848(93)90005-9.
22. Hoffmann B, Gross CR, Jöckel KH, Kröger K. Trends in mortality of pulmonary embolism–an international comparison. Thromb Res. 2010;125:303–8. https://doi.org/10.1016/j.thromres.2009.06.015.
23. OECD (2013), Health at a Glance 2013: OECD Indicators, OECD Publishing. https://doi.org/10.1787/health_glance-2013-en.
24. WHO Regional Office for Europe (2014). Health for All database [online/offline database]. Copenhagen, WHO Regional Office For Europe (http://data.euro.who.int/hfadb, accessed 2 November 2014).
25. Kentikelenis A, Karanikolos M, Papanicolas I, Basu S, McKee M, Stuckler D. Health effects of financial crisis: omens of a Greek tragedy. Lancet. 2011;378: 1457–8. https://doi.org/10.1016/S0140-6736(11)61556-0.
26. Zavras D, Tsiantou V, Pav E, Mylona K, Kyriopoulos J. Impact of economic crisis and other demographic and socio-economic factors on self-rated health in Greece. Eur J Pub Health. 2013;23:206–10. https://doi.org/10.1093/eurpub/cks143.
27. Economou C, Kaitelidou D, Kentikelenis A, Maresso A, Sissouras A. The impact of the crisis on the health system and health in Greece. Economic crisis, health systems and health in Europe: Country experience [Internet]. EuropeanObservatoryonHealthSystemsandPolicies, 2015.
28. Bonovas S, Nikolopoulos G. High-burden epidemics in Greece in the era of economic crisis. Early signs of a public health tragedy. J Prev Med Hyg. 2012;53:169 71.

29. Ministry of Health and Social Solidarity. ESYnet database. Athens, 2012a.
30. Ministry of Health and Social Solidarity. Ministry of Health and Social Solidarity. Report on the outcomes of Ministry of Health and its health units, 2011. Athens, Dionikos, March 2012 [inGreek], 2012b.
31. Jiménez D, de Miguel-Díez J, Guijarro R, et al. Trends in the management and outcomes of acute pulmonary embolism: analysis from the RIETE registry. J Am Coll Cardiol. 2016;67:162–70. https://doi.org/10.1016/j.jacc.2015.10.060.

25

A case-report of widespread pulmonary embolism in a middle-aged male seven weeks after asymptomatic suspected COVID-19 infection

Mats Beckman[1,2], Sven Nyrén[1,2] and Anna Kistner[2,3]* ⓘ

Abstract

Background: Pulmonary embolism (PE) is seen in high frequency in hospital-treated patients with Covid-19. We present a case of suspected Covid-19 with long-term dyspnea and widespread PE.

Case presentation: A 51- year old male, with no prior medical history, no medication, and non-smoker arrived at the emergency department with exercise induced dyspnea during 4–5 weeks and for the last 48 h dyspnea at rest. Seven weeks before hospitalization, he felt difficulties taking deep breaths for some days but no other symptoms. Oxygen saturation at rest was 93%. Troponin T was 1200 mg/L (ref < 15 mg/L). CT angiography revealed widespread bilateral segmental pulmonary embolism. Additional findings were ground glass opacities that could match Covid-19. The patient tested negative for SARS -CoV-2. Full dose tinzaparin was given for 2 days in hospital, followed by apixaban for 6 months. Recovery has been uneventful so far.

Conclusions: Long-term breathing difficulties might be relatively common after non-hospitalized symptomatic Covid-19. The frequency of PE in this group is unknown. We report a case of suspected covid-19 with widespread PE and a long history of dyspnea but no other symptoms. In our case slight hypoxia and laboratory testing indicated significant disease, which was proven with contrast angiography. This case shows that PE is a differential diagnosis in non-hospitalized symptomatic Covid-19 with persisting breathing problems.

Keywords: Pulmonary embolism, Covid-19, Male, Ground-glass

Background

Pulmonary embolism (PE) has been shown to be common in hospitalized Covid-19 patients with a 30% incidence [1]. In Sweden, infected subjects treated at home were not tested. Falling ill with fever and cough were regarded as typical Covid-19 infection and the recommendations from the Public Health Authority (FHM) in Sweden was "stay at home until you feel healthy and 48 hours thereafter" [2]. We report a case of suspected Covid-19 infection with widespread pulmonary embolism in a patient with no previous symptoms and severe pulmonary embolism.

Case presentation

A 51- year old male, with no prior medical history, no medication, non-smoker and without risk factors for venous thrombo-embolism arrived at the end of April to the emergency department with exercise induced dyspnea during 4–5 weeks and for the last 48 h

* Correspondence: anna.kistner@sll.se
2Department of Molecular Medicine and Surgery, Karolinska Institutet, Stockholm, Sweden
3Medical Radiation Physics and Nuclear Medicine, Imaging and Physiology, Karolinska University Hospital, Stockholm, Sweden
Full list of author information is available at the end of the article

dyspnea also at rest. Prior to the onset of symptoms, he had lived socially isolated with his wife from mid-March, approximately 40 days, both working from home and with their two children home from school. He described a short period in the beginning of March, 7 weeks before hospitalization, when he felt difficulties taking deep breaths for a couple of days but no other symptoms like cough, fever or feeling of malaise. Following that episode he experienced a gradually increased fatigue on his regular run and in the beginning of April he had to start walking when running uphill. During the last 5 weeks before hospitalization his wife and daughter had noticed signs of heavy breathing when he walked up the stairs.

Physical examination was normal, examination of the heart and lungs revealed no discrepancies, no swollen legs or other signs of cardiac decompensation. The bodyweight of the patient was 90 kg and his height was 1.88 m, body mass index (BMI) was 25,5 kg/m^2. He had normal temperature and a regular heart rate of 80 beats/min. He had a blood pressure of 180/65 mmHg and an oxygen saturation of 93% breathing ambient air. High sensitivity Troponin T was markedly elevated, 1200 (reference < 15 mg/L) and also B-type natriuretic peptide was increased, 737 (reference < 125 ng/L). He had a slightly increased C-reactive protein of 15 (reference < 5 mg/L) and modest leukocytosis 11,7 (normal range 3,5–8,8 × 10^9/L). ECG showed incomplete right-sided branch block. Computerized Tomography Angiography (CTA) of the chest was performed as pulmonary embolism was suspected. The CTA revealed widespread bilateral segmental pulmonary embolism (Fig. 1) and an additional area of consolidation in the right upper lobe consistent with infarction. Additional findings of ground glass opacities that could match Covid-19 were also found (Fig. 2). The patient tested negative for SARS -CoV-2 (polymerase chain reaction SARS

-CoV-2, GeneXpert, Cepheid, Sunnyvale, CA, United States) at two consecutive nasopharynx tests. No antibody test was performed. The patient was given oxygen and subcutaneous low molecular weight heparin (LWMH), tinzaparin 18,000 units daily during 2 days of hospitalization and was discharged with apixaban 5 mg, twice daily, with a treatment recommendation for 6 months.

Echocardiography revealed dilated right chamber, midventricular diameter of 5 cm and left septum deviation, light to moderate insufficiency of the tricuspid valve with a velocity max of 4,2 m/s. Vena cava inferior showed normal width and breathing variation. Severe pulmonary hypertension with a systolic pulmonary pressure of approximately 75–80 mmHg (normal upper limit 35 mmHg) was present. No significant amount of pericardial fluid was present.

Discussion and conclusions

This case of suspected asymptomatic Covid-19 infection with widespread pulmonary embolism 7 weeks after possible infection proves the complex nature of this disease. It indicates the importance of informing individuals with or without a previously suspected Covid-19 to be aware of the risk for complications during a long time period. It is of importance that subjects seek care if suffering dyspnea or swollen legs. Healthcare workers need to be informed about pulmonary embolism as a possible late complication in subjects not severely affected by the disease. A weakness of this study is that we do not have the definite diagnosis. However, nasopharynx-and serology tests are seldom performed on individuals without clinical symptoms. A negative virus test 7 weeks after a possible infection is to be anticipated. A commercial antibody test (Abbott Architect SARS-CoV-2 IgG, North Chicago, Illinois, United States) taken 10 weeks after hospital discharge was negative. T cell immunity,

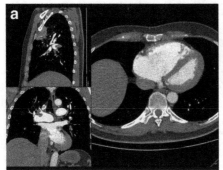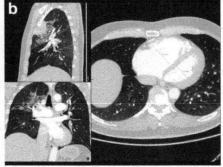

Fig. 1 a and **b** Widespread bilateral pulmonary embolism with right ventricular affection and a right ventricular to left ventricular quotient of 1,7 (ref < 0,9), as well as consolidation in the ventral part of the right upper lobe consistent with a suspected infarction

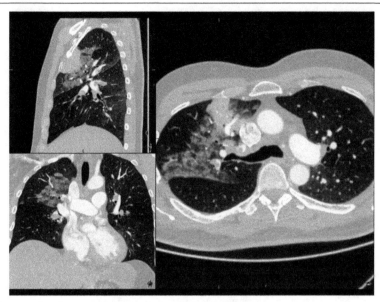

Fig. 2 Ground glass opacities as well as the area of infarction in the right upper lobe

that has been shown to be robust in convalescent individuals with asymptomatic or mild Covid-19 [3], was not investigated.

From the combination of very light respiratory symptoms 7 weeks before the examination and Covid-19 typical consolidations on the CTA we find it very probable that the patient had a Covid-19 infection almost 2 months before the acute illness and a widespread pulmonary embolism.

Longitudinal studies in medically ill patients have shown that the majority of venous thrombosis events occur in the posthospital setting within 6 weeks of hospitalization [4]. Consensus is emerging and recommendations at the moment say that hospitalized patients with Covid-19 should receive anticoagulants. The present practice guidelines recommend thromboprophylaxis with subcutaneous LMWH twice daily at prophylactic or intermediate doses, to reduce thrombotic risk [5, 6]. Security considerations are important with dose reduction in renal insufficiency etc. Patients hospitalized with severe Covid-19 pneumonia, especially if obese (BMI $> 30 \, \mathrm{kg/m^2}$), might be at further increased risk for thombosis and now often receive full dose (therapeutic) anticoagulation from hospital admission [7]. Thus treatment and recommended doses has changed over time.

After hospital discharge from Covid-19, extended prophylaxis with LMWH or novel oral anticoagulants (NOAC) can reduce the risk of venous thrombosis event [8] and treatment with NOAC during 2 to 4 weeks after hospital discharge is common practice according to region Stockholm expert committee guidelines (janusinfo.se), sometimes for longer period. If venous thromboembolism

has been detected during hospitalization, a treatment period of 3 to 6 months is recommended. The possible value of anticoagulants to non-hospitalized patients with Covid-19 is subject to investigation. The case discussed in this paper indicates a possible value of such antithrombotic treatment. It also shows that PE could be a differential diagnosis in non-hospitalized symptomatic Covid-19 with persisting breathing difficulties.

Abbreviations
PE: Pulmonary embolism; FMH: Public Health Authority; CTA: Computerized Tomography Angiography; BMI: Body mass index; LWMH: Low molecular weight heparin; NOAC: Novel oral anticoagulants

Acknowledgements
We want to express our gratitude to Dr. Jens Frick, Head of the Radiology Department, Nyköpings Lasarett, Sweden for help and support.

Declarations
The research was conducted in accordance with the ethical standards of all applicable national and institutional committees and the World Medical Association's Helsinki Declaration.

Authors' contributions
AK performed the acquisition, AK, MB and SN contributed in the analysis and interpretation of data; AK and MB drafted the work and SN revised it. The author(s) read and approved the final manuscript.

Authors' information
not applicable

Author details
[1]Department of Radiology, Imaging and Physiology, Karolinska University Hospital, Stockholm, Sweden. [2]Department of Molecular Medicine and Surgery, Karolinska Institutet, Stockholm, Sweden. [3]Medical Radiation Physics and Nuclear Medicine, Imaging and Physiology, Karolinska University Hospital, Stockholm, Sweden.

References

1. Leonard-Lorant I, Delabranche X, Severac F, Helms J, Pauzet C, Collange O, et al. Acute pulmonary embolism in COVID-19 patients on CT angiography and relationship to D-dimer levels. Radiology. 2020;296:E189. https://doi.org/10.1148/radiol.2020201561.

2. Swedish Public Health Authority. Guidance for criteria of assessment of freedom of infection at Covid-19. (Publication in Swedish) 2020. Published July 20 2020.

3. Sekine T, Perez-Potti A, Rivera-Ballesteros O, Strålin K, Gorin J-B, Olsson A, et al. Robust T cell immunity in convalescent individuals withasymptomatic or mild COVID-19. Cell. 2020. https://doi.org/10.1016/j.cell.2020.08.017.

4. Spyropoulos AC, Ageno W, Cohen AT, Gibson CM, Goldhaber SZ, Raskob G. Prevention of venous thromboembolism in hospitalized medically ill patients: a U.S. perspective. Thromb Haemost. 2020;120(6):924–36.

5. Spyropoulos AC, Levy JH, Ageno W, Connors JM, Hunt BJ, Iba T, et al. Scientific and standardization committee communication: clinical guidance on the diagnosis, prevention and treatment of venous thromboembolism in hospitalized patients with COVID-19. J Thromb Haemost. 2020;18:1859.

6. Cohoon KP, Mahe G, Tafur AJ, Spyropoulos AC. Emergence of institutional antithrombotic protocols for coronavirus 2019. Res Pract Thromb Haemost. 2020;4:510–7.

7. Susen S, Tacquard CA, Godon A, Mansour A, Garrigue D, Nguyen P, et al. Prevention of thrombotic risk in hospitalized patients with COVID-19 and hemostasis monitoring. Crit Care. 2020;24(1):364.

8. Bikdeli B, Madhavan MV, Jimenez D, Chuich T, Dreyfus I, Driggin E, et al. COVID-19 and thrombotic or thromboembolic disease: implications for prevention, antithrombotic therapy, and follow-up: JACC state-of-the-art review. J Am Coll Cardiol. 2020;75(23):2950–73.

26

Low molecular weight heparins use in pregnancy: A practice survey from Greece

E. Papadakis[1]* ⓘ, A. Pouliakis[2], A. Aktypi[3], A. Christoforidou[4], P. Kotsi[5], G. Anagnostou[6], A. Foifa[7] and E. Grouzi[8]

Abstract

Background: Use of LMWH in pregnancy is not only limited to VTE management, but it extends, to the management of vascular gestational complications and the optimization of IVF pregnancies despite the lack of concrete scientific evidence. In this context, we conducted the present study aiming to gain insights regarding the use of LMWH during pregnancy and puerperium. We recorded indication for use, diagnostic work-up as well as the safety and efficacy of the treatment, trying to elucidate the clinical practice in our country.

Methods: We analyzed data regarding 818 pregnant women received LMWH during 2010–2015.Our cohort had a median age of 33.9 years and a BMI of 23.6.There were 4 groups: those with a history of VTE [Group-A: 76], those with pregnancy complications [Group-B: 445], those undergoing IVF [Group-C: 132] and those carrying prothrombotic tendency (thrombophilia, family history of VTE, other) [Group-D: 165]. Mean duration of LMWH administration was 8.6 ± 1.5 months. Out of the total number, 440 received LMWH in fixed prophylactic dose, 272 in higher prophylactic-weight adjusted dose and 106 in therapeutic dose. Moreover, 152 women received in addition low-dose acetylsalicylic acid (ASA). 93.8% of pregnancies were single and 6.2% were multiple ones. Live births occurred in 98.7% of pregnancies.

Results: Anticoagulation was efficacious and well tolerated. Seventeen VTE events were recorded; 7 of them antepartum and 10 postpartum. No major bleeding events were observed while 13 clinical relevant non-major bleeding events were recorded. Regarding gestational vascular complications, 28 IUGR events were recorded, as well as 48 cases of preterm labor of which 12 were concomitant with IUGR (25%). Six early pregnancy losses were recorded; there were 3 fetal deaths and 3 cases of pre-eclampsia/eclampsia.

Conclusions: LMWHs are used extensively during pregnancy and puerperium in Greece for VTE treatment and prophylaxis and for a variety of other indications as well. Although the drug has been shown to be both safe and efficacious, its use for some indications has no proven scientific evidence. In order to clearly define the role of LMWHs in pregnancy, beyond thromboprophylaxis, large prospective studies are required, which could be based on the conclusions of this study.

Keywords: Low molecular weight heparin, Pregnancy, Venous thromboembolism, Pregnancy complications

* Correspondence: emmpapadoc@yahoo.com
[1]Hemostasis Unit-Hematology Department Papageorgiou Hospital, Thessaloniki Ringroad 56403 Nea Efkarpia, Thessaloniki, Greece
Full list of author information is available at the end of the article

Introduction

It is well known that pregnancy alters the haemostatic system into a hypercoagulable state, which increases throughout pregnancy and is maximal around term. These physiological changes are important for minimizing intra-partum blood loss, but they entail an increased risk of thromboembolism during pregnancy and the post-partum period [1]. For the mother, this risk begins from the time of conception and continues well into the postnatal period, with recent data suggesting that the risk could extend to 12 weeks postpartum [2].

The pro-coagulant state of pregnancy could also contribute to the occurrence of gestational vascular complications (GVCs) (pre-eclampsia, placental abruption, fetal growth restriction (FGR), late and recurrent early miscarriage, intrauterine death and stillbirth), especially in the presence of acquired or inherited thrombophilia [3–5]. There is some evidence suggesting that placental thrombosis could play a role in the pathogenesis of pregnancy loss [6]. On the other hand, other GVCs, such as pre-eclampsia or FGR, have been suggested at least partly due to placental insufficiency, possibly as a result of inappropriate coagulation activation [7].

Anticoagulation with low molecular weight heparins (LMWHs) is a well-established antithrombotic practice for primary and secondary thromboprophylaxis during pregnancy. There has been evidence that heparin and its derivatives could exert a beneficial effect in preventing gestational vascular complications [3, 8]. However, the published data on the role of LMWH were obtained mostly from women with thrombophilia [9]. Low dose aspirin (ASA) and LMWH have proven their effectiveness in increasing live birth rates in the setting of gestational antiphospholipid syndrome. However, their use in the context of inherited thrombophilia and pregnancy complications is less well established.

There is increasing evidence in favor of the use of heparin in women with pregnancy complications mediated by the placenta, selected by previous pregnancy outcome and not by thrombophilic defect [10]. Due to their excellent safety record, LMWHs have been offered to women at high risk of an adverse pregnancy outcome in advance of scientific evidence. The administration of LMWHs in the prevention of preeclampsia and small for gestational age (SGA) fetuses is based on biological plausibility and extrapolation from antiphospholipid syndrome [11].

An increasing number of women undergoing assisted reproductive technology (ART) receives LMWHs due to its possible role in increasing the possibility of a successful implantation of the developing embryo in in vitro ART, through modulating a wide variety of proteins involved [12]. It has been suggested that heparins can improve the apposition of the blastocyst and interfere with the apoptosis occurring during the implantation stage of a pregnancy [13]. Two systematic reviews [12, 14] found that the administration of LMWH may increase clinical pregnancy and live birth rates in women undergoing in vitro fertilization (IVF) or intra cell sperm injection (ICSI); authors concluded that, due to the wide heterogeneity of protocols used and the small sample size of women randomized, these results need to be further confirmed in 'ad hoc' studies.

In this context, in an attempt to elucidate the clinical practice in our country, we conducted the present cohort study aiming to gain insights regarding the use of LMWHs during pregnancy and puerperium, describing the indications for use, the diagnostic work-up as well as the safety and efficacy of the treatment.

Patients and methods

A multicenter, retrospective study that addressed the issue of LMWH use in pregnancy in Greece, was performed including pregnant women receiving LMWH for prophylaxis either due to personal history of thromboembolic events, mainly venous thromboembolism (VTE) (group A), or history of GVCs, with the majority of them being less than 3 early pregnancy losses, (group B), or because they were undergoing IVF (group C). A number of women who received LMWH due to family history of VTE, thrombophilia and other, not specified reasons, were also included (Group D). Participants were recruited from seven Hematological Centers all over Greece. The following data were collected for each participant: age, BMI, indication for using LMWH, type and dose of LMWH (fixed-prophylactic dose, higher prophylactic – weight adjusted or therapeutic dose) according to RCOG guidelines, as well as thrombophilia factors [FV Leiden, FII mutation, LAC, antipospholipid antibodies (APLA) (lupus anticoagulant and/ or anticardiolipin and/or β2-glycoprotein-1 antibodies), antithrombin (AT), protein C (PC) and protein S (PS) concentrations]. In addition, low dose ASA (80–100 mg) use was assessed. High risk thrombophilia was defined as the presence of AT deficiency, compound heterozygosity for FV Leiden and FII mutations or homozygosity for FV Leiden or FII mutations and PC and PS deficiencies [15]. All pregnant women receiving thromboprophylaxis were eligible to be included and no exclusion criteria were applied. This was a retrospective study, data were retrieved from women' medical records and missing data were retrieved via additional contact.

All women were followed-up until the end of puerperium (6 weeks after birth) in order to monitor safety and efficacy of anticoagulation recording any thrombotic or bleeding events. We tracked down VTEs and superficial thromboses objectively confirmed during gestation and puerperium and we noticed any bleeding episode during the same period and classified it according to the definitions as proposed by the ISTH [16, 17]. Data for adverse events that would led to discontinuation or modification of treatment were recorded. Furthermore we recorded any gestational vascular complication and the pregnancy outcome.

Statistics

Statistical analysis was performed by the SAS for Windows 9.4 software platform [18] (SAS Institute Inc., NC, U.S.A.). Demographic and clinical/prognostic data of the patients at baseline were described with numerical and categorical summary statistics. Statistics were expressed as the mean value along with the standard deviation (SD). In addition, for the sake of completeness, the median value and the values for 25 and 75% quartiles were also reported. Comparisons between two or more groups for the categorical parameters were performed by means of the chi-square test [19]. For the parameters expressed in numerical form (such as the women's age, their BMI, the duration of treatment with LMWH or ASA, etc.) normality was not always ensured, therefore, non-parametric tests were preferred; more specifically the Kruskal-Wallis test was applied [18]. The significance level (p-value) was set to 0.05, thus statistically significant difference between the parameters compared for the groups under study was for $p < 0.05$.

Results

In total 818 women (mean age 33.9 SD ± 4.9 years) that used LWMH during pregnancy and puerperium were studied. 76 (9.3%) women used LMWH due to personal history of VTE (Deep Vein Thrombosis (DVT), Pulmonary Embolism (PE)) (group A), 445 (54.4%) used LWMH due to pregnancy (early or late) complications (group B), 132 (16.1%) used LMWH after undergoing IVF (group C) and 165 (20.2%) used LMWH for other reasons (group D). The Baseline Characteristics of all patients are presented in Table 1 (and in more details in Table 4 in Appendix), while the summary and comparison of the parameters studied for each group are presented in Table 2 (and in a higher detail in Table 5 in Appendix).

The LMWH compounds that were administered were the following: tinzaparin (innohep®) to 651 women (79.6%, CI: 76.7–82.2%), enoxaparin (Clexane®) to another 140 (17.1%, CI: 14.7–19.8%) and Bemiparin (Ivor®) to 27 (3.3%, CI: 2.3–4.8%) of pregnant women. The mean duration of LMWH administration was 8.6 ± 1.5 months. Among them 440 (53.8%, CI: 50.4–57.2%) received LMWH in fixed

Table 1 Baseline Characteristics of the cohort/all patients

Characteristic	$N = 818$
Age (mean ± SD)	33.9 ± 4.9
BMI (mean ± SD)	24.5 ± 4
No. of fetuses at observed gestation (N, %)	
1	767 (93.8)
≥ 2	51 (6.2)
Delivery by CS (N, %)	644 (78.7)
Reason for enrolling in the study	
Group A: History of VTE (DVT/SVT/Arterial thrombosis/Arterial Ischemia)	76 (9.3%)
Group B: History of Pregnancy complications	445 (54.4%)
Group C: IVF	132 (16.1%)
Group D: Other reasons	165 (20.2%)
Mean Duration of LMWH (months) (mean ± SD)	8.6 ± 1.5
Concomitant Use of ASA (N, %)	152 (18.6)
Mean Duration of ASA (months) (mean ± SD)	6.2 ± 2.7

prophylactic dose, 272 (33.3%, CI: 30.1–36.6%) received higher prophylactic LMWH dose and 106 (13.0%, CI: 10.8–15.4%) received a therapeutic LMWH dose. Moreover, 152 (18.6%, CI: 16.1–21.4%) women received concomitantly low-dose ASA.

In our cohort, live births were recorded in 807 (98.7%, CI: 97.6–98.7%) pregnancies. Anticoagulation during pregnancy was efficacious and well tolerated. One allergic effect on injection site required intervention. Seventeen VTE events were recorded; 7 (0.8%) of them antepartum and 10 (1.2%) postpartum. Interestingly, no major bleeding events were observed while 13 (1.6%) clinically relevant non major (CRNM) bleeding events were recorded (Table 3). The majority of bleedings [11] were observed antepartum, 10 of them were vaginal blood dripping and 1 was an epistaxis episode. All of them were self-limited but were managed with temporary withhold of anticoagulant treatment, and no-dose adjustment was necessary. Regarding postpartum bleeding we observed 2 episodes. One was CRNM bleeding of the gastric varices in a woman with paroxysmal nocturnal hemoglobinuria and portal vein thrombosis. In her case no transfusion was necessitated but we withhold LMWH and we reduced for 72 h the dose by 50%. The second postpartum bleeding was surgical bleeding from the caesarian section site that was managed by omission of 1 dose of LMWH. One can wonder how we did not observe any major postpartum hemorrhages. That can be attributed to the fact that nearly all women underwent planned cesarean section and LMWH was withhold for 24–48 h. Another possibility could be that the Obstetricians were meticulous since they were coping with high risk pregnancies. All in all we did not record

Table 2 Baseline characteristics and studied parameters of the four groups along with statistical comparison

	Group A N = 76	Group B N = 445	Group C N = 132	Group D N = 165	p-value*
Age (mean ± SD)	33.0 ± 4.3	33.5 ± 4.6	37.2 ± 5.1	32.5 ± 4.4	<.0001
BMI (mean, SD)	25.0 ± 4.3	24.4 ± 3.9	24.7 ± 3.8	24.4 ± 4.3	0.2607
No. of foetuses at the observed gestation (N. %)					
1	73, 96.1%	434, 97.5%	102, 77.3%	158, 95.8%	<.0001
≥ 2	3, 4.0%	11, 2.5%	30, 22.7%	7, 4.2%	
Mean Duration of LMWH (months)	8.7 ± 1.7	8.7 ± 1.3	8.7 ± 1.7	8.3 ± 1.6	<.0001
ASA Duration (months) (N of patients)	6.7 ± 2.8 (N = 11)	6.1 ± 2.4 (N = 79)	5.5 ± 2.8 (N = 39)	7.9 ± 2.0 (N = 19)	0.0068
Fixed Prophylactic Dose	34.2%	58.9%	50%	52.1%	<.0001
Weight Adjusted prophylactic dose	21.1%	32.4%	38.6%	37.0%	
Therapeutic dose of LMWH	44.7%	8.8%	11.4%	10.9%	
Concomitant Use of ASA	14.5%	18.2%	30.3%	12.1%	0.0006
Caesarian	80.3%	79.7%	91.7%	65.5%	<.0001
Live Birth	97.4%	99.1%	97.0%	99.4%	0.1632
High risk Thrombophilia (positive cases)	25%	10.1%	9.9%	10.3%	0.0018
APA status (total successful tests N = 363) (% positive cases within group)	29.6%	29.1%	27.1%	20.4%	0.6264

*p-value is for Kruskal-Wallis test for numerical parameters and for x-square test for categorical parameters

any major postpartum hemorrhage (according to ISTH definition) and no transfusion was needed peripartum. One pregnant developed painful skin rash in her first week of LMWH treatment which was managed with a switch to another LMWH compound, albeit the 30% risk of cross-reactivity. Eventually she underwent an uneventful pregnancy and delivery.

Regarding GVCs, 28 (3.4%) intrauterine growth restriction (IUGR) events were recorded, as well as 48 (5.9%) cases of preterm labor – of which 12 were concomitant with IUGR (25%). Six early (< 10 weeks of gestation) pregnancy losses were recorded (0.7%); there were 3 fetal deaths (0.4%) and 3 cases of pre-eclampsia/eclampsia (0.4%).

As was expected, women in **Group A** more often received LMWH at higher doses (67.1%, $p < .0001$) and had a higher percentage of known high risk

thrombophilia (25%, $p = 0.0018$), (Table 2). In **Group B**, the largest group of our cohort, the main reason of LMWH administration was early pregnancy losses ($N = 396$ women, 89%). In more detail the major pregnancy complications considered to include these women in group B (see Table 4 in Appendix) were early pregnancy loss (89%), fetal death (6%), IUGR (2%) and eclampsia/pre-eclampsia (2%). Notably, 27% of these women had simultaneously additional history (secondary reasons), such as: retrograde pregnancy (9%), early pregnancy loss and fetal death (3%). Concerning abnormal pregnancy loss, 66% of women had one incident, 22% two incidents and 12% three or more incidents. That was the group in which the majority of women (58.9%) received fixed prophylactic doses of LMWH. In **Group C**, women that received LMWH for IVF optimization, the mean age

Table 3 Events recorded in the cohort and in each of the four groups

	Group A N = 76	Group B N = 445	Group C N = 132	Group D N = 165	Total N = 818	p*
VTE [VTE postpartum]	3 (3.9%) [1 (1.3%)]	3 (0.7%) [3 (0.7%)]	0 [1 (0.8%)]	1 (0.6%) [5 (3.0%)]	7 (0.8%) [10 (1.2%)]	0.0008
Bleeding	1 (1.3%)	6 (1.3%)	5 (3.8%)	1 (0.6%)	13 (1.6%)	0.151
Gestational vascular complications	12 (15.8%)	37 (8.3%)	23 (17.4%)	16 (9.7%)	88 (10.8%)	0.0064
IUGR	2 (2.6%)	13 (2.9%)	8 (6.1%)	5 (3.0%)	28 (3.4%)	0.8784
Preterm Labor	7 (9.2%)	19 (9.1%)	12 (9.1%)	10 (6.1%)	48 (5.9%)	
Fetal Death	1 (1.3%)	1 (0.2%)	1 (0.8%)		3 (0.4%)	
Early pregnancy loss/abortion	1 (1.3%)	3 (0.7%)	2 (1.5%)		6 (0.7%)	
Pre-eclampsia/eclampsia	1 (1.3%)	1 (0.2%)		1 (0.6%)	3 (0.4%)	

* p-value is for chi-square test

$(37.2 \pm 5.1 \text{ years})$ was higher $(p < .0001)$ and multiple pregnancy was observed more often $(22.7\%, \ p < .0001)$. Furthermore, the vast majority of them $(91, 7\%)$ delivered by caesarian section (CS). In **Group D**, a quite heterogeneous cluster, the mean duration of LMWH use was the shortest among all the groups; this was also the group where the higher percentage of vaginal delivery (VD) $(34.6\%, \ p < .0001)$ was noted (Table 5 in Appendix).

Within the population under study investigation for the presence of APLA was performed in 363 women (44.4%), out of whom 100 were found positive and 263 negative for APLA. Considering the APLA status in relation to ASA treatment, within our sample, it was found that 53 women out of the 263 with negative APA were treated with ASA (20.2% of the normal APLA population) and 39 women out of the 100 with abnormal APLA status were treated with ASA (39% of the number of women who had tested positive for APLA). Therefore, about twice as many women who tested positive for APLA were simultaneously treated with ASA compared to women who tested negative for APLA (OR: 2.5, 95% CI: 1.5–4.2, $p = 0.0002$). Furthermore the highest percentage of positive APLA was found in the women of Group B who received a therapeutic dose of LMWH $(p < .0024$, Table 6 in Appendix).

In our study cohort, from the baseline characteristics per dosage used it seems that a higher mean age at enrollment, a higher BMI and a presence of high risk thrombophilia were the key drivers for the administration of higher doses (Table 6 in Appendix). Also, there was an association between the personal history of VTE and the dose of LMWH received. Bleeding events, antepartum or postpartum, were not correlated $(p = 0.82)$ with higher LMWH doses (Table 7 in Appendix).

Although pregnancy complications were noted in 10.8% of pregnancies only 1.1% of them resulted in fetal loss. It is worth mentioning that the most frequently observed complication was preterm labor in 5.9% of the cases (Table 3).

Discussion

VTE in pregnancy is an important cause of maternal morbidity and mortality in developed countries. In addition to hemostatic changes occurring during normal pregnancy, several risk factors, including hereditary and acquired thrombophilia, have been identified. Pregnant women are 4 to 5 times more likely to develop VTE than non-pregnant women of a similar age [20]. The components of Virchow's triad (hypercoagulability, venous stasis and vascular damage) are all affected during pregnancy until the postpartum period [21]. Increases in coagulation factors and decreases in natural anticoagulants during pregnancy lead to a hypercoagulable state. Venous stasis occurs as a result of a diminution in venous return caused by the pressure from the gravid uterus on the iliac veins and vena

cava [22]; trauma to the venous system could occur in the course of vaginal delivery (VD) and the risk can be exacerbated by cesarean section (CS). In a recent meta-analysis, the risk of VTE was four times greater following CS than following VD; this seemed independent of other VTE risk factors and was greater following emergency CS than following elective CS [23].

Apart from hereditary thrombophilia certain conditions have been associated with an increased risk of pregnancy related VTE. These include a previous history of thrombosis, antiphospholipid syndrome, lupus and other co-morbidities [24]. Other independent risk factors are age (older than 35 years), null parity, multiple gestation, obesity, smoking and immobility - all these factors represent an 1.5–2-fold increase in the risk [24, 25]. More recently, in pregnancies following IVF, several observational studies [26–29] have reported a higher risk of VTE, independently of the occurrence of ovarian hyper-stimulation syndrome (OHSS) compared to the spontaneous pregnancies. However, in these women, OHSS represents the main factor involved in the VTE occurrence, with a 100-fold increase in risk [26, 30].

Therefore, a careful evaluation, using a validated numerical risk assessment model, of all known preexisting, pregnancy-related and transient risk factors in both antepartum and postpartum periods is crucial to identify moderate–/high-risk women who could benefit from antithrombotic prophylaxis. The RCOG guidelines on antenatal and postnatal thromboprophylaxis [15] recommends a documented risk assessment for VTE in early pregnancy or pre-pregnancy. The assessment needs to be repeated if the woman is hospitalized or in the case of other intercurrent problems occur; and in the intrapartum or peripartum phase as well. These guidelines take into consideration the risk associated with intercurrent problems, obstetric factors and transient risk factors for VTE.

Also, depending on the level of risk it is recommended that, if the decision is made to use antepartum prophylaxis, this should be done from the earliest possible stages of pregnancy, due to the early activation of the hemostatic system [31, 32]. Similarly, as the VTE risk is increased during the first 6–12 weeks postpartum [2], prophylaxis should be extended until 6 weeks after delivery [15, 33, 34]. In most cases the benefits of anticoagulation outweigh its risks.

LMWHs represent the anticoagulant of choice for VTE prophylaxis and treatment in pregnancy, with a clear consensus among the guideline documents reviewed [15, 35, 36]. Compared with UFH, LMWH has a better bioavailability, longer plasma half-life, more predictable dose–response, and improved safety profile with respect to osteoporosis and HIT -heparin induced thrombocytopenia- [15, 35]. As far as the breast-feeding phase is concerned, LMWH as well as UFH and oral anticoagulants (Vitamin K Antagonists (VKA) - not

DOACs) have proven safety in breast-feeding women, due to their limited transfer into breast milk [37]. Although LMWHs represent the anticoagulant of choice for VTE prophylaxis in pregnancy [38], the question of optimal dosage and molecules to be used or the weight of each risk factor in predicting the recurrence of VTE are only addressed in a limited way in the literature.

Recurrent miscarriage affects 1–2% of pregnant women, and nearly 50% of these women have idiopathic recurrent miscarriages [39]. Apart from VTE, the procoagulant state during pregnancy can be involved in the occurrence of GVCs (i.e., early or late pregnancy loss, intrauterine growth restriction, pre-eclampsia, placental abruption, etc.). It has been hypothesized that in some cases, a thrombotic or an inflammatory process could be partly involved in their origin. Inherited thrombophilia [factor V Leiden (FV G1691A), activated protein C resistance (APCR), prothrombin G20210A gene mutation (FII G20210A), protein C (PC) or S (PS) deficiencies or antithrombin deficiency (AT)] have all been studied in epidemiological studies exploring an association with adverse pregnancy outcomes [6]. The association of APLA with adverse pregnancy outcomes has been recognized and included in the Sapporo diagnostic criteria for antiphospholipid syndrome (APS) [40].

Antithrombotic drugs, such as heparins or low doses of ASA, have been suggested to prevent the recurrence of GVCs. Unfortunately, there is a paucity of high-quality evidence from randomized trials in this field, and current recommendations are based on observational studies or evidence gathered from studies in the non-pregnant population.

In a recent review [38] it is concluded, as an expert opinion, that ASA is effective in preventing GVCs in women at risk for pre-eclampsia and in those with APS. Heparins could also confer benefits to women at risk of GVCs (early pregnancy loss in APS, intrauterine fetal death in APS, intrauterine fetal death associated with inherited thrombophilia, pre-eclampsia, small for gestational age newborn, pregnancy loss after an ART attempt) and/or pregnancy-related VTE.

ART has been widely used in couples with fertility problems. According to RCOG, IVF is considered a transient risk factor, thus women with an IVF pregnancy and three other risk factors should be considered for thromboprophylaxis with LMWH starting in the first trimester [15]. In a Norwegian case–control study [41], it was shown that there is an additive effect when ART is performed after multiple pregnancies and a Swedish study showed that IVF increases the risk of VTE by a factor of four and the risk of PE by a factor of seven in the first trimester compared to natural conception [27].

Many studies have investigated the effects of low-dose ASA or LMWH to improve ART outcomes. The biological plausibility of antithrombotic prophylaxis may be represented by a beneficial effect in counteracting existing or developing at risk pro-thrombotic conditions. However, the data are controversial. It has been shown that heparin and its derivatives have a beneficial effect on implantation. Heparins play a role in embryonic implantation and placentation, and contribute to the development of a normal pregnancy. This effect is achieved through the interaction of heparins with coagulation factors, anticoagulation proteins, their effect on the expression of adhesion molecules, matrix degrading enzymes and trophoblast phenotype and apoptosis - all important components in the process of embryonic implantation and placentation. In recurrent implantation failures (RIF) heparins demonstrated a beneficial effect that could be attributed to the effects of this molecule on enhancing endometrial receptivity and trophoblast invasion due to the regulation of heparin-binding factors, adhesion molecules or inhibition of complement activation [8].A meta-analysis of RCTs showed that in women with ≥3 RIF, the addition of LMWH to IVF/ICSI treatment resulted in a 79% improvement in the Live Birth Rate [42]. In addition, a meta-analysis of observational studies showed a significant increase both in the clinical pregnancy rate (RR: 1.83, 95% CI: 1.04–3.23, $p = 0.04$) and in live birth rate (RR: 2.64, 95% CI: 1.84–3.80, $p < 0.0001$) after IVF/ICSI cycles [43]. Additional results suggest that in the case of women with RIF the use of LMWH may have a beneficial effect in improving pregnancy outcomes especially when the outcome "live-birth" was considered [44, 45]. However, in a recent Greek RCT [46] comparing the effects of the administration of LMWH in sub-fertile patients with two or more unsuccessful IVF/ICSI cycles, no evidence was found in support of the standard addition of LMWH in patients with two or more unsuccessful IVF /ICSI cycles.

The present study enrolled a number of pregnant women ($N = 818$) and was conducted in seven hematologic centers all over the country. In this cohort, we aimed at investigating the efficacy and safety of antithrombotic prophylaxis in pregnant women with a history of VTE, in pregnant women with prior recurrent GVCs, or undergoing IVF. Our aim was to assess the occurrence of thrombosis, as well as, explore the utility of LMWH for the prevention of GVCs, for improving pregnancy outcomes and for improving success rates of ART.

The enrollment of pregnant women was heterogeneous since they were selected on the basis of history of VTE, previous pregnancy or IVF outcome. They were also heterogeneous in terms of risk factors, treatment dosage and preparation. Routine thrombophilia screening had been performed to the majority of pregnant women (87%) albeit it had not been complete in all of them. Investigation for the presence of APLA was carried out in 363 out of the 818 women. Thus, some of these women maybe have been classified as low risk for VTE, although they may actually have belonged to the high risk group.

In Group A the use of LMWH during pregnancy and puerperium due to personal history of VTE is well supported by studies and recommended by existing guidelines. As was expected, in our study, this was the group that received higher doses of LMWH more often than the other groups. According to our results thromboprophylaxis was efficacious with 4 (5.3%) DVT events and no fatal event. DVTs in our cohort were mainly noticed (Table 3), $p < .0008$), in Group A, a finding which suggests that personal history of VTE stands out among other thrombotic risk factors in pregnancy. What is quite noticeable is the percentage of high risk thrombophilia in Group A which reached 25% which is well above the average in the Greek population [47].

In Group B the evidence in favor of the use of LMWH prophylaxis during pregnancy to prevent recurrent GVCs is supported by limited and conflicting evidence [48] and thus, it is not recommended at present by guidelines with the exception of women with APLA. Most studies in pregnancy were non-randomized and retrospective, with a minority of prospective studies generally limited to small sample sizes. Although the use of LMWH in women with a history of GVCs is not supported by hard evidence, the analysis of Group B shows a live birth rate of 99% while 3 events of fetal loss were recorded (0.7%). On the basis of this finding one could argue that the use of LMWH might have a beneficial effect on pregnancy outcome. On the other hand, the majority of the women in this group were enrolled due to early pregnancy losses. In a considerable percentage of women, LMWHs were prescribed in women with single pregnancy loss which weakens the strength of our results.

In Group C, although the causes of IVF failure are not very clear, the data from our study seem to support the use of LMWH in women undergoing IVF, since there was a really high live birth rate with practically no VTE events. Although for the women on IVF and the ones with history of GVCs, there is no clear recommendation, the results from our study suggest that LMWH use in these categories of women is safe and effective even if a fixed prophylactic or a higher dosage scheme is selected. Noticeably, in this group thrombotic risk factors clustering was observed such as older age, (> 6 years more), multiple pregnancy and delivery by CS.

In Group D, the inherited thrombophilia by itself does not necessitate thromboprophylaxis during pregnancy and puerperium. Indications for thromboprophylaxis of asymptomatic thrombophilia carriers in pregnancy, vary throughout international guidelines, but they are dependent on the type of thrombophilia (high risk vs low risk) and on family history for VTE.

Recent studies have been consistent with a higher risk of pregnancy-related VTE in women who are antithrombin, protein C or S deficient or who are homozygous for factor V Leiden, the prothrombin gene mutation, or are compound heterozygotes for factor V Leiden and the prothrombin gene mutation [49–52]. Family history by itself, in the absence of an identifiable thrombophilic tendency, is associated with an increased risk of VTE. It may be reasonable to consider cases of high-risk thrombophilic families and of asymptomatic pregnant women with a family history of VTE in a first-degree relative aged under 50 years, where the episode has been unprovoked or provoked by pregnancy, combined oral contraceptive exposure or the presence of a minor risk factor [53, 54]. In light of the above, women should be stratified according to both the level of risk associated with their thrombophilia and the presence or absence of a family history or other risk factors [55].

Although not well documented, over prescription of LMWHs in pregnant women with a history of GVCs represents the current clinical practice throughout our country and beyond. This is a practice not adequately supported by scientific data and guidelines that does not taking into account the costs and the side effects of LMWHs but misconceptionally accepts the usefulness of LMWH in women with GVC history as an axiom. LMWHs are used extensively during pregnancy for a plethora of indications, a considerable majority of which has no proven scientific basis. Since the first studies exploring the use of LMWHs to prevent fetal losses produced encouraging results [56], there is a popular misconception among women, many of whom seem to believe that LMWHs use during pregnancy is 'the shot that prevents miscarriage'. This belief has inadvertently affected the physicians' practice and has led to inappropriate prescription of antithrombotics in pregnancy. Out of our cohort of 818 women 160 had a clear indication to receive anticoagulants during pregnancy (history of VTE and gestational APS). In another 75 women (carriers of high risk thrombophilia) the use of LMWH is justified by guidelines - albeit not uniformly. Another relevant finding is the increased co-prescription of ASA with LMWH. In our cohort, while 110 women required ASA administration (classical, gestational APS and pre-eclampsia history), actually 152 women were treated with a combination of ASA and LMWH. In a recent Cochrane analysis [57] ASA did not confer a beneficial effect in studies at low risk of bias when combined with LMWH in women with unexplained recurrent miscarriage (with or without inherited thrombophilia). The effect of anticoagulants in women with unexplained recurrent miscarriage and inherited thrombophilia needs to be assessed in further randomized controlled trials. One could argue though that the population that received LMWH without a clear indication was actually in need of thromboprophylaxis due to increased thrombotic risk. This study resulted in the construction of a scoring model for thrombotic risk factors in pregnancy that is based on the latest RCOG guidelines and is currently available as a prognostic calculus throughout Greece for Physicians. It is a digital VTE-risk assessment tool (PAT-pregnancy associated thrombosis-risks) accessible at www.PATrisks.com. Using PAT-risks we evaluated the women of the present cohort for thrombotic risk retrospectively (unpublished data). It is worth mentioning that a considerable percentage of women treated in Groups B, C and D were already at a high VTE-risk according to PAT-risks and the administration of LMWH may have had the additional benefit of preventing thromboembolic events.

Another worrying conclusion is that in the vast majority of women in our cohort, CS was the preferred delivery method. This is due on the one hand to the fact that CS is a well-controlled method of delivery for women under anticoagulation treatment, and on the other that in our country the rate of women who opt for CS is in any case very high [58, 59]. According to published data this is between 48 and 53%, with a higher percentage observed in women having their first child. This fact is stressed by the WHO who point out that "over half the births in the country occur by CS, putting Greece among countries with the highest CS rates in the world" [60]. Given that all the women were in high risk of bleeding due to anticoagulation, this may well account for such a high rate of CS even though it actually carries greater thrombotic risk than the natural vaginal delivery.

In our study the administration of three different LMWHs was recorded. The popularity of tinzaparin could be explained by scientific evidence and data supporting its use in diverse clinical scenarios in pregnancy necessitating VTE prophylaxis. An international, retrospective study of the safety and efficacy profile of tinzaparin use in pregnancy included 1267 pregnancies, making it the largest report of a single LMWH in pregnancy [61]. The above-mentioned study provided reassuring maternal and fetal outcome information in pregnancies exposed to tinzaparin.

Conclusions

In conclusion, LMWHs are used extensively during pregnancy and puerperium in Greece for VTE treatment and prophylaxis and for a variety of other indications as well. This study is the first national survey regarding LMWHs use in pregnancy and demonstrates the safety and efficacy of the drug in a high risk pregnancy setting. It is of great concern that over prescription of LMWHs in pregnant women with a history of GVCs, despite the lack of solid scientific data, represents the current clinical practice throughout our country and beyond. The study limitations are its non-controlled, retrospective nature, and the heterogeneity of indications for LMWHs administration. The inappropriate use of these drugs should be prevented by establishing and implementing

diagnostic and therapeutic guidelines and providing the necessary education for healthcare professionals. In order to clearly define the role of LMWHs in pregnancy, beyond thromboprophylaxis, large prospective studies are required, which could be based on the conclusions of this study.

Appendix
Detailed results of the study

Table 4 Baseline Characteristics of the cohort/all patients

Characteristic	N = 818
Age (mean ± SD, median, q25-q75)	33.86 ± 4.85, 34, 31–37
BMI (mean ± SD, median, q25-q75)	24.5 ± 4, 23.64, 21.87–26.18
No. of foetuses at observed gestation (N, % and 95 CI)	
1	767 (93.77%, CI: 91.90–95.23%)
≥ 2	51 (6.23%, CI: 4.77–8.10%)
Delivery by CS (N, %)	644 (78.7)
Reason for enrolling in the study	
Group A: History of VTE (DVT/SVT/Arterial thrombosis/Arterial Ischemia)	76 (9.29%, CI: 7.49–11.47%)
Group B: History of Pregnancy complications	445 (54.40%, CI: 50.97–57.78%)
Early pregnancy losses	396 (88.99%, CI: 85.74–91.57%)
Pregnancy losses < 3–3 or more	348–48
IUGR	10 (2.25%, CI: 1.23–4.09%)
Fetal death	28 (6.29, CI: 4.39–8.94%)
Pre-eclampsia/eclampsia	10 (2.25%, CI: 1.23–4.09%)
Preterm labor/placenta abruption	1 (0.22%, CI: 0.04–1.25%)
Group C: IVF	132 (16.14%, CI: 13.78–18.82%)
Group D: Other reasons	165 (20.17%, CI: 17.56–23.06%)
Family History of VTE	73 (44.24%, CI: 36.88–51.96%)
Asymptomatic Hereditary Thrombophilia	45 (27.27%, CI: 21.05–34.52%)
Increased resistance in uterine arteries	2 (1.21%, CI: 0.03–4.31%)
Reasons not specified	45 (27.27%, CI: 21.05–34.52%)
Mean Duration of LMWH (months) (mean ± SD, median, q25-q75)	8.63 ± 1.49, 9, 9–9.5
Concomitant Use of ASA (N, % and 95 CI)	152 (18.58%, CI: 16.06–21.39%)
Mean Duration of ASA (months) (mean ± SD, median, q25-q75)	6.21 ± 2.56, 7, 3–8

Table 5 Baseline characteristics and studied parameters of the four groups along with statistical comparison

	Group A N=76	Group B N=445	Group C N=132	Group D N=165	p-value*
Age (mean ± SD, median, q25-q75, N)	32.96 ± 4.26, 32.5, 30-36, N=76	33.54 ± 4.59, 34, 31-36, N=445	37.17 ± 5.1, 37, 34-41, N=132	32.48 ± 4.43, 32, 32-35, N=165	<.0001
BMI (mean, SD)	24.98 ± 4.29, 23.88, 21.85-27.48, N=76	24.38 ± 3.91, 23.51, 21.87-25.95, N=445	24.69 ± 3.75, 24.16, 21.84-26.81, N=130	24.44 ± 4.32, 23.51, 23.51-25.86, N=165	0.2607
No. of foetuses at the observed gestation (N. %)					
1	73, 96.05%	434, 97.53%	102, 77.27%	158, 95.76%	<.0001
≥ 2	3, 3.95%	11, 2.47%	30, 22.73%	7, 4.24%	
Mean Duration of LMWH (months)	8.67 ± 1.7, 9, 9-9.5, N=74	8.73 ± 1.32, 9, 9-9.5, N=445	8.69 ± 1.7, 9, 9-9.5, N=131	8.31 ± 1.61, 9, 9-9, N=162	<.0001
ASA Duration	6.73 ± 2.76, 8, 6-9, N=11	6.1 ± 2.38, 7, 3-8, N=79	5.46 ± 2.79, 7, 3-8, N=39	7.89 ± 1.97, 8, 8-9, N=19	0.0068
Fixed Prophylactic Dose	26, 34.21%	262, 58.88%	66, 50%	86, 52.12%	<.0001
Weight Adjusted prophylactic dose	16, 21.05%	144, 32.36%	51, 38.64%	61, 36.97%	
Therapeutic dose of LMWH	34, 44.74%	39, 8.76%	15, 11.36%	18, 10.91%	
Concomitant Use of ASA (N, % women rceived ASA within the group)	11, 14.47%	81, 18.2%	40, 30.3%	20, 12.12%	0.0006
Caesarian	61, 80.26%	354, 79.73%	121, 91.67%	108, 65.45%	<.0001
Live Birth	74, 97.37%	441, 99.1%	128, 96.97%	164, 99.39%	0.1632
High risk Thrombophilia (positive cases)	19, 25%	45, 10.11%	13, 9.85%	17, 10.3%	0.0018
APA status (total successful tests N=363) (positive cases, % within group))	16, 29.63%	57, 29.08%	16, 27.12%	11, 20.37%	0.6264

* p-value is for Kruskal-Wallis test for numerical parameters and for x-square test for categorical parameters

Table 6 Baseline characteristics per dosage used for each group

Group A*

	Fixed prophylactic dose (n = 26)	Higher prophylactic (weight/anti-Xa-adjusted) (n = 16)	Full treatment dose (n = 34)	p-value
Mean age at enrolment	32.23 ± 4.39, 32, 30–35	33.94 ± 3.94, 32.5, 31–37	33.06 ± 4.31, 33, 30–36	0.5021
BMI	23.02 ± 2.85, 22.86, 20.76–23.88	26.03 ± 3.62, 25.37, 23.66–28.65	25.98 ± 5.01, 24.45, 21.88–29.38	0.0101
Mean duration of LMWH use	8.82 ± 1.46, 9.5, 9–9.5	9.17 ± 1.25, 9, 9–10	8.34 ± 1.98, 9, 8–9.5	0.1560
No of foetuses at the observed gestation	1.04 ± 0.2, 1, 1–1	1.06 ± 0.25, 1, 1–1	1.03 ± 0.17, 1, 1–1	0.8560
High risk thrombophilia (Positives,% in group)	4, 15.38%	3, 18.75%	12, 35.29%	0.1706
APA status (successful tests N = 54) (N positive/N negative, % in treatment type)	7/22, 31.82%	2/11, 18.18%	7/21, 33.33%	0.6440
History of VTE				
Unprovoked	6	5	8	0.4238
Provoked by combined oral contraceptives	20	11	26	
Concomitant ASA use (Positives,% in group)	3, 11.54%	3, 18.75%	5, 14.71%	0.8111

Group B*

	Fixed dose prophylactic (n = 262)	Higher prophylactic (n = 144)	Therapeutic (n = 39)	p-value
Mean age at enrolment	33.43 ± 4.43, 34, 31–36	34.08 ± 4.75, 34, 31–37	32.31 ± 4.92, 33, 29–36	0.2326
BMI	23.58 ± 3.19, 23.18, 21.67–24.46	25.45 ± 4.6, 24.94, 21.87–28.28	25.77 ± 4.22, 24.57, 23.18–27.18	<.0001
No of foetuses at the observed gestation	1.02 ± 0.16, 1, 1–1	1.04 ± 0.2, 1, 1–1	1.03 ± 0.16, 1, 1–1	0.2657
Mean duration of LMWH use	8.51 ± 1.53, 9, 8–9	9.09 ± 0.87, 9, 9–10	8.86 ± 0.83, 9, 9–9.5	0.0001
High risk thrombophilia (Positives,% in group)	23, 8.78%	18, 12.50%	4, 10.26%	0.4924
APA status (successful tests N = 196) (N positive/N negative, % in treatment type)	30/126, 23.81%	17/55, 30.91%	10/15, 66.67%	0.0024
History of early pregnancy loss (Positives,% in group)	228, 87.02%	132, 91.67%	36, 92.31%	0.7271
History of IUGR (Positives,% in group)	5, 1.91%	4, 2.78%	1, 2.56%	
History of intrauteral fetal death (Positives,% in group)	20, 7.63%	6, 4.17%	2, 5.13%	
History of pre-eclampsia/eclampsia	8, 3.05%	2, 1.39%	0	
History of placenta abruption/preterm delivery (Positives,% in group)	1, 0.38%	0	0	
Concomitant ASA use (Positives,% in group)	34, 12.98%	41, 28.47%	6, 15.38%	0.0005

Group C*

	Fixed dose prophylactic (n = 66)	Higher prophylactic (n = 51)	Therapeutic (n = 15)	p-value
Mean age at enrolment	36.18 ± 4.95, 36, 34–39	38.55 ± 5.01, 38, 35–42	36.87 ± 5.3, 37, 32–42	0.0559
BMI	23.71 ± 3.71, 22.86, 21.05–24.978	25.48 ± 3.87, 24.83, 23.03–28.604765	26.34 ± 2.27, 26.3, 24.91–27.89	0.0003
No of foetuses at the observed gestation	1.15 ± 0.36, 1, 1–1	1.27 ± 0.49, 1, 1–2	1.47 ± 0.52, 1, 1–2	0.0278
Mean duration of LMWH use	8.18 ± 2.12, 9, 8.5–9	9.23 ± 1, 9, 9–10	9.17 ± 0.45, 9, 9–9.5	0.0007
High risk thrombophilia (Positives,% in group)	5, 7.58%	5, 9.80%	3, 20.00%	0.3456
APA status (successful tests N = 59) (N positive/N	10/33, 30.30%	6/20, 30.00%	0/6, 0%	0.2885

Table 6 Baseline characteristics per dosage used for each group (*Continued*)

	Fixed dose prophylactic (n = 86)	Higher prophylactic (n = 61)	Therapeutic (n = 18)	p-value
negative, % in treatment type				
Concomitant ASA use (Positives,% in group)	18, 27.27%	20, 39.22%	2, 13.33%	0.1194
Group D*				
Mean age at enrolment	31.33 ± 4.38, 31, 29–34	33.49 ± 4.35, 34, 31–36	34.61 ± 3.42, 34.5, 32–37	0.0007
BMI	23.68 ± 2.68, 23.57, 21.87–25.65	24.09 ± 4.26, 23.12, 21.21–25.34	29.3 ± 7.21, 27.59, 24.51–33.13	0.0004
No of foetuses at the observed gestation	1.02 ± 0.15, 1, 1–1	1.07 ± 0.25, 1, 1–1	1.06 ± 0.24, 1, 1–1	0.4385
Mean duration of LMWH use	8.15 ± 1.63, 9, 8–9	8.6 ± 1.37, 9, 9–9	8.06 ± 2.17, 9, 9–9	0.0521
High risk thrombophilia (Positives,% in group)	7, 8.14%	7, 11.48%	3, 16.67%	0.5181
APA status (successful tests N = 54) (N positive/N negative, % in treatment type)	3/26, 11.54%	8/26, 30.77%	0/2, 0%	0.1742
Family History of VTE (Positives,% in group)	48, 55.81%	21, 34.43%	4, 22.22%	0.0003
Asymptomatic Thrombophilia	22, 25.58%	21, 34.43%	2, 11.11%	
Increased resistance in uterine arteries (Positives,% in group)	2, 2.33%	0	0	
Reasons not specified (Positives,% in group)	14, 16.28%	19, 31.15%	12, 66.67%	
Concomitant ASA use (Positives,% in group)	7, 8.14%	13, 21.31%	0	0.0136

* p-value is a) for Kruskal-Wallis for the numerical parameters or b) chi-square for categorical parameters, numerical parameters are reported as: Mean ± SD, Median, 25% quantile –75% quantile75, categorical parameters are reported as N (positive cases), % of positive cases within the treatment type group

Table 7 Events in the total cohort and per group for each dose

Group A		Fixed dose prophylactic (n = 26)	Higher prophylactic (n = 16)	Therapeutic (n = 34)	p
	VTE (pre or postpartum)	3, 11.54%	0	3, 8.82%	0.3894
	Bleeding	0	0	1, 2.94%	0.5348
	Adverse pregnancy complications	2, 7.69%	2, 12.50%	8, 23.53%	0.2295
	IUGR	*1, 3.85%*	*0*	*1, 2.94%*	*0.5193*
	Preterm Labor	*0*	*2, 12.50%*	*5, 14.71*	
	Fetal Death	*0*	*0*	*1, 2.94%*	
	Early pregnancy loss/abortion	*1, 3.85%*	*0*	*0*	
	Pre-eclampsia/eclampsia	*0*	*0*	*1, 2.94%*	
Group B		Fixed dose prophylactic (n = 262)	Higher prophylactic (n = 144)	Therapeutic (n = 39)	p
	VTE (pre or postpartum)	1, 0.38%	1, 0.69%	3, 7.69%	0.0002
	Bleeding	5, 1.91%	1, 0.69%	o	0.4462
	Adverse pregnancy complications	18, 6.87%	11, 2.47%	3, 7.69%	0.952
	IUGR	*2, 0.76%*	*6, 4.17%*	*0*	*0.315*
	Preterm Labor	*12, 4.58%*	*5, 3.47%*	*2, 5.13%*	
	Fetal Death	*1, 0.38%*	*0*	*0*	
	Early pregnancy loss/abortion	*2, 0.76%*	*0*	*1, 2.56%*	
	Pre-eclampsia/eclampsia	*1, 0.38%*	*0*	*0*	
Group C		Fixed dose prophylactic (n = 66)	Higher prophylactic (n = 51)	Therapeutic (n = 15)	p
	VTE (pre or postpartum)	0	1, 1.96%	0	0.4492
	Bleeding	2, 3.03%	3, 5.88%	0	0.5199
	Adverse pregnancy complications	8, 12.12%	10, 19.61%	2, 13.33%	0.5226
	IUGR	*1, 1.52%*	*4, 7.84%*	*0*	*0.4374*
	Preterm Labor	*5, 7.58%*	*5, 9.80%*	*2, 13.33%*	
	Fetal Death	*0*	*1, 1.96%*	*0*	
	Early pregnancy loss/abortion	*2, 3.03%*	*0*	*0*	
	Pre-eclampsia/eclampsia	*0*	*0*	*0*	
Group D		Fixed dose prophylactic (n = 86)	Higher prophylactic (n = 61)	Therapeutic (n = 18)	p
	VTE (pre or postpartum)	1, 1.16%	5, 8.20%	0	0.055
	Bleeding	0	1, 1.64%	0	0.4242
	Adverse pregnancy complications	5, 5.81%	6, 9.84%	1, 5.56%	*0.7414*
	IUGR	*0*	*1, 1.64%*	*0*	
	Preterm Labor	*5, 5.81%*	*4, 6.56%*	*1, 5.56%*	
	Fetal Death	*0*	*0*	*0*	
	Early pregnancy loss/abortion	*0*	*0*	*0*	
	Pre-eclampsia/eclampsia	*0*	*1, 1.64%*	*0*	
All Groups		Fixed dose prophylactic (n = 440)	Higher prophylactic (n = 272)	Therapeutic (n = 106)	p
	VTE (pre or postpartum)	5, 1.14%	7, 2.57%	6, 5.66%	0.0151
	Bleeding	7, 1.59%	5, 1.84%	1, 0.94%	0.8226
	Adverse pregnancy complications	33, 7.50%	29, 10.66%	14, 13.21%	0.1218
	IUGR	*4, 0.91%*	*11, 4.04%*	*1, 0.94%*	*0.0592*
	Preterm Labor	*22, 5.00%*	*16, 5.88%*	*10, 9.43%*	
	Fetal Death	*1, 0.23%*	*1, 0.37%*	*1, 0.94%*	
	Early pregnancy loss/abortion	*5, 1.14%*	*0*	*1, 0.94%*	
	Pre-eclampsia/eclampsia	*1, 0.23%*	*1, 0.37%*	*1, 0.94%*	

Abbreviations
APCR: Activated protein C resistance; APLA: Antiphospholipid antibodies; APS: Antiphospholipid syndrome; ART: Assisted reproduction techniques; ASA: Acetylsalicylic acid; AT: Antithrombin; BMI: Body mass index; CRNM: Clinically relevant non major; CS: Caesarian section; DVT: Deep venous thrombosis; FGR: Fetal growth restriction; GVCs: Gestational vascular complications; HIT: Heparin induced thrombocytopenia; ICSI: Intracytoplasmic sperm injection; IUGR: Intrauterine growth retardation; IVF: In vitro fertilization; LAC: Lupus anticoagulant; LMWH: Low molecular weight heparin; OHSS: Ovarian hyper-stimulation syndrome; PAT: Pregnancy associated thrombosis; PE: Pulmonary embolism; RCOG: Royal college of Obstetricians and Gynecologists; RIF: Recurrent implantation failures; SD: Standard deviation; SGA: Small for gestational age; UFH: Unfractionated heparin; VD: Vaginal delivery; VTE: Venous thromboembolism

Acknowledgments
N/A

Author's contributions
EP, AA, AC, PK, GA, AF, EG designed the study and enrolled patients and patient data. EP, EG, AP wrote the first draft of the manuscript and the final version. AP performed the statistical analysis and constructed the tables and the graphs of the manuscript. All authors read and approved the final manuscript.

Author details
[1]Hemostasis Unit-Hematology Department Papageorgiou Hospital, Thessaloniki Ringroad 56403 Nea Efkarpia, Thessaloniki, Greece. [2]2nd Department of Pathology, National and Kapodistrian University of Athens, "ATTIKON" University Hospital, Rimini 1 Haidari, Athens, Greece. [3]OLYMPION General Clinic, Volou-Patras, 26443 Patras, Greece. [4]University Hospital of Alexandroupolis, Dragana Site 68100 Nea Chili, Alexandroupoli, Greece. [5]Blood Transfusion Unit, National Ref. Centre for Congenital Bleeding Disorders, Hemostasis Unit, Laiko General Hospital, Ag. Thoma, 17 11527 Athens, Greece. [6]Head of Transfusion Service and Clinical Haemostasis, Henry Dunant Hospital Center, Mesogion 107, 115 26 Athens, Greece. [7]IASO, General Maternity and Gynecology Clinic, 37-39, Kifissias Avenue, 151 23 Maroussi, Athens, Greece. [8]"St Savvas" Oncology Hospital, Alexandras Avenue 171, 11522 Ambelikipoi, Athens, Greece.

References
1. Bremme KA. Haemostatic changes in pregnancy. Best Pract Res Clin Haematol. 2003;16(2):153–68.
2. Kamel H, Navi BB, Sriram N, Hovsepian DA, Devereux RB, Elkind MS. Risk of a thrombotic event after the 6-week postpartum period. N Engl J Med. 2014; 370(14):1307–15.
3. Aracic N, Roje D, Jakus IA, Bakotin M, Stefanovic V. The impact of inherited thrombophilia types and low molecular weight heparin treatment on pregnancy complications in women with previous adverse outcome. Yonsei Med J. 2016;57(5):1230–5.
4. Middeldorp S. Pregnancy failure and heritable thrombophilia. Semin Hematol. 2007;44(2):93–7.
5. Rai R, Regan L. Recurrent miscarriage. Lancet. 2006;368(9535):601–11.
6. Duffett L, Rodger M. LMWH to prevent placenta-mediated pregnancy complications: an update. Br J Haematol. 2015;168(5):619–38.
7. Dodd JM, McLeod A, Windrim RC, Kingdom J. Antithrombotic therapy for improving maternal or infant health outcomes in women considered at risk of placental dysfunction. Cochrane Database Syst Rev. 2013;7:CD006780.
8. Quaranta M, Erez O, Mastrolia SA, Koifman A, Leron E, Eshkoli T, et al. The physiologic and therapeutic role of heparin in implantation and placentation. PeerJ. 2015;3:e691.
9. Greer IA, Nelson-Piercy C. Low-molecular-weight heparins for thromboprophylaxis and treatment of venous thromboembolism in pregnancy: a systematic review of safety and efficacy. Blood. 2005;106(2): 401–7.
10. Rodger MA, Carrier M, Le Gal G, Martinelli I, Perna A, Rey E, et al. Meta-analysis of low-molecular-weight heparin to prevent recurrent placenta-mediated pregnancy complications. Blood. 2014;123(6):822–8.
11. Greer IA, Brenner B, Gris JC. Antithrombotic treatment for pregnancy complications: which path for the journey to precision medicine? Br J Haematol. 2014;165(5):585–99.
12. Akhtar MA, Sur S, Raine-Fenning N, Jayaprakasan K, Thornton JG, Quenby S. Heparin for assisted reproduction. Cochrane Database Syst Rev. 2013;8: CD009452.
13. Luley L, Schumacher A, Mulla MJ, Franke D, Lottge M, Fill Malfertheiner S, et al. Low molecular weight heparin modulates maternal immune response in pregnant women and mice with thrombophilia. Am J Reprod Immunol. 2015;73(5):417–27.
14. Dentali F, Grandone E, Rezoagli E, Ageno W. Efficacy of low molecular weight heparin in patients undergoing in vitro fertilization or intracytoplasmic sperm injection. J Thromb Haemost. 2011;9(12):2503–6.
15. RCOG. Reducing the Risk of Venous Thromboembolism during Pregnancy and the Puerperium. RCOG Green-top Guideline No. 37a. London: Royal College of Obstetricians and Gynaecologists; 2015. p. 1–40. Available from: https://www.rcog.org.uk/globalassets/documents/guidelines/gtg-37a.pdf.
16. Schulman S, Kearon C. Subcommittee on control of anticoagulation of the S, standardization Committee of the International Society on T, Haemostasis. Definition of major bleeding in clinical investigations of antihemostatic medicinal products in non-surgical patients. J Thromb Haemost. 2005;3(4):692–4.
17. Kaatz S, Ahmad D, Spyropoulos AC, Schulman S. Subcommittee on control of a. definition of clinically relevant non-major bleeding in studies of anticoagulants in atrial fibrillation and venous thromboembolic disease in non-surgical patients: communication from the SSC of the ISTH. J Thromb Haemost. 2015;13(11):2119–26.
18. DiMaggio C. SAS for epidemiologists: applications and methods. New York: Springer; 2013. p. 258.
19. Stokes ME, Davis CS, Koch GG. Categorical data analysis using the SAS system. 2nd ed. Cary: SAS Institute; 2000. p. 626.
20. Heit JA, Kobbervig CE, James AH, Petterson TM, Bailey KR, Melton LJ 3rd. Trends in the incidence of venous thromboembolism during pregnancy or postpartum: a 30-year population-based study. Ann Intern Med. 2005; 143(10):697–706.
21. Gray G, Nelson-Piercy C. Thromboembolic disorders in obstetrics. Best Pract Res Clin Obstet Gynaecol. 2012;26(1):53–64.
22. Gherman RB, Goodwin TM, Leung B, Byrne JD, Hethumumi R, Montoro M. Incidence, clinical characteristics, and timing of objectively diagnosed venous thromboembolism during pregnancy. Obstet Gynecol. 1999; 94(5 Pt 1):730–4.
23. Blondon M, Casini A, Hoppe KK, Boehlen F, Righini M, Smith NL. Risks of venous thromboembolism after cesarean sections: a meta-analysis. Chest. 2016;150(3):572–96.
24. James AH, Jamison MG, Brancazio LR, Myers ER. Venous thromboembolism during pregnancy and the postpartum period: incidence, risk factors, and mortality. Am J Obstet Gynecol. 2006;194(5):1311–5.
25. Jacobsen AF, Skjeldestad FE, Sandset PM. Incidence and risk patterns of venous thromboembolism in pregnancy and puerperium--a register-based case-control study. Am J Obstet Gynecol. 2008;198(2):233 e1–7.
26. Rova K, Passmark H, Lindqvist PG. Venous thromboembolism in relation to in vitro fertilization: an approach to determining the incidence and increase in risk in successful cycles. Fertil Steril. 2012;97(1):95–100.

27. Henriksson P, Westerlund E, Wallen H, Brandt L, Hovatta O, Ekbom A. Incidence of pulmonary and venous thromboembolism in pregnancies after in vitro fertilisation: cross sectional study. BMJ. 2013;346:e8632.

28. Hansen AT, Kesmodel US, Juul S, Hvas AM. Increased venous thrombosis incidence in pregnancies after in vitro fertilization. Hum Reprod. 2014;29(3):611–7.

29. Villani M, Dentali F, Colaizzo D, Tiscia GL, Vergura P, Petruccelli T, et al. Pregnancy-related venous thrombosis: comparison between spontaneous and ART conception in an Italian cohort. BMJ Open. 2015;5(10):e008213.

30. Chan WS. The 'ART' of thrombosis: a review of arterial and venous thrombosis in assisted reproductive technology. Curr Opin Obstet Gynecol. 2009;21(3):207–18.

31. McLean KC, Bernstein IM, Brummel-Ziedins KE. Tissue factor-dependent thrombin generation across pregnancy. Am J Obstet Gynecol. 2012;207(2):135 e1–6.

32. Dargaud Y, Hierso S, Rugeri L, Battie C, Gaucherand P, Negrier C, et al. Endogenous thrombin potential, prothrombin fragment 1+2 and D-dimers during pregnancy. Thromb Haemost. 2010;103(2):469–71.

33. James A. Committee on practice B-O. practice bulletin no. 123: thromboembolism in pregnancy. Obstet Gynecol. 2011;118(3):718–29.

34. Chan WS, Rey E, Kent NE, et al. Venous thromboembolism and antithrombotic therapy in pregnancy. J Obstet Gynaecol Can. 2014;36(6):527–53.

35. Bates SM, Greer IA, Middeldorp S, Veenstra DL, Prabulos AM, Vandvik PO. VTE, thrombophilia, antithrombotic therapy, and pregnancy: antithrombotic therapy and prevention of thrombosis, 9th ed: American College of Chest Physicians Evidence-Based Clinical Practice Guidelines. Chest. 2012;141(2 Suppl):e691S–736S.

36. Bates SM, Middeldorp S, Rodger M, James AH, Greer I. Guidance for the treatment and prevention of obstetric-associated venous thromboembolism. J Thromb Thrombolysis. 2016;41(1):92–128.

37. Villani M, Ageno W, Grandone E, Dentali F. The prevention and treatment of venous thromboembolism in pregnancy. Expert Rev Cardiovasc Ther. 2017;15(5):397–402.

38. Grandone E, Villani M, Tiscia GL. Aspirin and heparin in pregnancy. Expert Opin Pharmacother. 2015;16(12):1793–803.

39. de Jong PG, Goddijn M, Middeldorp S. Antithrombotic therapy for pregnancy loss. Hum Reprod Update. 2013;19(6):656–73.

40. Miyakis S, Lockshin MD, Atsumi T, Branch DW, Brey RL, Cervera R, et al. International consensus statement on an update of the classification criteria for definite antiphospholipid syndrome (APS). J Thromb Haemost. 2006;4(2):295–306.

41. Jacobsen AF, Skjeldestad FE, Sandset PM. Ante- and postnatal risk factors of venous thrombosis: a hospital-based case-control study. J Thromb Haemost. 2008;6(6):905–12.

42. Potdar N, Gelbaya TA, Konje JC, Nardo LG. Adjunct low-molecular-weight heparin to improve live birth rate after recurrent implantation failure: a systematic review and meta-analysis. Hum Reprod Update. 2013;19(6):674–84.

43. Seshadri S, Sunkara SK, Khalaf Y, El-Toukhy T, Hamoda H. Effect of heparin on the outcome of IVF treatment: a systematic review and meta-analysis. Reprod BioMed Online. 2012;25(6):572–84.

44. Grandone E, Villani M, Dentali F, Tiscia GL, Colaizzo D, Cappucci F, et al. Low-molecular -weight heparin in pregnancies after ART -a retrospective study. Thromb Res. 2014;134(2):336–9.

45. Urman B, Ata B, Yakin K, Alatas C, Aksoy S, Mercan R, et al. Luteal phase empirical low molecular weight heparin administration in patients with failed ICSI embryo transfer cycles: a randomized open-labeled pilot trial. Hum Reprod. 2009;24(7):1640–7.

46. Siristatidis C, Dafopoulos K, Salamalekis G, Galazios G, Christoforidis N, Moustakarias T, et al. Administration of low-molecular-weight heparin in patients with two or more unsuccessful IVF/ICSI cycles: a multicenter cohort study. Gynecol Endocrinol. 2018;34(9):747–51.

47. Yapijakis C, Serefoglou Z, Nixon AM, Vylliotis A, Ragos V, Vairaktaris E. Prevalence of thrombosis-related DNA polymorphisms in a healthy Greek population. In Vivo. 2012;26(6):1095–101.

48. Skeith L, Rodger M. Anticoagulants to prevent recurrent placenta-mediated pregnancy complications: is it time to put the needles away? Thromb Res. 2017;151(Suppl 1):S38–42.

49. Bramham K, Retter A, Robinson SE, Mitchell M, Moore GW, Hunt BJ. How I treat heterozygous hereditary antithrombin deficiency in pregnancy. Thromb Haemost. 2013;110(3):550–9.

50. Rogenhofer N, Bohlmann MK, Beuter-Winkler P, Wurfel W, Rank A, Thaler CJ, et al. Prevention, management and extent of adverse pregnancy outcomes in women with hereditary antithrombin deficiency. Ann Hematol. 2014;93(3):385–92.

51. Jacobsen AF, Dahm A, Bergrem A, Jacobsen EM, Sandset PM. Risk of venous thrombosis in pregnancy among carriers of the factor V Leiden and the prothrombin gene G20210A polymorphisms. J Thromb Haemost. 2010;8(11):2443–9.

52. van Vlijmen EF, Veeger NJ, Middeldorp S, Hamulyak K, Prins MH, Buller HR, et al. Thrombotic risk during oral contraceptive use and pregnancy in women with factor V Leiden or prothrombin mutation: a rational approach to contraception. Blood. 2011;118(8):2055–61 quiz 375.

53. Baglin T, Gray E, Greaves M, Hunt BJ, Keeling D, Machin S, et al. Clinical guidelines for testing for heritable thrombophilia. Br J Haematol. 2010;149(2):209–20.

54. SIGN. Prevention and management of venous thromboembolism a national clinical guideline. Edinburgh: Scottish Intercollegiate Guidelines Network; 2010. Available from: https://www.sign.ac.uk/assets/sign122.pdf

55. Chunilal SD, Bates SM. Venous thromboembolism in pregnancy: diagnosis, management and prevention. Thromb Haemost. 2009;101(3):428–38.

56. Brenner B, Hoffman R, Carp H, Dulitsky M, Younis J, Investigators L-E. Efficacy and safety of two doses of enoxaparin in women with thrombophilia and recurrent pregnancy loss: the LIVE-ENOX study. J Thromb Haemost. 2005;3(2):227–9.

57. de Jong PG, Kaandorp S, Di Nisio M, Goddijn M, Middeldorp S. Aspirin and/or heparin for women with unexplained recurrent miscarriage with or without inherited thrombophilia. Cochrane Database Syst Rev. 2014;7:CD004734.

58. Mossialos E, Allin S, Karras K, Davaki K. An investigation of caesarean sections in three Greek hospitals: the impact of financial incentives and convenience. Eur J Pub Health. 2005;15(3):288–95.

59. Vassilaki M, Chatzi L, Rasidaki M, Bagkeris E, Kritsotakis G, Roumeliotaki T, et al. Caesarean deliveries in the mother-child (Rhea) cohort in Crete, Greece: almost as frequent as vaginal births and even more common in first-time mothers. Hippokratia. 2014;18(4):298–305.

60. World Health Organisation. Greece commits to addressing excessive reliance on caesarean sections: WHO; 2016. [cited 2019 28 June]. Available from: http://www.euro.who.int/en/countries/greece/news/news/2016/11/greece-commits-to-addressing-excessive-reliance-on-caesarean-sections

61. Nelson-Piercy C, Powrie R, Borg JY, Rodger M, Talbot DJ, Stinson J, et al. Tinzaparin use in pregnancy: an international, retrospective study of the safety and efficacy profile. Eur J Obstet Gynecol Reprod Biol. 2011;159(2):293–9.

27

The effect of civil and military flights on coagulation, fibrinolysis and blood flow: Insight from a rat model

Anna Levkovsky[1,2†], Rima Dardik[3†], Daniel Barazany[4], David M. Steinberg[5], Mark Dan Kirichenko[4], Sara Apter[6,7], Edna Peleg[2,8], Daniel Silverberg[2,9], Ehud Grossman[2,10†] and Ophira Salomon[1,2*†] [iD]

Abstract

Background: Air travel thrombosis continues to be a controversial topic. Exposure to hypoxia and hypobaric conditions during air travel is assumed a risk factor. The aim of this study is to explore changes in parameters of coagulation, fibrinolysis and blood flow in a rat model of exposure to hypobaric conditions that imitate commercial and combat flights.

Methods: Sixty Sprague-Dawley male rats, aged 10 weeks, were divided into 5 groups according to the type and duration of exposure to hypobaric conditions. The exposure conditions were 609 m and 7620 m for 2 and 12 h duration. Blood count, thrombin– antithrombin complex, D-dimer, interleukin-1 and interleukin-6 were analyzed. All rats went through flight angiography MRI at day 13-post exposure.

Results: No effect of the various exposure conditions was observed on coagulation, fibrinolytic system, IL-1 or IL-6. MRI angiography showed blood flow reduction in lower limb to less than 30% in 50% of the rats. The reduction in blood flow was more pronounced in the left vessel than in the right vessel ($p = 0.006$, Wilcoxon signed rank test). The extent of occlusion differed across exposure groups in the right, but not the left vessel ($p = 0.002$, $p = 0.150$, respectively, Kruskal-Wallis test). However, these differences did not correlate with the exposure conditions.

Conclusion: In the present rat model, no clear correlation between various hypobaric conditions and activation of coagulation was observed. The reduction in blood flow in the lower limb also occurred in the control group and was not related to the type of exposure.

Keywords: D-dimer, Hypobaric conditions, IL-6, MRI, Thrombin–antithrombin

* Correspondence: ophira.Salomon@sheba.health.gov.il
†Anna Levkovsky, Rima Dardik, Ehud Grossman and Ophira Salomon contributed equally to this work.
[1]Thrombosis Unit Sheba Medical Center, Coagulation Institute, 52621 Tel Hashomer, Israel
[2]Sackler Faculty of Medicine, Tel Aviv University, Tel Aviv, Israel
Full list of author information is available at the end of the article

Introduction

Air travel thrombosis is a subgroup of thrombosis that occurs within 4 weeks following long haul air travel [1]. Exposure to hypoxia and hypobaric conditions during air travel are considered as risk factors, alongside immobilization, which is common to all land travel thrombosis cases [1–4].

Commercial airplanes usually fly at about 10,800 m (35,433 ft) above sea level, while compressing air to about 75.8 kPa (570 mmHg), which is essential to prevent hypoxia because of reduced barometric pressure at such an altitude. The cabin's pressure is kept equivalent to an altitude of 1500-2500 m with partial oxygen pressure of 16.7 kPa (125 mmHg). Oxygen saturation is reduced to 90–93% in healthy individuals, but it may drop even to 80% during the flight in patients with pulmonary and/or heart disease.

Combat aircraft may operate at altitudes of 7620 m (25,000 ft) and even more [5], and the grade of air pressurization is dependent on the altitude [3, 5, 6].

The phenomenon of air travel thrombosis as a concept continues to be a controversial topic since most studies were conducted on few participants with heterogeneous clinical characteristics, type of exposure and duration, with no pre- and post-exposure comparison of coagulation parameters and lack of a control group [3, 7]. Furthermore, there was inconsistency concerning the activation of coagulation and fibrinolytic pathways when fragment 1 + 2, thrombin-antithrombin (TAT) complex and D-dimers were measured [3, 7–10].

The incidence of deep vein thrombosis (DVT) in low risk travelers was 1.6% compared to 5% in those with additional risk factors [11, 12].

Concerning hypobaric conditions, there was a transient activation of coagulation factors in volunteers held in a hypobaric chamber [13]. In rabbits, the risk of DVT was augmented by exposure to hypobaric conditions following surgery of the femur, as compared to rabbits that were not exposed to a postoperative drop in air pressure [14].

Hypoxia has been demonstrated to decrease fibrinolytic activity and incite the formation of oxygen free radicals and nitric oxide by endothelial cells [7]. The latter causes relaxation of the venous vessels with decreased blood flow velocity and stasis, which may promote venous thromboembolism.

Direct evidence that would support or exclude the association between air travel and thrombosis would require a large number of participants due to the low incidence of air-travel thrombosis, and it is unlikely that airline companies or funding agencies would sponsor such studies.

Therefore, in this study we used a rat model of exposure to hypobaric conditions compatible with conditions present during commercial and combat flights to explore changes that may occur in the coagulation, fibrinolysis and blood flow.

Materials and methods
Animals

Sprague-Dawley male rats were purchased from Envigo RMS (Jerusalem, Israel) at the age of 10 weeks and weight 340–405 g. The rats were acclimated for 3 days before study initiation. Three rats per plastic cage were housed at a temperature of $22 \pm 2\,°C$ in a controlled room with alternating 12-h light/dark cycle, with regular chow diet and water available ad libitum before and after the exposure experiment. During exposure to hypobaric conditions, smaller cages, housing two rats each, were needed to adjust to the cabin settings. The rats received regular diet but no water as the water bottles were not adjusted to the hypobaric conditions. The control rats were also deprived of water for 12 h, which corresponded to their time of exposure. All rat procedures were carried out based on ethical approval and in accordance with The Animal Care and Use Committee of Sheba Medical Center, Tel-Hashomer (approval number 1046/16).

Study design

Groups of 12 rats each were assigned to the five groups defined by the type and duration of exposure to hypobaric conditions as shown in Table 1.

Hypobaric exposure

Rats were exposed to hypobaric conditions at the Israel Air Force Aeromedical Center's Hypobaric Training facility. The chamber, purchased from Vacudyne (Chicago, USA), was connected to a vacuum pump with controlled air inflow and outflow. The hypobaric conditions were launched by dropping the barometric pressure. The low altitude condition in the study was equivalent to 609 m and represents atmospheric pressure of 706 mmHg, and 148 mmHg oxygen partial pressure (effective oxygen 19.4%, by measurement). The high altitude condition was equivalent to 7620 m and represents atmospheric pressure of 282 mmHg and 59 mmHg oxygen partial pressure (effective oxygen 7.6%, by measurement).

Table 1 Characteristic of rats' group according to type and duration of exposure to hypobaric conditions

Groups	Height	Duration of exposure
1	609 m (2,000 ft)	2 h
2	609 m (2,000 ft)	12 h
3	7620 m (25,000 ft)	2 h
4	7620 m (25,000 ft)	12 h
5	Sea levels	12 h

Blood samples

Three mL blood was drawn from the retro-orbital sinus of each rat and divided into 3 tubes with 10% ethylenediaminetetraacetic acid (EDTA) following anesthesia (with 0.5 ml isoflurane), at day 4 before exposure to hypobaric conditions, at day 6 immediately post exposure and at day 21 a day before MRI was done. Blood count was performed using Beckman Coulter DxH900 analyzer (Farminpex N. V, USA).

Thrombin-Antithrombin (TAT) complex and D-dimer tests

Blood samples were centrifuged at 1000 x g for 15 min at room temperature, followed by additional centrifugation of the plasma at 10,000 x g for 15 min at 4 °C. Blood samples were processed within 1 h of blood withdrawal and stored at − 80 °C until analysis at the end of the study. Rat enzyme-linked immunosorbent assay (ELISA) kit (Mybiosource company, San Diego, USA) and rat D-dimer (D2D) competitive ELISA kit (Mybiosource company) were used for analyzing TAT complex and D-dimer, respectively, according to the manufacturer's instructions.

Cytokines

Interleukin-1 (IL-1) and interleukin- 6 (IL-6) were analyzed by rat interleukin-1β and rat IL-6 ELISA kit (Mybiosource company) according to the manufacturer's instructions.

MRA screening

All rats went through MRI angiography (MRA) scan at Strauss MRI Center, Tel Aviv University, 13 days after hypobaric exposure using a 7 T/30 Bruker Biospec scanner with a 72 mm cylinder transmit-receive coil. The rats were placed in prone position in the scanner with the back limbs secured by tape. Anesthesia was maintained with isoflurane (2–3% in pure O_2) and body temperature was kept at 38.5 °C by a heating pad during imaging. We used 2-dimensional Time of Flight (2D-TOF) angiography through TR/TE = 20 ms/2.25 ms, flip angle was 80°, 39 coronal slices of 1 mm with an in-plane resolution of 0.275 mm2 in a scan time of 7 min and 30 s. The 2D-TOF MRA images were acquired perpendicular to the orientation of the vessels' blood flow.

MRA score

TOF MRA produces an enhanced signal intensity stemming from flow of unsaturated blood into saturated area. The acquired signal intensity is correlated to the degree of blood, hence, TOF MRA technique is mostly used to demonstrate blood flow qualitatively. To quantify the flow reduction, the TOF signal intensity was standardized by division by a reference flow. The minimal standardized flow was recorded as an MRA score to measure and compare occlusion for both the right and left blood vessels.

Statistical methods

Data are summarized for all animals by mean values. Comparisons were performed using non-parametric statistical tests. Comparisons across groups were performed using the Kruskal-Wallis test and comparisons for paired data were performed using the Wilcoxon signed rank test. Pearson correlations were used to describe relationships between numerical variables.

Results

Clinical characteristics of the rats

Sixty rats were included in the study. Four rats died during exposure as follows: one rat following exposure to 609 m for 2 h and 3 rats following exposure to 7620 m for 12 h. One rat died immediately after exposure to 7620 m for 2 h and one control group rat died just before MRI. There was a consistent decrease in weight immediately following exposure to hypobaric conditions, with significant differences by group ($p < 0.00001$, Kruskal-Wallis test). The largest reduction, approximately 20 g on average, occurred in rats that were exposed for 12 h to hypobaric conditions. Weight returned to pre-exposure levels when measured 13 days later.

Blood counts

There were reductions in both hematocrit and hemoglobin. The reduction in hematocrit differed significantly among the groups ($p = 0.00016$, Kruskal-Wallis test), with the largest reduction observed in rats exposed to 609 m and 7620 m for 2 h as shown in Fig. 1a. There was a weak negative correlation between the change in weight and the change in hematocrit ($r = -0.27$). The number of platelets increased in 69% of the rats following exposure, with an average increase of 138.3 k/µL. There were no significant differences among the groups ($p = 0.32$, Kruskal-Wallis test) as seen in Fig. 1b.

TAT and D-dimer

The analysis of TAT complex revealed that five rats were positive at the time of acclimation before exposure to hypobaric conditions (mean ± SD for positive rats: 3020 ± 1692 pg/mL). Following exposure, TAT complex levels were elevated in 8 rats, 4 of which belonged to the control group. No differences in the level of TAT complex were observed between rats exposed to hypobaric conditions and the control group rats (mean ± SD for positive rats: 4900 ± 2125 pg/mL and 4875 ± 3147 pg/mL for control and hypobaric exposure groups, respectively). At 16 days, TAT complexes were elevated in 7 rats: two were exposed to 609 m for 2 h (mean ± SD: 6100 ± 2187 pg/mL), 4 were exposed to 609 m for 12 h (mean ± SD:

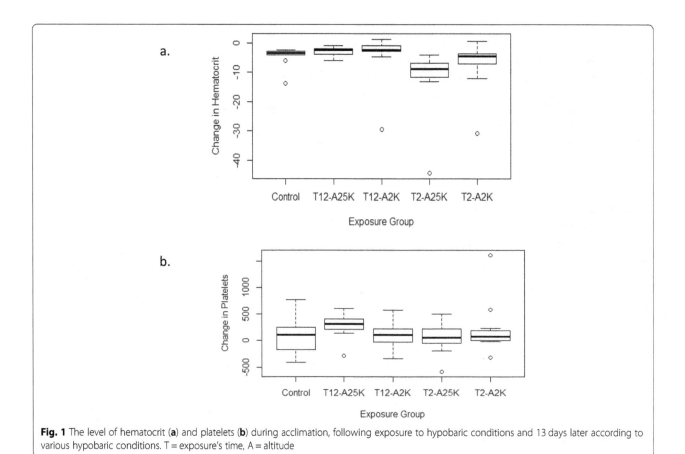

Fig. 1 The level of hematocrit (**a**) and platelets (**b**) during acclimation, following exposure to hypobaric conditions and 13 days later according to various hypobaric conditions. T = exposure's time, A = altitude

5625 ± 5648 pg/mL) and 1 rat was exposed to 7620 m for 2 h (3000 pg/mL). Dot plots of TAT levels at various exposure conditions are presented in supplemental Fig. 1.

D-dimer was negative in all rats during acclimation. Following hypobaric exposure slightly elevated D-dimer levels were observed at 16 days in only two rats (4 ng/ml [609 m for 2 h]; 8 ng/ml [609 m for 12 h]), both of which were negative for TAT complex at all 3 measurements.

Cytokines: IL-1 and IL-6 levels
The decrease in weight and hematocrit led us to measure IL-1 and IL-6, as both cytokines are known to be involved in inflammation and thrombosis. In 6 rats, the IL-1 levels were already high at the time of acclimation (mean ± SD: 70 ± 46.5 pg/mL). Following exposure, IL-1 was 40 pg/mL in one rat and 80 pg/mL in another one. At the end of the experiment, IL-1 increased in only 2 rats, with levels of 40 pg/mL each.

Elevated IL-6 was found in 4 rats during acclimation (mean ± SD: 238 ± 180 pg/mL). After exposure, IL-6 increased in 3 rats exposed to 609 m for 2 h (mean ± SD: 154 ± 87 pg/mL), in one rat exposed for 12 h (500 pg/mL) and in 2 control rats (300 and 400 pg/mL). At 16 days, IL-6 was elevated in 5 rats, 2 of which were control rats (range 150–400 pg/mL).

Taken together, the increment of IL-1 and IL-6 was not related to mode of exposure or time post-exposure.

MRA
MRA was performed in 54 rats, but could be evaluated in only 52 rats. Figure 2 presents an MRA taken from a representative rat with minimal blood flow in the

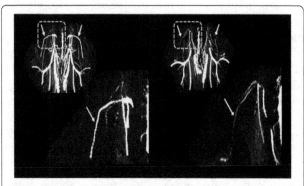

Fig. 2 2D-TOF MRI angiography images of the rat's abdomen area in the coronal view. Two representative rats (N1, N4) with intact and minimal blood flow are given (left and right respectively), with enlargement focusing on the left femoral veins (white arrows). Note the reduction of blood flow in bilateral femoral veins bilaterally, but with different severity

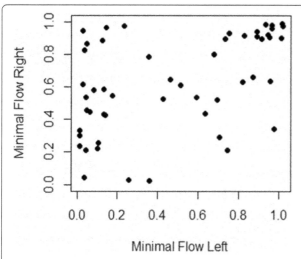

Fig. 3 Plot of minimum blood flow (as a fraction of reference flow) in the right vs. the left femur. The line is y = x. Most points are above the line indicating more obstruction in the left vessel. There is a modest positive correlation between the two femurs (r = 0.48). Animals with strong reduction in blood flow in the left femur often have little or no reduction in the right femur

femoral veins (white arrows) alongside a healthy rat with intact blood flow.

Note that the flow deficiency was observed in both right and left femoral veins, but with different severity. Figure 3 shows the modest correlation between minimal flow in the right versus left femoral vein (r = 0.48).

Greater flow reduction was observed in the left vessel in 65% of the rats. The median difference of the right vs left flow reduction scores was 0.11 and the differences were statistically different from 0 (p = 0.006, Wilcoxon signed rank test).

There were significant differences by exposure group for reduced flow in the right vessel, but not in the left vessel (p = 0.002, p = 0.150, respectively, Kruskal-Wallis test). The extent of flow reduction did not show any correlation with the exposure conditions. For the right vessel, the lowest median values were 0.36 (for the group exposed for 2 h at 609 m) and 0.46 (12 h at 7620 m). The median values for the other groups were 0.75 (12 h at 609 m), 0.87 (2 h at 7620 m) and 0.90 (control). The left vessel had larger flow reductions; the lowest median values were 0.13 (12 h at 7620 m), 0.14 (2 h at 609 m) and 0.28 (control). The median values for the other groups were 0.69 (2 h at 7620 m) and 0.82 (12 h at 609 m).

Half of the rats (26/52) had serious blood flow reduction to 0.3 or less in at least one of the two femoral veins. By group, these fractions ranged from 27% (3/11) in the 2 h, 7620 m group to 80% (8/10) in the 2 h, 609 m group, with 50% (5/10) in the control group.

Discussion

In this study of a rat model of exposure to different hypobaric conditions and duration, designed to mimic the conditions prevailing during civil flights or military aircraft missions, we found no laboratory indications for the activation of coagulation and fibrinolytic systems. Indeed, the amount of thrombin generated, which is often assessed by TAT complex, and the fibrinolytic system activity, which is reflected by increased D- dimer levels, were not elevated in most animals immediately following exposure or 13 days later.

In fact, when D-dimer was measured in cockpit crews who fly multiple short duration flights to rule out sub-clinical thrombotic events, there was no evidence for an increase [15]. Others assumed that the failure to detect raised concentration of D-dimer in passengers with positive ultrasound scans is related to the short half-life (about 6 h) of D-dimer and the long delay (up to 48 h) before blood was sampled upon return from travel [16]. Therefore, in our project, we withdrew blood immediately post exposure and after 13 days, taking into account the fact that the risk of DVT tends to increase in the first 2 weeks following the flight [4, 11].

Additionally, we found reductions in hemoglobin and hematocrit, despite the fact that the rats were water deprived. Similar observations were noticed in 20 volunteers after transatlantic flight, where hemoglobin decreased without signs of dehydration [7].

A significant weight loss was observed in rats immediately post-exposure, with weight regained when analyzed 13 days later. The loss of weight following hypobaric exposure is attributed to muscle atrophy caused by increased protein degradation rate through up regulation of the ubiquitin-proteasome pathway [17]. This mechanism cannot explain the regained weight we observed in our rat model at day 13-post exposure or the decrease in weight in the control group. This fact led us to assess IL-1 and IL-6, both inflammatory cytokines that may be involved in thrombosis, besides being involved in the regulation of body fat [18, 19].

The level of IL-1 and IL-6 increased post-exposure in a small number of rats, but it was not related to exposure conditions.

We speculated that by using a 7 T/30 MRA, we might reach higher diagnostic accuracy for detecting vessel occlusion in rats at 13 days post exposure. A significant reduction of blood flow to less than 30% in 26 rats (50%) was observed in the femoral vein. These reductions were not related to exposure conditions.

Furthermore, we compared the blood flow between the right and left side of the lower limbs in all the rats and in relation to their group to rule out some slow-down of the flow that may indicate the likelihood of imminent clot formation. Occlusion of the left femoral vein was significantly greater than that of the right. Occlusion only of the right vessel achieved statistically significant differences across groups, but the extent of occlusion in that vessel was again unrelated to the exposure conditions.

We realize that our rat model cannot replace a human being, but we found that the aircraft cabin environment with hypobaric conditions did not promote vessel occlusion. This may explain why the incidence of DVT in pilots is not increased, even if they fly more frequently than most passengers [20].

We are aware of the fact that we did not have real-time measurements of partial oxygen pressure during exposure to of 609 m and 7620 m, but used estimated pressures corresponding to the altitudes, reaching 19.4 and 7.6% respectively.

Since the coagulation and fibrinolysis pathways were not found to be activated, the degree of hypoxia should not alter our results.

Conclusion

In summary, our rat model points out that in hypobaric conditions simulating civil and combat flights to a certain degree, there was no evidence of substantial activation of coagulation, fibrinolysis, increased inflammatory cytokines or alteration of blood flow correlated with the type of exposure.

Abbreviations

TAT: thrombin-antithrombin; DVT: deep vein thrombosis; ELISA: enzyme-linked immunosorbent assay; 2D-TOF: 2-dimensional Time of Flight; MRA: MRI angiography

Acknowledgments

The authors thank Mrs. Zehava Shabtay for expert assistance in handling the rats.

Authors' contributions

Anna Levkovsky – Performed the experiment. Rima Dardik – Performed the experiment and approved the final version to be submitted. Daniel Barazany – Performed the experiments and analyzed the data. David M. Steinberg – Analyzed, interpreted the data and wrote the manuscript. Mark Dan Kirichenko – Performed the experiment. Sara Apter – Analyzed and interpreted the data. Edna Peleg – Performed the experiment. Daniel Silverberg - Analyzed the data. Ehud Grossman – Revised the manuscript critically for important intellectual content. Ophira Salomon – The conception and design of the study, analyzed and wrote the manuscript. The author(s) read and approved the final manuscript.

Author details

[1]Thrombosis Unit Sheba Medical Center, Coagulation Institute, 52621 Tel Hashomer, Israel. [2]Sackler Faculty of Medicine, Tel Aviv University, Tel Aviv, Israel. [3]National Hemophilia Center and Thrombosis Unit, Sheba Medical Center, Tel-Hashomer, Israel. [4]Strauss Computational Neuroimaging Center, Tel Aviv University, Tel Aviv, Israel. [5]Department of Statistics and Operations Research, Faculty of Exact Sciences, Tel Aviv University, Tel Aviv, Israel. [6]Department of Diagnostic Imaging, Sheba Medical Center, Tel-Hashomer, Israel. [7]Tel Aviv University, Tel Aviv, Israel. [8]Hypertension Unit, Sheba Medical Center, Tel-Hashomer, Israel. [9]Department of Vascular Surgery, Sheba Medical Center, Tel-Hashomer, Israel. [10]Internal Medicine Department, Sheba Medical Center, Tel Hashomer, Israel.

References

1. Sandor T. Travel thrombosis: Pathomechanisms and clinical aspects. Pathophysiology. 2008;15:243–52.
2. Toff WD, Jones CI, Ford I, Pearse RJ, Watson HG, Watt SJ, et al. Effect of hypobaric hypoxia, simulating conditions during long-haul air travel, on coagulation, fibrinolysis, platelet function, and endothelial activation. JAMA. 2006;295:2251–61.
3. Kuipers S, Schreijer AJ, Cannegieter SC, Büller HR, Rosendaal FR, Middeldorp S. Travel and venous thrombosis: a systematic review. J Intern Med. 2007; 262:615–34.
4. Brown HK, Simpson AJ, Murchison JT. The Influence of meteorological variables on the development of deep venous thrombosis. Thromb Haemost. 2009;102:676–82.
5. Cable GG. In-flight hypoxia incidents in military aircraft: causes and implications for training. Aviat Space Environ Med. 2003;74:169–72.
6. Keynan Y, Bitterman N, Bitterman H. Hypoxia-reoxygenation contributes to increased frequency of venous thromboembolism in air travelers. Med Hypotheses. 2006;66:165–8.
7. Schobersberger W, Fries D, Mittermayr M, Innerhofer P, Sumann G, Schobersberger B, et al. Changes of biochemical markers and functional tests for clot formation during long-haul flights. Thromb Res. 2002;108:19–24.
8. Boccalon H, Boneu B, Emmerich J, Thalamas C, Ruidavets JB. Long-haul flights do not activate hemostasis in young healthy men. J Thromb Haemost. 2005;3:1539–41.
9. Mannucci PM, Gringeri A, Peyvandi F, Di Paolantonio T, Mariani G. Short-term exposure to high altitude causes coagulation activation and inhibits fibrinolysis. Thromb Haemost. 2002;87:342–3.
10. von Känel R, Mills PJ, Fainman C, Dimsdale JE. Effects of psychological stress and psychiatric disorders on blood coagulation and fibrinolysis: a biobehavioral pathway to coronary artery disease? Psychosom Med. 2001; 63:531–44.
11. Aryal KR, Al-Khaffaf H. Venous thromboembolic complications following air travel: what's the quantitative risk? A literature review. Eur J Vasc Endovasc Surg. 2006;31:187–99.
12. Martinelli I, Taioli E, Battaglioli T, Podda GM, Passamonti SM, Pedotti P, et al. Risk of venous thromboembolism after air travel: interaction with thrombophilia and oral contraceptives. Arch Intern Med. 2003;163:2771–4.
13. Bendz B, Rostrup M, Sevre K, Andersen TO, Sandset PM. Association between acute hypobaric hypoxia and activation of coagulation in human beings. Lancet. 2000;356:1657–8.
14. Hoffmann R, Schimmer RC, Largiader F. Surgery and environmental influence as risk –factors for the development of deep vein thrombosis in animal experiments. Thromb Haemost. 1993;70:712–6.
15. Jacobson BF, Philippides M, Malherbe M, Becker P. Risk factors for deep vein thrombosis in short-haul cockpit crews: a prospective study. Aviat Space Environ Med. 2002;73:481–4.
16. Scurr JH, Machin SJ, Bailey-King S, Mackie IJ, McDonald S, Smith PD. Frequency and prevention of symptomless deep- vein thrombosis in long-haul flights: a randomised trial. Lancet. 2001;357:1485–9.
17. Chaudhary P, Suryakumar G, Prasad R, Singh SN, Ali S, Ilavazhagan G. Chronic hypobaric hypoxia mediated skeletal muscle atrophy: role of ubiquitin- proteasome pathway and calpain. Mol Cell Biochem. 2012;364: 101–13.

18. Chida D, Osaka T, Hashimoto O, Iwakura Y. Combined interleukin-6 and interleukin-1 deficiency causes obesity in young mice. Diabetes. 2006;55: 971–7.
19. Saghazadeh A, Rezaei N. Inflammation as a cause of venous thromboembolism. Crit Rev Oncol Hematol. 2016;99:272–85.
20. Johnston R, Evans A. Venous thromboembolic disease in pilots. Lancet. 2001;358:1734.

28

Multiple simultaneous embolic cerebral infarctions 11 months after COVID-19

Rajiv Advani[1,2], Torbjørn Austveg Strømsnes[1,3]*, Espen Stjernstrøm[4] and Sebastian T. Lugg[5]

Abstract

Background: The coronavirus disease (COVID-19) pandemic has led to an unprecedented worldwide burden of disease. However, little is known of the longer-term implications and consequences of COVID-19. One of these may be a COVID-19 associated coagulopathy that can present as a venous thromboembolism (VTE) and further, as multiple paradoxical cerebral emboli.

Case presentation: A 51 year old man presented to the emergency department with multiple simultaneous embolic cerebral infarctions 11 months after mild COVID-19. In the subacute phase of the COVID-19 illness the patient developed increasing shortness of breath and was found to have an elevated D-dimer and multiple bilateral segmental pulmonary emboli. He was subsequently treated with 3 months of anticoagulation for a provoked VTE. The patient then presented 11 months after the initial COVID-19 diagnosis with multiple simultaneous cerebral infarctions where no traditional underlying stroke etiology was determined. A patent foramen ovale (PFO) and an elevated D-dimer were found suggesting a paradoxical thromboembolic event due to an underlying coagulopathy.

Conclusions: This case report highlights the one of the potentially more serious complications of long-term COVID-19 where VTE due to a persistent coagulopathy is seen almost a year after the initial illness. Due to the highly prevalent nature of PFO in the general population, VTE due to COVID-19 associated coagulopathy could lead to ischemic stroke. This case report highlights the possibility for an underlying COVID-19 associated coagulopathy which may persist for many months and beyond the initial illness.

Keywords: COVID-19, Pulmonary Embolus, Stroke, Thrombolysis, Anticoagulation, Coagulopathy

Background

The longer-term implications and consequences of COVID-19 remain largely unmapped. One of the previously identified longer-term complications is a COVID-19 associated coagulopathy. This associated coagulopathy can present as a venous thromboembolism (VTE) and, as yet unreported, multiple paradoxical cerebral emboli. Furthermore, the temporal correlation of the emergence of a COVID-19 associated coagulopathy to the primary illness remains unknown. In cases of milder COVID-19 symptoms, an associated coagulopathy can remain undiagnosed and result in thromboembolic events after the initial illness.

Case presentation

A 51 year old man presented to the Emergency Department (ED) with acute onset left sided peripheral facial palsy and a complete right sided homonymous hemianopsia.

The patient was a Caucasian male of normal BMI with no prior history of hypertension, hypercholesterolemia, diabetes, smoking and or heart disease. He had been in good health until March 2020 when he returned from a group holiday to Austria. The patient started feeling unwell with a fever and was diagnosed with coronavirus

* Correspondence: t.a.austveg@gmail.com
[1]Stroke Unit, Department of Neurology, Oslo University Hospital, Oslo, Norway
[3]Department of Clinical Medicine, University of Bergen, Bergen, Norway
Full list of author information is available at the end of the article

disease (COVID-19) along with several members of the group that he had travelled with. A nasopharyngeal PCR swab confirmed the presence of SARS-CoV-2 RNA on the 22nd of March 2020. The patient was admitted the hospital on the 29th of March 2020 after increasing shortness of breath and onset of diarrhea and vomiting. The patient was febrile but had no oxygen requirement and was therefore diagnosed with mild COVID-19. He was admitted for observation, managed conservatively, and was discharged home 3 days later on the 1st of April 2020 after showing clinical improvement.

The patient was readmitted 2 days later on the 3rd of April 2020 with increasing shortness of breath. Clinically, pulmonary embolism (PE) was suspected with no signs of hemodynamic compromise. The diagnosis was confirmed by a CT Pulmonary Angiography (CTPA) (Fig. 1) which demonstrated multiple bilateral subsegmental PE with no signs of right sided heart strain. The CTPA also demonstrated bilateral ground glass and consolidation in the lungs in keeping with COVID-19 infection (Fig. 2). The CT examination was performed using the Siemens® Somatom Definition Flash using GE Healthcare® Omnipaque intravenous contrast and a standardized CTPA protocol. The patient had a D-dimer > 4.0 mg/L (normal range 0.2–0.6 mg/L). The Chest CT performed during the CTPA also shows the radiological extent of the COVID-19 illness in the lungs (Fig. 2). The patient was started on Low Molecular Weight Heparin (LMWH) with bridging to direct oral anticoagulation (DOAC) on a dose of 20 mg Rivaroxaban OD. The

patient continued DOAC treatment for a total of three months until the beginning of July 2020.

On the 26th of February 2021, approximately 11 months after being diagnosed with COVID-19, the patient contacted the emergency medical services due to acute onset visual field disturbances. The ambulance arrived on scene minutes after the onset of symptoms. A preliminary examination by the paramedics revealed as right sided visual field defect and a left sided facial palsy. The patient had a heart rate of 70 beats per minute and blood pressure of 147/89 mm Hg. The prehospital oxygen saturation was 98 % whilst breathing room air. Based on their initial findings, the paramedics suspected a stroke, and the patient was blue lighted to the ED.

On admission to the ED the patient was taken directly to the CT lab. The patient had a temperature of 35.5 ℃, ECG showing normal sinus rhythm, blood glucose of 5.8 mmol/L, a blood pressure of 157/99 mmHg and an oxygen saturation of 99 % on room air. A rapid neurological examination revealed a left sided peripheral facial palsy, right sided homonymous upper quadrantopia. A National Institutes of Health Stroke Scale (NIHSS) exam revealed a score of 3.

A CT scan was performed including a pre- and intracerebral angiography. A subsequent cerebral perfusion scan was also performed. The CT examination was performed using the Siemens® Somatom Definition Flash using GE Healthcare® Omnipaque intravenous contrast and standardized protocols for angiography and perfusion.

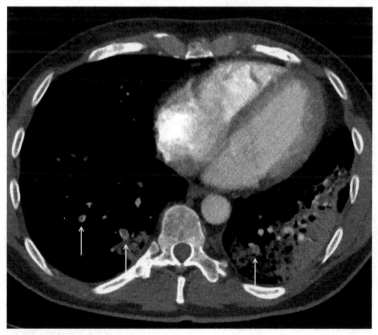

Fig. 1 CTPA showing multiple bilateral segmental pulmonary emboli

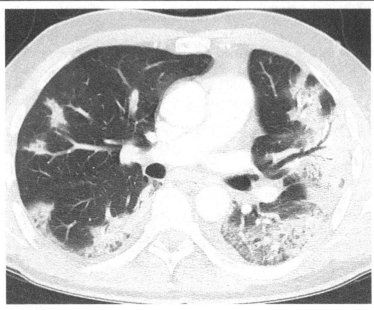

Fig. 2 Chest CT showing bilateral COVID-19 changes

The plain CT showed no signs of hemorrhage and based on the clinical suspicion of stroke the decision to treat with intravenous thrombolysis was made. Alteplase was administered at a dose of 0.9 mg/kg as per guidelines. The CT angiography three occluded intracerebral vessels, occlusions of the P2 and P3 segments of the left posterior cerebral artery (Fig. 3) and an occlusion of the

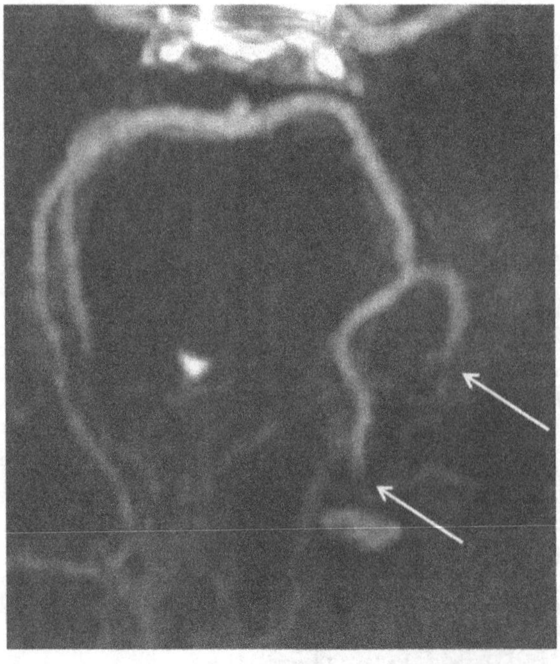

Fig. 3 CTA showing occlusions of the P2 and P3 segments of the left posterior cerebral artery

left superior cerebellar artery. The CT perfusion scan show increased time to drain (TTD) and reduced cerebral blood flow (CBF) in the afore mentioned occluded vascular territories (Fig. 4).

The patient was admitted to the stroke unit and showed neurological improvement after Alteplase administration. The following day the patient had a NIHSS of 0.

During hospital admission examinations were performed to determine ischemic stroke etiology. Ultrasound of the pre- and intra- cerebral vessels showed no significant stenoses or occlusions. Five day in-hospital cardiac rhythm monitoring showed sinus rhythm without any signs of atrial fibrillation and or other arrythmia. The patient underwent a Trans- Thoracic Echocardiography (TTE) which was normal and a Trans- Esophageal Echocardiography (TEE) where a patent foramen ovale was detected (PFO). The right to left shunting was visualized on color doppler and whilst using contrast (Fig. 5). A blood work up during admission showed a normal ESR, normal levels of Immunoglobulin G and M, normal levels of Protein C and S and normal Factor Xa activity. Immunological assays did not detect the presence of rheumatoid factor, ANCA, ANA, anti-CCP antibodies. Furthermore, no factor V Leiden mutation was detected nor the presence of Lupus anticoagulant. The only abnormal finding was an elevated D-dimer of 1.2 mg/L (normal range 0.2–0.6 mg/L). A full body CT was performed including a CTPA and a CT venography of the lower extremities. The full body CT showed no signs of malignancy. The CTPA showed no evidence of pulmonary embolus and the CT venography of the lower extremities ruled out deep vein thrombosis (DVT).

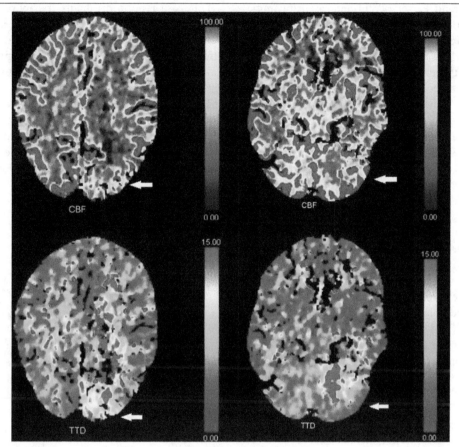

Fig. 4 CTP showing reduced CBF and increased TTD in P2 and P3 segments of the left posterior cerebral artery and the left superior cerebellar artery

The patient was discharged with a NIHSS of 0 following an Embolic Stroke of Unknown Source (ESUS). The patient is currently being treated with 20 mg Rivaroxaban OD, and atranscatheter closure of his PFO has been scheduled.

Discussion and conclusions

Patients with COVID-19 are frequently found to have underlying coagulopathy. This is demonstrated by evidence of microthrombosis/venous thrombus, elevated D-dimer and fibrinogen, activated complement system

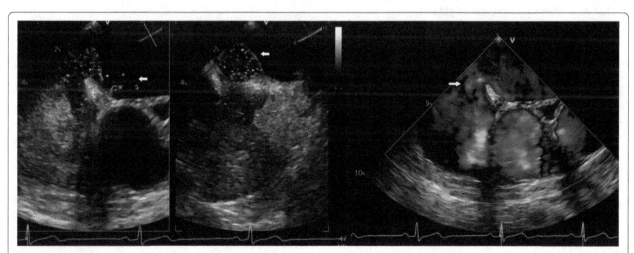

Fig. 5 Echocardiography showing a PFO using agitated sodium chloride contrast (left) and on colour doppler (right)

and von Willebrand Factor (vWF), increased inflammatory cytokines (IL-1β, IL-6) and antiphospholipid antibodies, as well as macrophage/endothelial cell dysfunction [1]. The resultant COVID-19 associated coagulopathy most commonly complicates in the form of venous thromboembolic event (VTE) such as PE or deep vein thrombosis. However, arterial thromboembolism in the form of acute ischemic stroke or acute coronary syndrome more rarely can occur.

Our case presented with VTE in the form of PE during the sub-acute phase of COVID-19 infection, then later, arterial thromboembolism in the form of acute ischemic stroke 11 months after COVID-19.

Large arterial vessel stroke can be a presenting feature of COVID-19 in young patients. This was demonstrated in early case series during the pandemic, of which the majority (4 of 5) had elevated levels of D-dimer at diagnosis [2]. There are however no published case reports to date of acute stroke as a presentation of suspected paradoxical thromboembolic recurrence in a patient with previous COVID-19 infection. As part of an extensive work up for the acute stroke the patient was found to have coagulopathy in the form of elevated D-dimer. Studies have previously shown D-dimer to be elevated in a sub-set of COVID-19 patients at follow up [3]. Up to 25 % of patients have shown to have elevated D-dimer levels 4 months after the initial infection [4], though the clinical significance of this remains unclear.

Of interest PFO was also found, which has previously been reported to complicate PE in the context of COVID-19 infection in a young female [5]. Underlying PFO has also been found in a young male with COVID-19 presenting with acute right cerebellar infarct [6]. Tough we are not certain, we suspect that the underlying long-term COVID-19 associated coagulopathy in the setting of a PFO led to paradoxical multiple simultaneous embolic cerebral infarctions in this young patient, with no other cause found after extensive investigations.

Venous thromboprophylaxis is now routinely considered for patients admitted with COVID-19 infection. There is little evidence to suggest that COVID-19 infection in the absence of clinically evident VTE warrants the use of therapeutic anticoagulation to address an underlying coagulopathy. There are similar short-term risks of both thrombosis and bleeding in these patients [7]. In the context of VTE, as in the early stages of this case, the patient was treated with a DOAC for 3 months which is a standard treatment duration for a provoked VTE [8]. There is however almost no evidence at present to suggest that these patients should be treated with DOAC over a prolonged period of time. Up to 35 % of the general population have a PFO. This combined with the unknown extent of COVID-19 related coagulopathy; a major challenge looms for stroke physicians worldwide [9].

This case reports highlights the more serious, longer term complications of COVID-19 where multiple embolic infarctions presented almost 1 year after the acute illness. The COVID-19 associated coagulopathy potentially persisting many months after diagnosis in patients with a milder clinical course of illness.

The long-term consequences of COVID-19 infection are only just beginning to surface potentially impacting a great number of individuals. More studies and reports are needed to map out the potential long-term consequences of COVID-19 associated coagulopathy.

Abbreviations
ED: Emergency Department; BMI: Body mass index; Covid-19: Coronavirus disease, sars-CoV-2; PCR: Polymearase chain reaction; PE: Pulmonary embolism; VTE: Venous thromboembolism; PFO: Patent foramen ovale; DVT: Deep vein Thrombosis; CT: Computer tomography; CTPA: CT pulmonary angiography; LMWH: Low Molecular Weight Heparin; DOAC: Direct oral anticoagulation; ECG: Electrocardiography; NIHSS |: National Institutes of Health Stroke Scale; TTD: Time to drain; CBF: Cerebral blood flow; ESR: Erythrocyte sedimentation rate; TEE: Trans- Esophageal Echocardiography; ANA: Anti nuclear antibodies; ANCA: Anti-neutrophil cytoplasmic antibodies; Anti-CCP: Anti- cyclic citrullinated peptides (CCP); ESUS: Embolic Stroke of Unknown Origin

Acknowledgements
None.

Authors' contributions
Rajiv Advani – Clinical management, Collection of clinical data, drafting the paper including critical revisions. Critical intellectual contribution approved the submitted version. Torbjørn Austveg Strømsnes – Clinical management, Collection of clinical data, reviewing and editing paper. Critical intellectual contributions approved the submitted version. Espen Stjernstrøm - Collection of clinical data, Interpretation of radiological findings. Critical intellectual contributions approved the submitted version. Sebastian Thomas Lugg - Critical intellectual contributions, Drafting and revising the paper including approved the submitted version.

Authors' information
None.

Author details
[1]Stroke Unit, Department of Neurology, Oslo University Hospital, Oslo, Norway. [2]Neuroscience Research Group, Stavanger University Hospital, Stavanger, Norway. [3]Department of Clinical Medicine, University of Bergen, Bergen, Norway. [4]Department of Radiology, Oslo University Hospital, Oslo, Norway. [5]Institute of Inflammation and Ageing, University of Birmingham, Birmingham, UK.

References

1. Iba T, Levy JH, Connors JM, Warkentin TE, Thachil J, Levi M. The unique characteristics of COVID-19 coagulopathy. Crit Care. 2020;24(1):360.
2. Oxley TJ, Mocco J, Majidi S, et al. Large-vessel stroke as a presenting feature of covid-19 in the young. N Engl J Med. 2020;382(20):e60.
3. Mandal S, Barnett J, Brill SE, et al. 'Long-COVID': a cross-sectional study of persisting symptoms, biomarker and imaging abnormalities following hospitalisation for COVID-19. Thorax 2020.
4. Townsend L, Fogarty H, Dyer A, et al. Prolonged elevation of D-dimer levels in convalescent COVID-19 patients is independent of the acute phase response. J Thromb Haemost 2021.
5. Fabre O, Rebet O, Carjaliu I, Radutoiu M, Gautier L, Hysi I. Severe acute proximal pulmonary embolism and COVID-19: a word of caution. Ann Thorac Surg. 2020;110(5):e409–11.
6. Ashraf M, Sajed S. Acute stroke in a young patient with coronavirus disease 2019 in the presence of patent foramen ovale. Cureus. 2020;12(9):e10233.
7. Patell R, Bogue T, Koshy A, et al. Postdischarge thrombosis and hemorrhage in patients with COVID-19. Blood. 2020;136(11):1342–6.
8. Kearon C, Akl EA, Ornelas J, et al. Antithrombotic Therapy for VTE Disease: CHEST Guideline and Expert Panel Report. Chest. 2016;149(2):315–52.
9. Fisher DC, Fisher EA, Budd JH, Rosen SE, Goldman ME. The incidence of patent foramen ovale in 1,000 consecutive patients. A contrast transesophageal echocardiography study. Chest. 1995;107(6):1504–9.

Permissions

The contributors of this book come from diverse backgrounds, making this book a truly international effort. This book will bring forth new frontiers with its revolutionizing research information and detailed analysis of the nascent developments around the world.

We would like to thank all the contributing authors for lending their expertise to make the book truly unique. They have played a crucial role in the development of this book. Without their invaluable contributions this book wouldn't have been possible. They have made vital efforts to compile up to date information on the varied aspects of this subject to make this book a valuable addition to the collection of many professionals and students.

This book was conceptualized with the vision of imparting up-to-date information and advanced data in this field. To ensure the same, a matchless editorial board was set up. Every individual on the board went through rigorous rounds of assessment to prove their worth. After which they invested a large part of their time researching and compiling the most relevant data for our readers.

The editorial board has been involved in producing this book since its inception. They have spent rigorous hours researching and exploring the diverse topics which have resulted in the successful publishing of this book. They have passed on their knowledge of decades through this book. To expedite this challenging task, the publisher supported the team at every step. A small team of assistant editors was also appointed to further simplify the editing procedure and attain best results for the readers.

Apart from the editorial board, the designing team has also invested a significant amount of their time in understanding the subject and creating the most relevant covers. They scrutinized every image to scout for the most suitable representation of the subject and create an appropriate cover for the book.

The publishing team has been an ardent support to the editorial, designing and production team. Their endless efforts to recruit the best for this project, has resulted in the accomplishment of this book. They are a veteran in the field of academics and their pool of knowledge is as vast as their experience in printing. Their expertise and guidance has proved useful at every step. Their uncompromising quality standards have made this book an exceptional effort. Their encouragement from time to time has been an inspiration for everyone.

The publisher and the editorial board hope that this book will prove to be a valuable piece of knowledge for researchers, students, practitioners and scholars across the globe.

List of Contributors

Osamah Al-Asadi
Department of Oncology, Milton Keynes University Hospital, Milton Keynes, UK
School of Medicine, University of Buckingham, Buckingham, UK
College of medicine, Al-Mustansiriyah University, Baghdad, Iraq

Hany Eldeeb
Department of Oncology, Milton Keynes University Hospital, Milton Keynes, UK
School of Medicine, University of Buckingham, Buckingham, UK

Manar Almusarhed
Department of Oncology, Milton Keynes University Hospital, Milton Keynes, UK
School of Medicine, University of Buckingham, Buckingham, UK
College of medicine, Babylon University, Babylon, Iraq

Russell Hull
Foothills Medical Centre and Thrombosis Research Unit, University of Calgary, Calgary, Canada

Roopen Arya
King's Thrombosis Centre, Department of Haematological Medicine, King's College Hospital NHS Foundation Trust, London, UK

Jan Beyer-Westendorf
Thrombosis Research Unit, Department of Medicine I, Division Hematology, University Hospital 'Carl Gustav Carus' Dresden, Dresden, Germany
King's Thrombosis Service, Department of Haematology, King's College London, London, UK

James Douketis
Department of Medicine, McMaster University, Hamilton, Ontario, Canada
Thrombosis and Atherosclerosis Research Institute, Hamilton, Ontario, Canada

Ismail Elalamy
Department of Obstetrics and Gynaecology, The First I.M. Sechenov Moscow State Medical University, Moscow, Russia
Hematology and Thrombosis Center, Tenon University Hospital, Sorbonne University, INSERM U938, Sorbonne University, Paris, France

Davide Imberti
Haemostasis and Thrombosis Center, Hospital of Piacenza, Piacenza, Italy

Zhenguo Zhai
Department of Pulmonary and Critical Care Medicine, Center of Respiratory Medicine, China-Japan Friendship Hospital, National Clinical Research Center for Respiratory Diseases, Beijing, China

Jing Loong Moses Loh
Department of Orthopaedic Surgery, Singapore General Hospital, 20 College Road, Academia, Level 4, Singapore 169865, Singapore

Stephrene Chan
Department of Haematology, Tan Tock Seng Hospital, Singapore, Singapore

Keng Lin Wong
Department of Orthopaedic Surgery, Sengkang General Hospital, Singapore, Singapore

Sanjay de Mel and Eng Soo Yap
Department of Hematology-Oncology, National University Cancer Institute, National University Hospital, Singapore, Singapore

Benjamin Brenner
Department of Hematology and Bone Marrow Transplantation, Rambam Health Care Campus, Haifa, Israel
Department of Obstetrics and Gynaecology, The First I.M. Sechenov Moscow State Medical University, Moscow, Russia

Olivia S. Costa and Craig I. Coleman
Department of Pharmacy Practice, University of Connecticut School of Pharmacy, 69 North Eagleville Road, Unit 3092, Storrs, CT 06269, USA
Evidence-Based Practice Center, Hartford Hospital, Hartford, CT, USA

Stanley Thompson
TeamHealth LifePoint Group, Southaven, MS, USA

Veronica Ashton
Real World Value and Evidence, Janssen Scientific Affairs LLC, Titusville, NJ, USA

Michael Palladino
Medical Affairs, Janssen Pharmaceuticals Inc., Titusville, NJ, USA

Thomas J. Bunz
Department of Pharmacoepidemiology, New England
Health Analytics LLC, Granby, CT, USA

Anadil Faqah, Fatima Tayyaab and Sahrish Khawaja
Department of Internal Medicine, Shaukat Khanam
Memorial Cancer Hospital & Research Centre, Lahore,
Pakistan

Hassan Sheikh
Department of Hematology and Oncology, Shaukat
Khanam Memorial Cancer Hospital & Research
Centre, Lahore, Pakistan

Muhammad Abu Bakar
Department of Cancer Registry, Shaukat Khanam
Memorial Cancer Hospital & Research Centre, Lahore,
Pakistan

Pascale Notten
Department of Vascular Surgery, Maastricht University
Medical Centre, Maastricht 6202 AZ, the Netherlands
CARIM, Cardiovascular Research Institute Maastricht,
School for Cardiovascular Diseases, Maastricht
University Medical Centre, Maastricht 6200 MD, the
Netherlands

Rob H. W. Strijkers and Irwin Toonder
Laboratory for Clinical Thrombosis and Hemostasis,
Maastricht University, Maastricht 6200 MD, the
Netherlands

Hugo ten Cate
CARIM, Cardiovascular Research Institute Maastricht,
School for Cardiovascular Diseases, Maastricht
University Medical Centre, Maastricht 6200 MD, the
Netherlands
Laboratory for Clinical Thrombosis and Hemostasis,
Maastricht University, Maastricht 6200 MD, the
Netherlands
Thrombosis Expertise Centre, Heart + Vascular Centre,
Maastricht University Medical Centre, Maastricht 6202
AZ, the Netherlands
Department of Internal Medicine, Maastricht University
Medical Centre, Maastricht, the Netherlands
Department of Biochemistry, Cardiovascular Research
Institute Maastricht, Maastricht, the Netherlands

Arina J. ten Cate-Hoek
CARIM, Cardiovascular Research Institute Maastricht,
School for Cardiovascular Diseases, Maastricht
University Medical Centre, Maastricht 6200 MD, the
Netherlands
Laboratory for Clinical Thrombosis and Hemostasis,
Maastricht University, Maastricht 6200 MD, The
Netherlands
Thrombosis Expertise Centre, Heart + Vascular Centre,
Maastricht University Medical Centre, Maastricht 6202
AZ, the Netherlands
Thrombosis Expertise Centre, Heart + Vascular Centre,
Maastricht University Medical Centre, P. Debyelaan
25, Maastricht 6229 HX, the Netherlands

**Wen Hu, Dong Xu, Juan Li, Cheng Chen, Yuan Chen,
Fangfang Xi, Feifei Zhou, Xiaohan Guo, Baihui Zhao
and Qiong Luo**
Department of Obstetrics, Women's Hospital, Zhejiang
University, School of Medicine, 1st Xueshi Road,
Hangzhou 310006, Zhejiang, China

**C. J. MacDonald, M. Canonico, A. Fournier and M.
C. Boutron-Ruault**
INSERM (Institut National de la Santé et de la
Recherche Médicale) U1018, Center for Research in
Epidemiology and Population Health (CESP), Institut
Gustave Roussy, Villejuif, France
Université Paris-Saclay, Université Paris-Sud, Villejuif,
France

A. L. Madika
INSERM (Institut National de la Santé et de la
Recherche Médicale) U1018, Center for Research in
Epidemiology and Population Health (CESP), Institut
Gustave Roussy, Villejuif, France
Université Paris-Saclay, Université Paris-Sud, Villejuif,
France
Université de Lille, CHU Lille, EA 2694 - Santé
publique: épidémiologie et qualité des soins, F-59000
Lille, France

M. Lajous
Center for Research on Population Health, INSP
(Instituto Nacional de Salud Pública), Cuernavaca,
Mexico
Department of Global Health and Population, Harvard
T.H. Chan School of Public Health, Boston, MA, USA

**Archrob Khuhapinant, Tarinee Rungjirajittranon,
Bundarika Suwanawiboon, Yingyong Chinthammitr
and Theera Ruchutrakool**
Division of Hematology, Department of Medicine,
Faculty of Medicine Siriraj Hospital, Mahidol
University, 2 Wanglang Road, Bangkok Noi, Bangkok
10700, Thailand

**Vahideh   Takhviji,   Sanaz   Hommayoun,
Mohammadreza Tabatabaei and Abbas Khosravi**
Transfusion Research center, High Institute for
Research and Education in Transfusion, Tehran, Iran

Kazem Zibara
PRASE and Biology Department, Faculty of Sciences, Lebanese University, Beirut, Lebanon

Asma Maleki
Department of hematology, School of Allied Medical Sciences, Tehran University of Medical Sciences, Tehran, Iran

Ebrahim Azizi and Maral Soleymani
Faculty of Medicine, Ahvaz Jundishapur University of Medical Sciences, Ahvaz, Iran

Seyed Esmaeil Ahmadi and Omid Kiani Ghalesardi
Department of Hematology and Blood Banking, Faculty of Allied Medicine, Iran University of Medical Sciences, Tehran, Iran

Mina Farokhian
Hematology Department, Tarbiat Modares University, Tehran, Iran

Afshin Davari
School of Public Health, Tehran University of Medical Sciences, Tehran, Iran

Pouria Paridar
Islamic Azad University, North-Tehran Branch, Tehran, Iran

Anahita Kalantari
Department of Anesthesiology, Golestan Hospital, Ahvaz Jundishapur University of Medical Sciences, Ahvaz, Iran

Wei Xiong, Yanmin Wang and Xuejun Guo
Department of Pulmonary and Critical Care Medicine, Xinhua Hospital, Shanghai Jiaotong University School of Medicine,Shanghai, No. 1665, Kongjiang Road, Yangpu District, Shanghai 200092, China

Yunfeng Zhao
Department of Pulmonary and Critical Care Medicine, Punan Hospital, Pudong New District, Shanghai, China

He Du
Department of Medical Oncology, Shanghai Pulmonary Hospital, Tongji University School of Medicine, Shanghai, China

Mei Xu
Department of General Medicine, North Bund Community Health Service Center, Hongkou District, Shanghai, China

Qiyan Cai and Hong Chen
Department of Pulmonary and Critical Care Medicine, the First Affiliated Hospital of Chongqing Medical University, No.1 Youyi Road, Yuzhong District, Chongqing 400016, China

Xin Zhang
Respiratory Disease Department, Xinqiao Hospital, Chongqing, China

Mauricio Castillo-Perez, Alejandra Castro-Varela, Ray Erick Ramos-Cazares, Jose Alfredo Salinas-Casanova, Abigail Montserrat Molina-Rodriguez, Arturo Adrián Martinez-Ibarra, Yoezer Z Flores-Sayavedra, Jaime Alberto Guajardo-Lozano, Hector Lopez-de la Garza, Hector Betancourt-del Campo and Daniela Martinez-Magallanes
Tecnologico de Monterrey. Escuela de Medicina y Ciencias de la Salud., Nuevo Leon, San Pedro Garza Garcia, Mexico

Jose Gildardo Paredes-Vazquez
Tecnologico de Monterrey. Escuela de Medicina y Ciencias de la Salud., Nuevo Leon, San Pedro Garza Garcia, Mexico
Instituto de Cardiologia y Medicina Vascular, TecSalud, Escuela de Medicina y Ciencias de la Salud, Tecnologico de Monterrey, Batallón San Patricio 112, Real de San Agustin, Nuevo Leon 66278 San Pedro Garza Garcia, Mexico

Eduardo Vazquez-Garza
Tecnologico de Monterrey. Escuela de Medicina y Ciencias de la Salud., Nuevo Leon, San Pedro Garza Garcia, Mexico
Centro de Investigacion Biomedica del Hospital Zambrano Hellion, TecSalud, Escuela de Medicina y Ciencias de la Salud, Tecnologico de Monterrey, Nuevo Leon, San Pedro Garza Garcia, Mexico

Mario Alejandro Fabiani
Instituto de Cardiologia y Medicina Vascular, TecSalud, Escuela de Medicina y Ciencias de la Salud, Tecnologico de Monterrey, Batallón San Patricio 112, Real de San Agustin, Nuevo Leon 66278 San Pedro Garza Garcia, Mexico

Jathniel Panneflek
Centro de Investigacion Biomedica del Hospital Zambrano Hellion, TecSalud, Escuela de Medicina y Ciencias de la Salud, Tecnologico de Monterrey, Nuevo Leon, San Pedro Garza Garcia, Mexico

Carlos Jerjes-Sanchez
Tecnologico de Monterrey. Escuela de Medicina y Ciencias de la Salud., Nuevo Leon, San Pedro Garza Garcia, Mexico
Centro de Investigacion Biomedica del Hospital Zambrano Hellion, TecSalud, Escuela de Medicina y Ciencias de la Salud, Tecnologico de Monterrey, Nuevo Leon, San Pedro Garza Garcia, Mexico
Instituto de Cardiologia y Medicina Vascular, TecSalud, Escuela de Medicina y Ciencias de la Salud, Tecnologico de Monterrey, Batallón San Patricio 112, Real de San Agustin, Nuevo Leon 66278 San Pedro Garza Garcia, Mexico
Tecnologico de Monterrey, Escuela de Medicina y Ciencias de la Salud, Av. Ignacio Morones Prieto 3000, N.L. CP, 64718 Monterrey, Mexico

Jiali Li, Jiao Qin, Lingyan He, Cao Dai and Rui Wen
Department of Rheumatology and Immunology, University of South China Affiliated Changsha Central Hospital, 161 South Shaoshan Road, Changsha 410008, Hunan, China

Mingming Yan
Department of Orthopaedic Surgery, The Second Xiangya Hospital of Central South University, Changsha, Hunan, China

Myrthe M. van der Bruggen
Department of Internal Medicine, Maastricht University Medical Centre, Maastricht, the Netherlands

Bram Kremers
Department of Internal Medicine, Maastricht University Medical Centre, Maastricht, the Netherlands
Department of Biochemistry, Cardiovascular Research Institute Maastricht, Maastricht, the Netherlands

Rene van Oerle
Department of Biochemistry, Cardiovascular Research Institute Maastricht, Maastricht, the Netherlands
Clinical Diagnostic Laboratory, Maastricht University Medical Center, Maastricht, the Netherlands

Robert J. van Oostenbrugge
Department of Neurology, Maastricht University Medical Centre, Maastricht, the Netherlands

Sarah Kelliher and Karl Ewins
Department of Haematology, Mater Misericordiae University Hospital, Eccles St, Dublin 7, Ireland

Patricia Hall and Tomás Breslin
Department of Emergency Medicine, Mater Misericordiae University Hospital, Eccles St, Dublin 7, Ireland

Barry Kevane
Department of Haematology, Mater Misericordiae University Hospital, Eccles St, Dublin 7, Ireland
Department of Haematology, Rotunda Hospital, Dublin 1, Ireland

Daniela Dinu
Department of Haematology, Mater Misericordiae University Hospital, Eccles St, Dublin 7, Ireland
Department of Emergency Medicine, Mater Misericordiae University Hospital, Eccles St, Dublin 7, Ireland

Peter MacMahon
Department of Radiology, Mater Misericordiae University Hospital, Eccles St, Dublin 7, Ireland

Fionnuala Ní Áinle
Department of Haematology, Mater Misericordiae University Hospital, Eccles St, Dublin 7, Ireland
Department of Haematology, Rotunda Hospital, Dublin 1, Ireland
School of Medicine, University College Dublin (UCD), Dublin 4, Ireland
UCD Conway Institute SPHERE Research Group, UCD, Dublin 4, Ireland

Na Cui, Chunguo Jiang, Liming Zhang and Xiaokai Feng
Department of Pulmonary and Critical Care Medicine, Beijing Chao-Yang Hospital, Capital Medical University, No. 8, Gongti South Road, Chaoyang District, Beijing 100020, People's Republic of China
Beijing Institute of Respiratory Medicine, Beijing 100020, People's Republic of China

Hairong Chen
Department of Intensive Care Unit, Shandong Provincial Qianfoshan Hospital, The First Affiliated Hospital of Shandong First Medical University, Ji'nan, People's Republic of China

Ahmed M. Elzanaty, Mohammed T. Awad and Ashu Acharaya
Internal Medicine Departement, University of Toledo, 3000 Arlington Avenue, Toledo, OH 43614, USA

Ebrahim Sabbagh and Moshrik AbdAlamir
Cardiology Departement, University of Toledo, Toledo, Ohio, USA

Eman Elsheikh
Cardiology Departement, Tanta University Hospital, Tanta, Egypt

Budi Setiawan, Eko Adhi Pangarsa, Damai Santosa and Catharina Suharti
Division of Hematology and Medical Oncology, Department of Internal Medicine, Medical Faculty of Diponegoro University and Dr. Kariadi Hospital, Semarang, Indonesia

Cecilia Oktaria Permatadewi, Baringin de Samakto and Ashar Bugis
Department of Internal Medicine, Medical Faculty of Diponegoro University and Dr. Kariadi Hospital, Semarang, Indonesia

Ridho M. Naibaho
Division of Hematology and Medical Oncology, Department of Internal Medicine, Medical Faculty of Diponegoro University and Dr. Kariadi Hospital, Semarang, Indonesia
Fellow in Hematology and Medical Oncology, Department of Internal Medicine, Medical Faculty of Mulawarman University, Parikesit General Hospital, Kutai Kartanegara, Indonesia

Takahisa Mori and Kazuhiro Yoshioka
Department of Stroke Treatment, Shonan Kamakura General Hospital, Okamoto 1370-1, 247-8533 Kamakura City, Kanagawa, Japan

Yuhei Tanno
Department of Stroke Treatment, Shonan Kamakura General Hospital, Okamoto 1370-1, 247-8533 Kamakura City, Kanagawa, Japan
Department of Neurology, Nakatsugawa Municipal General Hospital, Komaba 1522-1, Gifu 508-8502 Nakatsugawa City, Japan

Yan-ping Zhang, Bin Lin, Yuan-yuan Ji, Ya-nan Hu, Yi Tang, Jian-hui Zhang, Shao-jie Wu, Sen-lin Cai, Yan-feng Zhou, Ting Chen and Zhu-ting Fang
Shengli Clinical Medical College of Fujian Medical University, Fuzhou 350001, China
Department of Interventional Radiology, Fujian Provincial Hospital, Fuzhou 350001, China

Xin-fu Lin
Shengli Clinical Medical College of Fujian Medical University, Fuzhou 350001, China
Department of Pediatrics, Fujian Provincial hospital, Fuzhou 350001, China

Jie-wei Luo
Shengli Clinical Medical College of Fujian Medical University, Fuzhou 350001, China
Department of Traditional Chinese Medicine, Fujian Provincial Hospital, Fuzhou 350001, China

Kaoru Fujieda, Akie Watanabe and Keiko Shi
Tsukuba Medical Center Hospital, Tsukuba, Ibaraki, Japan
Department of Obstetrics and Gynecology, Faculty of Medicine, University of Tsukuba, 1-1-1 Tennoudai, Tsukuba, Ibaraki 305-8575, Japan

Akiko Nozue and Ken Nishide
Tsukuba Medical Center Hospital, Tsukuba, Ibaraki, Japan

Hiroya Itagaki, Yoshihiko Hosokawa, Keiko Nishida, Nobutaka Tasaka and Toyomi Satoh
Department of Obstetrics and Gynecology, Faculty of Medicine, University of Tsukuba, 1-1-1 Tennoudai, Tsukuba, Ibaraki 305-8575, Japan

Dimitrios G. Raptis, Konstantinos I. Gourgoulianis and Zoe Daniil
Respiratory Medicine Department, School of Medicine, University of Thessaly, Larissa, Greece

Foteini Malli
Respiratory Medicine Department, School of Medicine, University of Thessaly, Larissa, Greece
Anatomy and Phsyiology Lab, Nursing Department, University of Thessaly, Larissa, Greece

Mats Beckman and Sven Nyrén
Department of Radiology, Imaging and Physiology, Karolinska University Hospital, Stockholm, Sweden
Department of Molecular Medicine and Surgery, Karolinska Institutet, Stockholm, Sweden

Anna Kistner
Department of Molecular Medicine and Surgery, Karolinska Institutet, Stockholm, Sweden
Medical Radiation Physics and Nuclear Medicine, Imaging and Physiology, Karolinska University Hospital, Stockholm, Sweden

E. Papadakis
Hemostasis Unit-Hematology Department Papageorgiou Hospital, Thessaloniki Ringroad 56403 Nea Efkarpia, Thessaloniki, Greece

A. Pouliakis
2nd Department of Pathology, National and Kapodistrian University of Athens, "ATTIKON" University Hospital, Rimini 1 Haidari, Athens, Greece

A. Aktypi
OLYMPION General Clinic, Volou-Patras, 26443 Patras, Greece

A. Christoforidou
University Hospital of Alexandroupolis, Dragana Site 68100 Nea Chili, Alexandroupoli, Greece

P. Kotsi
Blood Transfusion Unit, National Ref. Centre for Congenital Bleeding Disorders, Hemostasis Unit, Laiko General Hospital, Ag. Thoma, 17 11527 Athens, Greece

G. Anagnostou
Head of Transfusion Service and Clinical Haemostasis, Henry Dunant Hospital Center, Mesogion 107, 115 26 Athens, Greece

A. Foifa
IASO, General Maternity and Gynecology Clinic, 37-39, Kifissias Avenue, 151 23 Maroussi, Athens, Greece

E. Grouzi
"St Savvas" Oncology Hospital, Alexandras Avenue 171, 11522 Ambelikipoi, Athens, Greece

Anna Levkovsky and Ophira Salomon
Thrombosis Unit Sheba Medical Center, Coagulation Institute, 52621 Tel Hashomer, Israel
Sackler Faculty of Medicine, Tel Aviv University, Tel Aviv, Israel

Rima Dardik
National Hemophilia Center and Thrombosis Unit, Sheba Medical Center, Tel-Hashomer, Israel

Daniel Barazany and Mark Dan Kirichenko
Strauss Computational Neuroimaging Center, Tel Aviv University, Tel Aviv, Israel

David M. Steinberg
Department of Statistics and Operations Research, Faculty of Exact Sciences, Tel Aviv University, Tel Aviv, Israel

Sara Apter
Department of Diagnostic Imaging, Sheba Medical Center, Tel-Hashomer, Israel
Tel Aviv University, Tel Aviv, Israel

Edna Peleg
Sackler Faculty of Medicine, Tel Aviv University, Tel Aviv, Israel
Hypertension Unit, Sheba Medical Center, Tel-Hashomer, Israel

Daniel Silverberg
Sackler Faculty of Medicine, Tel Aviv University, Tel Aviv, Israel
Department of Vascular Surgery, Sheba Medical Center, Tel-Hashomer, Israel

Ehud Grossman
Sackler Faculty of Medicine, Tel Aviv University, Tel Aviv, Israel
Internal Medicine Department, Sheba Medical Center, Tel Hashomer, Israel

Rajiv Advani
Stroke Unit, Department of Neurology, Oslo University Hospital, Oslo, Norway
Neuroscience Research Group, Stavanger University Hospital, Stavanger, Norway

Torbjørn Austveg Strømsnes
Stroke Unit, Department of Neurology, Oslo University Hospital, Oslo, Norway
Department of Clinical Medicine, University of Bergen, Bergen, Norway

Espen Stjernstrøm
Department of Radiology, Oslo University Hospital, Oslo, Norway

Sebastian T. Lugg
Institute of Inflammation and Ageing, University of Birmingham, Birmingham, UK

Index